Castrate-Resistant Prostate Cancer

Editor

ADAM S. KIBEL

UROLOGIC CLINICS
OF NORTH AMERICA

www.urologic.theclinics.com

Consulting Editor
SAMIR S. TANEJA

November 2012 • Volume 39 • Number 4

ELSEVIER

1600 John F. Kennedy Blvd. • Suite 1800 • Philadelphia, PA 19103-2899

http://www.theclinics.com

UROLOGIC CLINICS OF NORTH AMERICA Volume 39, Number 4
November 2012 ISSN 0094-0143, ISBN-13: 978-1-4557-4903-4

Editor: Stephanie Donley

Urologic Clinics of North America (ISSN 0094-0143) is published quarterly by Elsevier Inc., 360 Park Avenue South, New York, NY 10010-1710. Months of issue are February, May, August, and November. Business and Editorial Offices: 1600 John F. Kennedy Blvd., Suite 1800, Philadelphia, PA 19103-2899. Periodicals postage paid at New York, NY and additional mailing offices. Subscription prices are $339.00 per year (US individuals), $561.00 per year (US institutions), $396.00 per year (Canadian individuals), $687.00 per year (Canadian institutions), $492.00 per year (foreign individuals), and $687.00 per year (foreign institutions). Foreign air speed delivery is included in all *Clinics* subscription prices. All prices are subject to change without notice. **POSTMASTER:** Send address changes to *Urologic Clinics of North America*, Elsevier Health Sciences Division, Subscription Customer Service, 3251 Riverport Lane, Maryland Heights, MO 63043. Customer Service: 1-800-654-2452 (US). From outside the United States, call 1-314-447-8871. Fax: 1-314-447-8029. E-mail: JournalsCustomerServiceusa@elsevier.com (for print support) and JournalsOnlineSupport-usa@elsevier.com (for online support).

Reprints. For copies of 100 or more, of articles in this publication, please contact the Commercial Reprints Department, Elsevier Inc., 360 Park Avenue South, New York, New York 10010-1710. Tel.: 212-633-3813; Fax: 212-462-1935; E-mail: reprints@elsevier.com.

Urologic Clinics of North America is covered in MEDLINE/PubMed (*Index Medicus*), *Excerpta Medica*, *Current Contents/Clinical Medicine*, *Science Citation Index*, and *ISI/BIOMED*.

Printed and bound by CPI Group (UK) Ltd, Croydon, CR0 4YY

Transferred to digital print 2012

GOAL STATEMENT

The goal of *Urologic Clinics of North America* is to keep practicing urologists and urology residents up to date with current clinical practice in urology by providing timely articles reviewing the state of the art in patient care.

ACCREDITATION

The *Urologic Clinics of North America* is planned and implemented in accordance with the Essential Areas and Policies of the Accreditation Council for Continuing Medical Education (ACCME) through the joint sponsorship of the University of Virginia School of Medicine and Elsevier. The University of Virginia School of Medicine is accredited by the ACCME to provide continuing medical education for physicians.

The University of Virginia School of Medicine designates this enduring material activity for a maximum of 15 *AMA PRA Category 1 Credit*(s)™ for each issue, 60 credits per year. Physicians should claim only the credit commensurate with the extent of their participation in the activity.

The American Medical Association has determined that physicians not licensed in the US who participate in this CME enduring material activity are eligible for a maximum of 15 *AMA PRA Category 1 Credit*(s)™ for each issue, 60 credits per year.

Credit can be earned by reading the text material, taking the CME examination online at http://www.theclinics.com/home/cme, and completing the evaluation. After taking the test, you will be required to review any and all incorrect answers. Following completion of the test and evaluation, your credit will be awarded and you may print your certificate.

FACULTY DISCLOSURE/CONFLICT OF INTEREST

The University of Virginia School of Medicine, as an ACCME accredited provider, endorses and strives to comply with the Accreditation Council for Continuing Medical Education (ACCME) Standards of Commercial Support, Commonwealth of Virginia statutes, University of Virginia policies and procedures, and associated federal and private regulations and guidelines on the need for disclosure and monitoring of proprietary and financial interests that may affect the scientific integrity and balance of content delivered in continuing medical education activities under our auspices.

The University of Virginia School of Medicine requires that all CME activities accredited through this institution be developed independently and be scientifically rigorous, balanced and objective in the presentation/discussion of its content, theories and practices.

All authors/editors participating in an accredited CME activity are expected to disclose to the readers relevant financial relationships with commercial entities occurring within the past 12 months (such as grants or research support, employee, consultant, stock holder, member of speakers bureau, etc.). The University of Virginia School of Medicine will employ appropriate mechanisms to resolve potential conflicts of interest to maintain the standards of fair and balanced education to the reader. Questions about specific strategies can be directed to the Office of Continuing Medical Education, University of Virginia School of Medicine, Charlottesville, Virginia.

The faculty and staff of the University of Virginia Office of Continuing Medical Education have no financial affiliations to disclose.

The authors/editors listed below have identified no professional or financial affiliations for themselves or their spouse/partner:
Faris Azzouni, MD; Heather H. Cheng, MD, PhD; Stephanie Donley, (Acquisitions Editor); Terence W. Friedlander, MD; Michael Xiang Lee, MD, MPH; Brian Lewis, MD; Jianqing Lin, MD; Yohann Loriot, MD; James Mohler, MD; Alicia K Morgans, MD, MPH; David F. Penson, MD, MPH; Mark Pomerantz, MD; Michael W. Rabow, MD; Matthew R. Smith, MD, PhD; Eliezer M. Van Allen, MD; and Amina Zoubeidi, PhD.

The authors/editors listed below identified the following professional or financial affiliations for themselves or their spouse/partner:
Emmanuel S. Antonarakis, MD is a consultant and is on the Advisory Board for Dendreon, Sanofi-Aventis, and Janssen.
Mario A. Eisenberger, MD is the Co-founder Oncology Trials Insights, and receives research support from Sanofi, Agensys, and Genentech.
Martin E. Gleave, MD is founder and CSO of OncoGenex; receives research funding from AstraZeneca, OncoGenex, Pfizer, Inc., and Takeda; and is a consultant and is on the Advisory Board for AstraZeneca, Jansen, Astellas, and Sanofi.
Philip W. Kantoff, MD is a consultant for Amgen USA, Bayer, Bellicum, BN Immunotheraputics, Dendreon, Genentech, Progenics Pharmaceuticals, Inc., Janssen, and Tokai; is on the Advisory Board for BIND Biosciences, Inc., and Metamark; and is on the Monitoring Board for Celgene, Takeda/Millenium, and Oncogenex.
William K. Kelly, DO is on the Advisory Committee for Dendreon.
Adam S. Kibel, MD (Guest Editor) is a consultant and is on the Advisory Board for Dendreon and Sanofi-Aventis.
Daniel W. Lin, MD is on the Speakers' Bureau for Dendreon.
Sumanta K. Pal, MD receives research support from GSK, is on the Speakers' Bureau for Pfizer, Inc., and Novartis, and is on the Advisory Committee for Novartis.
Matthew J. Resnick, MD is on the Advisory Board for Bayer Healthcare.
Charles J. Ryan, MD receives research support from Janssen, Medivation, Aragon, and Millenium; is a consultant for Millenium; and receives honorarium from Astellas.
Oliver Sartor, MD is a consultant for Algeta, Amgen, Bayer, Bellicum, Bristol-Myers Squibb, Celgene, Dendreon, Exelixis, GSK, Johnson & Johnson, Medivation, Oncogenex, Sanofi-Aventis, and Takeda; and receives grant/research support from Algeta, AstraZeneca, Bayer, Cougar, Johnson & Johnson, Sanofi-Aventis, Takeda, and Exelixis.
Guru Sonpavde, MD is on the Advisory Board for Dendreon and Astellas, is on the Speakers' Bureau for Janssen, Sanofi-Aventis, and Amgen, and receives research support from Bellicum Pharmaceuticals.
William Steers, MD (Test Author) is on the Advisory Borad for NIH and FDA, and is an industry funded investigator for Allergan.
Samir S. Taneja, MD (Consulting Editor) is a consultant for Eigen, Gtx, and Steba Biotech, is an industry funded research/investigator for Gtx and Steba Biotech, and is on the Speakers' Bureau for Janssen.
Evan Y. Yu, MD is on the Advisory Board for Amgen, Astellas, Dendreon, GTx, and Janssen, is a consultant for Astellas, Bristol Myers-Squibb, Janssen, and Millennium, and receives research support from Astra Zeneca, Bristol Myers-Squibb, Cougar, Dendreon, GTx, ImClone, and OncoGeneX.

Disclosure of Discussion of Non-FDA Approved Uses for Pharmaceutical Products and/or Medical Devices.
The University of Virginia School of Medicine, as an ACCME provider, requires that all faculty presenters identify and disclose any off-label uses for pharmaceutical and medical device products. The University of Virginia School of Medicine recommends that each physician fully review all the available data on new products or procedures prior to clinical use.

TO ENROLL

To enroll in the Urologic Clinics of North America Continuing Medical Education program, call customer service at 1-800-654-2452 or visit us online at www.theclinics.com/home/cme. The CME program is available to subscribers for an additional fee of $207.00.

GOAL STATEMENT

The goal of UroOnc (Clinics of North) America is to keep practicing urologists and urology residents up to date with current clinical practice in urology by providing timely articles reviewing the state of the art in patient care.

ACCREDITATION

The University School of Medicine is planned and implemented in accordance with the Essential Areas and Policies of the Accreditation Council for Continuing Medical Education (ACCME) through the joint sponsorship of the University of Virginia School of Medicine and Elsevier. The University of Virginia School of Medicine is accredited by the ACCME to provide continuing medical education for physicians.

The University of Virginia School of Medicine designates this enduring material activity for a maximum of 15 AMA PRA Category 1 Credit(s)™ for each issue, 90 credits per year. Physicians should claim only the credit commensurate with the extent of their participation in the activity.

The American Medical Association has determined that physicians not licensed in the US who participate in this CME enduring material activity are eligible for a maximum of 15 AMA PRA Category 1 Credit(s)™ for each issue, 90 credits per year.

Credit can be earned by reading the text material, taking the CME examination online at http://www.theclinics.com/home/cme, and completing the evaluation. After taking the test, you will be required to review any and all incorrect answers. Following completion of the test and evaluation, your credit will be awarded and you may print your certificate.

FACULTY DISCLOSURE/CONFLICT OF INTEREST

The University of Virginia School of Medicine, as an ACCME accredited provider, endorses and strives to comply with the Accreditation Council for Continuing Medical Education (ACCME) Standards of Commercial Support, Commonwealth of Virginia statutes, University of Virginia policies and procedures, and associated federal and private regulations and guidelines on the need for disclosure and monitoring of proprietary and financial interests that may affect the scientific integrity and balance of content delivered in continuing medical education activities under our auspices.

The University of Virginia School of Medicine requires that all CME activities accredited through this institution be developed independently and be scientifically rigorous, balanced and objective in the presentation/discussion of its content, topics and issues.

All authors/editors participating in an accredited CME activity are expected to disclose to the readers relevant financial relationships with commercial entities occurring within the past 12 months (such as grants or research support, employee, consultant, stock holder, member of speakers bureau, etc.). The University of Virginia School of Medicine will employ appropriate mechanisms to resolve potential conflicts of interest to maintain the standards of fair and balanced education to the reader. Questions about specific strategies can be directed to the Office of Continuing Medical Education, University of Virginia School of Medicine, Charlottesville, Virginia.

The faculty and staff of the University of Virginia Office of Continuing Medical Education have no financial affiliations to disclose.

The authors/editors listed below have identified no professional or financial affiliations for themselves or their spouse/partner:

Paul L. Acosta, MD; Hualing H. Chang, MD, PhD; Stephanie Donley; [names illegible]...; and Arlene Elizabeth, PhD.

The authors/editors listed below identified the following professional or financial affiliations for themselves or their spouse/partner:

[body text largely illegible]

Disclosure of Discussion of Non-FDA Approved Uses for Pharmaceutical Products and/or Medical Devices

The University of Virginia School of Medicine, as an ACCME provider, requires that all faculty presenters identify and disclose any off-label uses for pharmaceutical and medical device products. The University of Virginia School of Medicine recommends that each physician fully review all the available data on new products or procedures prior to clinical use.

TO ENROLL

To enroll in the Urologic Clinics of North America Continuing Medical Education program, call customer service at 1-800-654-2452 or visit us online at www.theclinics.com/home/cme. The CME program is available to subscribers for an additional fee of $235.00.

Contributors

CONSULTING EDITOR

SAMIR S. TANEJA, MD
The James M. Neissa and Janet Riha Neissa
Professor of Urologic Oncology; Professor of
Urology and Radiology; Director, Division of
Urologic Oncology; Co-Director, Smilow
Comprehensive Prostate Cancer Center,
Department of Urology, NYU Langone Medical
Center, New York, New York

GUEST EDITOR

ADAM S. KIBEL, MD
Professor of Surgery, Harvard Medical School;
Chief of Urology, Brigham and Women's
Hospital, Boston, Massachusetts

AUTHORS

EMMANUEL S. ANTONARAKIS, MD
Assistant Professor of Oncology, The Sidney
Kimmel Comprehensive Cancer Center, The
Johns Hopkins University, Baltimore, Maryland

FARIS AZZOUNI, MD
Department of Urology, Roswell Park Cancer
Institute, Buffalo, New York

HEATHER H. CHENG, MD, PhD
Division of Medical Oncology, Department
of Medicine, University of Washington; Clinical
Research Division, Fred Hutchinson Cancer
Research Center, Seattle, Washington

MARIO A. EISENBERGER, MD
R. Dale Hughes Professor of Oncology,
The Sidney Kimmel Comprehensive Cancer
Center, The Johns Hopkins University,
Baltimore, Maryland

TERENCE W. FRIEDLANDER, MD
Assistant Clinical Professor of Medicine,
Division of Genitourinary Medical Oncology,
Helen Diller Family Comprehensive Cancer
Center, University of California, San Francisco,
California

MARTIN E. GLEAVE, MD
Liber Ero BC Leadership Chair in Prostate
Cancer Research; Director, Vancouver
Prostate Centre; Distinguishable Professor,
Department of Urologic Sciences, University
of British Columbia, Vancouver, British
Columbia, Canada

PHILIP W. KANTOFF, MD
Lank Center for Genitourinary Oncology,
Dana-Farber Cancer Institute, Harvard Medical
School, Boston, Massachusetts

WILLIAM K. KELLY, DO
Professor, Department of Medical Oncology
and Urology; Director, Division of Solid Tumor
Oncology; Associate Director, Translation
Research, Jefferson Kimmel Cancer Center,
Thomas Jefferson University, Philadelphia,
Pennsylvania

MICHAEL XIANG LEE, MD, MPH
Fellow, Division of Clinical Hematology/
Oncology, Department of Medicine, University
of California San Francisco, San Francisco,
California

BRIAN LEWIS, MD
Department of Medicine, Tulane University School of Medicine, New Orleans, Louisiana

DANIEL W. LIN, MD
Department of Urology, University of Washington, Seattle, Washington

JIANQING LIN, MD
Assistant Professor, Department of Medical Oncology, Jefferson Kimmel Cancer Center, Thomas Jefferson University, Philadelphia, Pennsylvania

YOHANN LORIOT, MD
Research Fellow, Vancouver Prostate Centre, University of British Columbia, Vancouver, British Columbia, Canada

JAMES MOHLER, MD
Department of Urology, Roswell Park Cancer Institute, Buffalo, New York

ALICIA K. MORGANS, MD
Fellow, Department of Hematology/Oncology, Massachusetts General Hospital Cancer Center, Boston, Massachusetts

SUMANTA K. PAL, MD
Department of Medical Oncology & Experimental Therapeutics, City of Hope Comprehensive Cancer Center, Duarte, California

DAVID F. PENSON, MD, MPH
Ingram Professor of Cancer Research, Department of Urologic Surgery; Director, Center for Surgical Quality and Outcomes Research, Vanderbilt University; VA Tennessee Valley Geriatric Research, Education, and Clinical Center (GRECC), Nashville, Tennessee

MARK POMERANTZ, MD
Department of Medical Oncology, Dana-Farber Cancer Institute, Boston, Massachusetts

MICHAEL W. RABOW, MD
Director, Symptom Management Service, Helen Diller Family Comprehensive Cancer Center; Professor of Clinical Medicine, University of California San Francisco, San Francisco, California

MATTHEW J. RESNICK, MD
Instructor, Department of Urologic Surgery, Center for Surgical Quality and Outcomes Research, Vanderbilt University; Fellow, VA National Quality Scholars Program, VA Tennessee Valley Geriatric Research, Education, and Clinical Center (GRECC), Nashville, Tennessee

CHARLES J. RYAN, MD
Associate Professor of Medicine, Division of Genitourinary Medical Oncology, Helen Diller Family Comprehensive Cancer Center, University of California, San Francisco, California

OLIVER SARTOR, MD
Laborde Professor of Cancer Research, Departments of Medicine and Urology, Tulane University School of Medicine; Medical Director, Tulane Cancer Center, Tulane Medical School, New Orleans, Louisiana

MATTHEW R. SMITH, MD, PhD
Professor of Medicine, Department of Hematology/Oncology, Massachusetts General Hospital Cancer Center, Boston, Massachusetts

GURU SONPAVDE, MD
Section of Medical Oncology, Department of Medicine, University of Alabama at Birmingham (UAB) Comprehensive Cancer Center, Birmingham, Alabama

ELIEZER M. VAN ALLEN, MD
Department of Medical Oncology, Dana-Farber Cancer Institute, Boston, Massachusetts; The Broad Institute of Harvard and MIT, Cambridge, Massachusetts

EVAN Y. YU, MD
Division of Medical Oncology, Department of Medicine, University of Washington; Clinical Research Division, Fred Hutchinson Cancer Research Center, Seattle, Washington

AMINA ZOUBEIDI, PhD
Research Scientist, Vancouver Prostate Centre; Assistant Professor, Department of Urologic Sciences, University of British Columbia, Vancouver, British Columbia, Canada

Contents

> Although androgen-deprivation therapy is the standard therapy for advanced and metastatic prostate cancer, this treatment is only palliative. Prostate cancer recurs then grows despite low circulating testicular androgens, using several mechanisms that remain dependent on androgen-receptor signaling in most cases. This article reviews the diversity of mechanisms used for growth by castration-recurrent prostate cancer.

> Androgen receptor (AR)-mediated signaling is critical to the growth and survival of prostate cancer. Although medical castration and antiandrogen therapy can decrease AR activity and lower PSA, castration resistance eventually develops. Recent work exploring the molecular structure and evolution of AR in response to hormonal therapies has revealed novel mechanisms of progression of castration-resistant prostate cancer and yielded new targets for drug development. This review focuses on understanding the mechanisms of persistent AR signaling in the castrate environment, and highlights new therapies either currently available or in clinical trials, including androgen synthesis inhibitors and novel direct AR inhibitors.

> The improved survival with sipuleucel-T, an autologous antigen-presenting cell–based agent, for the treatment of patients with metastatic asymptomatic and minimally symptomatic castration-resistant prostate cancer supports immunotherapy as a valid approach. Also, multiple novel immunotherapeutic approaches are undergoing vigorous investigation. T-lymphocyte checkpoint blockade and poxvirus-based prime-boost approaches are in phase III evaluation. Other immunotherapeutic platforms undergoing early investigation include radioimmunoconjugates and adenovirus-based, DNA-based, and Listeria-based approaches. The development of predictive markers for immune response that translate into improved long-term outcomes is important. This article reviews the emerging data and the unique strengths and weaknesses of these approaches.

In men, prostate cancer is the most common non-cutaneous malignancy and the second most common cause of cancer death. Skeletal complications occur at various points during the disease course, either due to bone metastases directly, or as an unintended consequence of androgen deprivation therapy (ADT). Bone metastases are associated with pathologic fractures, spinal cord compression, and bone pain and can require narcotics or palliative radiation for pain relief. ADT results in bone loss and fragility fractures. This review describes the biology of bone metastases, skeletal morbidity, and recent advances in bone-targeted therapies to prevent skeletal complications of prostate cancer.

Antiangiogenic therapy has been successful for the treatment of solid tumors. Several strategies have been used to target angiogenesis in prostate cancer. These strategies include blocking proangiogenic factors via monoclonal antibodies or small molecule inhibitors targeting downstream signaling effector pathways, or using agents with immune-modulatory effects. This review examines the general concepts of tumor angiogenesis and the key clinical trials that have used these agents and other novel biologics in prostate cancer. Targeting angiogenesis is still a promising treatment strategy in prostate cancer with a rational trial design and combination approach.

The classification of clinical disease states within advanced prostate cancer is set apart from other solid tumors largely through measurement of prostate-specific antigen in the blood. This testing has allowed the distinction between the castration-sensitive and the castration-resistant states, to complement radiographic distinction within advanced prostate cancer. This has paved the way for advances in prognostication and treatment of patients within a heterogeneous disease group. Currently used clinical classifications have limitations and continue to evolve. The authors define the current disease states and discuss implications for prognosis and treatment decisions, as well as the limitations of existing classifications and emerging discoveries.

This article reviews the initial experience with chemotherapy in metastatic castration-resistant prostate cancer (mCRPC) and outlines some of the ongoing clinical trials in this area. In addition, the authors outline current knowledge on outcomes of patients treated with taxane-based chemotherapy on retrospective analysis of randomized trials. These data are intended to provide physicians and patients with a general idea on the outcomes of men with mCRPC that may facilitate clinical decisions as well as the design and evaluation of clinical trials.

The treatment of metastatic castration-resistant prostate cancer has evolved since the approval of docetaxel-based therapy. Since docetaxel approval, three new agents have gained approval for this indication: sipuleucel-T, cabazitaxel, and abiraterone. Recent Phase III trials have also demonstrated survival benefits for MDV-3100 and radium-223 though regulatory approval ispending. Practicing physicians face the challenge of determining the optimal sequencing of these new agents. This dilemma is particularly relevant to the post-docetaxel setting, in which the indication for several of these agents overlaps. This article details the efficacy and safety of these agents to provide a framework for their clinical use.

UROLOGIC CLINICS OF NORTH AMERICA

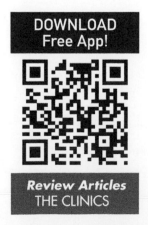

DOWNLOAD Free App!

Review Articles
THE CLINICS

NOW AVAILABLE FOR YOUR iPhone and iPad

UROLOGIC CLINICS OF NORTH AMERICA

FORTHCOMING ISSUES

February 2013
The Multidisciplinary Management of Urinary Stone Disease
Ojas Shah, MD, Guest Editor

May 2013
Diagnosis, Evaluation, and Treatment of Non-Muscle Invasive Bladder Cancer
Sam Chang, MD, Guest Editor

August 2013
Urologic Trauma and Reconstruction
Alan F. Morey, MD, and Steven J. Hudak, MD, Guest Editors

RECENT ISSUES

August 2012
Controversies in Female Pelvic Reconstruction
Roger Dmochowski, MD, and Mickey Karram, MD, Guest Editors

May 2012
Evolving Treatment Paradigms for Renal Cancer
William C. Huang, MD, and Samir S. Taneja, MD, Guest Editors

February 2012
Men's Health
Steven A. Kaplan, MD, Guest Editor

Foreword

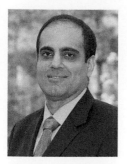

Samir S. Taneja, MD
Consulting Editor

The care of prostate cancer has long been the job of practicing urologists. Even before the transforming discoveries of Huggins in the 1950s, men with advanced prostate cancer were cared for by the urologist. With the advent of androgen deprivation therapy, this care became more than simple palliation of local symptoms and pain. Through hormonal deprivation, the longevity of men with metastatic prostate cancer improved, and the responsibilities of urologists caring for these men grew to include the management of local symptoms of disease, side effects of therapy including bone health, and counseling regarding the anticipation of end of life. In many ways, prostate cancer created urologists as oncologists, and from this the true discipline of urologic oncology arose.

Although prostate cancer patients have formed long-lasting relationships with their urologists historically, there has always been the frustration of having little to offer at the time of castration-resistance progression. In the contemporary era, new therapies have arisen, and now multiple therapies are approved for the care of castration-resistant disease. This has shifted the paradigm from one of "nothing to offer" to "which therapy to offer first." Within a previously empty therapeutic cupboard have arrived approved or evolving chemotherapies, immunotherapy, second-line hormonal agents, and targeted biologic agents. Management that used to be purely palliative is now a complex decision process dependent on disease state and patient characteristics.

In this issue of the *Urologic Clinics*, Dr Adam Kibel, our guest editor, has assembled a group of articles that beautifully present the multidisciplinary decision process that occurs in the management of men with castration-resistant prostate cancer.

These expert authors have provided great insight into the biologic rationale of current therapeutics, the selection of candidates for therapy, and the perspective of various disciplines in the care of these patients. We are extremely indebted to Dr Kibel and our contributing authors for the care with which this issue was prepared.

It has been a great concern of mine, in recent years, that urologists have confined their interest and focus to the techniques of treating early stage prostate cancer while relegating the care of patients with adverse pathology, advanced and recurrent disease, or disease-related symptoms to other disciplines with whom we collaborate. Not only does this stand against the conventional paradigm of prostate cancer care, but it risks isolation and has the potential of limiting urologists to the role of a technician with little to no input in overall patient care. It remains critically important for the practicing and training urologist to be the most knowledgeable individual in the hospital about every aspect of prostate cancer biology, epidemiology, and clinical care. This issue goes a long way toward stressing this to our community. I hope you will all use this as a tool and springboard toward continuing our specialty's excellence in the care of prostate cancer patients.

Samir S. Taneja, MD
Division of Urologic Oncology
Smilow Comprehensive Prostate Cancer Center
Department of Urology
NYU Langone Medical Center
150 East 32nd Street, Suite 200
New York, NY 10016, USA

E-mail address:
samir.taneja@nyumc.org

Urol Clin N Am 39 (2012) xiii
http://dx.doi.org/10.1016/j.ucl.2012.09.003
0094-0143/12/$ – see front matter © 2012 Elsevier Inc. All rights reserved.

Preface

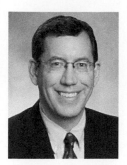

Adam S. Kibel, MD
Guest Editor

Barely 10 years ago, our primary treatment for metastatic prostate cancer revolved completely around surgical or medical castration. Once a patient failed, there was little to offer them. The state of prostate cancer treatment has shifted dramatically over the past decade. With the FDA's approval of docetaxel for the treatment of hormone refractory prostate cancer, the era of nihilism toward advanced prostate cancer ended. It has been replaced by a much more complex landscape, which, while offering the promise of prolongation of life, is often confusing to both physician and patient. Instead of having nothing to offer, we have an array of choices. Which should be offered to our patient is a question we wrestle with every day.

In this edition of *Urologic Clinics*, experts in the field define the different disease states and what is the best treatment for each. First and foremost are reviews of the biology of advanced prostate cancer. While we have moved beyond castration, the hormonal axis clearly remains the most important therapeutic target. Beyond the hormonal axis, there are multiple novel agents ranging from standard chemotherapy to bone-targeting agents. Each has a population that has been demonstrated in randomized trials to benefit.

As we strive to manage patients with advanced disease, it is important to recognize that the treatments still only offer extended life, not cure. As such, palliation and quality of life must be balanced against tumor response. Next, we must look to the future, when we may cure patients. How are we going to sequence our treatments, so that patients only receive the treatment that will cure them and are spared the toxicity of those that are unlikely to provide benefit? Last, small molecule therapy has revolutionized the treatment of many malignancies including renal cell carcinoma. The hope is that these novel agents will soon be used in the treatment of prostate carcinoma, offering cure with fewer side effects.

While cure is currently beyond our reach, reading this edition of *Urologic Clinics* will make you realize it is closer than we think. Increasingly the urologist will be serving as a guild to the patient, making sure they get the right treatment at the right time. These articles will provide the framework for advocating for the best treatment in our patients.

Adam S. Kibel, MD
Professor of Surgery
Harvard Medical School
Chief of Urology
Brigham and Women's Hospital
45 Francis Street
Boston, MA 02115, USA

E-mail address:
akibel@partners.org

Biology of Castration-Recurrent Prostate Cancer

Faris Azzouni, MD*, James Mohler, MD

KEYWORDS

- Prostate cancer • Castration resistant • Castration recurrent • Biology • Mechanism

KEY POINTS

- Castration-recurrent prostate cancer is androgen-stimulated.
- The clinical terms hormone-refractory and androgen-independent are obsolete and should be abandoned.
- Castration-recurrent prostate cancer is androgen stimulated, and remains dependent on androgen-receptor signaling in most cases.
- Several mechanisms are used by castration-recurrent prostate cancer cells to grow despite castrate serum androgens levels. These mechanisms include the hypersensitive, the intracrine androgen synthesis, the promiscuous, the outlaw, the bypass, and the stem-cell pathways.
- Many promising therapeutic agents are becoming available for treatment of castration-recurrent prostate cancer because of better understanding of the molecular processes that fuel the growth of castration-recurrent prostate cancer.

INTRODUCTION

Prostate cancer (CaP) is the second leading cause of death from cancer in American men. Almost all cases of CaP mortality occur as a result of metastatic disease. More than 7 decades ago, Huggins and Hodges[1] demonstrated the benefits of androgen-deprivation therapy (ADT) for metastatic CaP. On initiation of ADT, most men experience significant clinical, biochemical, and radiologic remission. However, this response is only temporary and almost all patients experience disease recurrence, hence the term castration-recurrent (castration-resistant) CaP (CRCaP), which is fatal in 80% of patients. Until recently, CRCaP was inaccurately labeled as hormone-refractory or androgen-independent. However; recent advances have shown that CRCaP remains dependent on androgen receptor (AR) signaling in most cases.[2] This article reviews the diversity of mechanisms used for growth by CRCaP (**Table 1**).

THE ANDROGEN RECEPTOR

The biological effects of androgens are mediated through AR, a member of the nuclear steroid hormone receptor superfamily. The AR gene is located on the X chromosome (Xq11–12), spans approximately 180 kb of DNA, and has 8 exons (exons A–H).[3] The AR protein is composed of 919 amino acids and is divided into 4 domains: an amino-terminal transactivation domain (NTD), a DNA-binding domain (DBD), a hinge region, and a ligand-binding domain (LBD) (**Fig. 1**).[3]

The AR NTD, encoded by exon A, constitutes about half of the AR protein and is responsible for the majority of the AR transcriptional activities and AR coactivator interaction.[4] The AR NTD is composed of 2 transcription activation units (TAU): TAU-1 (amino acids 1–485), required for full ligand-stimulated, wild-type AR activity, and TAU-5 (amino acids 360–528), which confers constitutive ligand-independent AR activity.[5]

Disclosures: None.
Department of Urology, Roswell Park Cancer Institute, Elm and Carlton streets, Buffalo, NY 14263, USA
* Corresponding author.
E-mail address: faris.azzouni@roswellpark.org

Urol Clin N Am 39 (2012) 435–452
http://dx.doi.org/10.1016/j.ucl.2012.07.002

Table 1
Mechanisms of CRCaP growth

Pathway	Ligand Availability	AR Dependence	Components
Hypersensitive	Testicular androgens	Yes	1. AR overexpression 2. Increased AR sensitivity to low androgen levels
Intracrine testicular androgen synthesis	Testicular androgens	Yes	1. De novo synthesis of testicular androgens from ubiquitous substrates, eg, cholesterol, acetate, and adrenal androgens 2. Upregulated expression of genes encoding steroidogenic enzymes
Promiscuous	Testicular and adrenal androgens, corticosteroids, estradiol, progesterone, antiandrogens	Yes	Widened AR specificity via AR mutations or altered coregulator profiles
Outlaw	No	Yes	1. AR activation by growth factors or cytokines 2. AR splice variants (constitutively active)
Bypass	No	No	1. Inhibition of apoptosis 2. Neuroendocrine differentiation 3. Estrogen receptors
Stem cell	No	No	Prostate cancer stem cells

Unique to AR is the variable-length polyglutamine repeat (polyQ) in the NTD. Shorter polyQ appears to increase AR transcriptional activity, and has been linked to increased CaP incidence and aggressiveness in some[6–8] but not other studies.[9,10] Long polyQ (>40) causes spinal bulbar muscular atrophy (Kennedy disease).[11]

The AR DBD is composed of 2 zinc-finger motifs, which are encoded by exons B and C, respectively. The first zinc finger mediates DNA recognition through interaction with specific base pairs in response elements, which facilitates binding of AR to the major groove of DNA.[12] The second zinc finger stabilizes DNA binding and mediates AR dimerization.[13] The hinge region, encoded by part of exon D, contains a bipartite nuclear localization signal as well as important sites for phosphorylation, acetylation, and degradation.[14,15] The LBD, encoded by part of exon D and exons E to H, mediates ligand binding.[16] The AR LBD has 12 conserved α-helices that form a ligand-binding pocket.[17] Agonist binding induces a conformational change in the LBD and the folding of helix 12 across the ligand-binding pocket, which forms the activation function 2 (AF2) surface. The AF2 surface mediates interaction with the FQNLF peptide of the AR NTD and can bind coregulators containing similar sequences.[18] In the absence of ligand binding, AR is present diffusely throughout the cytoplasm and held in an inactive state in association with chaperones, such as heat-shock proteins (HSPs). The minimal chaperone complex required for efficient folding and stabilization of AR consists of Hsp70 (hsc70), Hsp40 (Ydj1), Hop (p60), Hsp90, and p23.[19,20] Ligand binding releases AR from HSPs, and is followed by nuclear translocation, homodimer formation, binding to AR response element DNA (target genes), and recruitment of AR coregulators (coactivators and/or corepressors), which regulate gene transcription.[21,22] The best characterized AR target gene is Kallikrein-related peptidase 3 gene (KLK3), which encodes the prostate-specific antigen (PSA) protein.

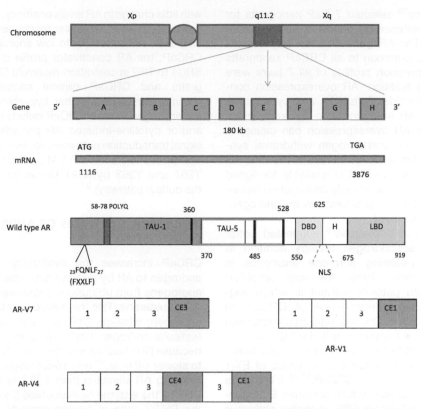

Fig. 1. Wild-type AR and the 3 most common AR splice variants. ATG, translation start site; CE, cryptic exon containing a premature stop codon; DBD, DNA-binding domain; H, hinge region; LBD, ligand-binding domain; NLS, nuclear localization signal; TGA, stop codon.

THE HYPERSENSITIVE PATHWAY

CRCaP can increase its sensitivity to available low androgen levels by increasing AR synthesis and/or increasing AR sensitivity.

AR Gene Amplification and AR Overexpression

AR gene amplification was first reported in 1995.[23] Early studies reported AR gene amplification in 28% to 30% of CRCaP patients.[23,24] AR gene amplification seemed important because no AR gene amplification was found in primary CaP in eugonadal patients (androgen-stimulated CaP [AS-CaP]). AR gene amplification was detected mainly in CRCaP that had initially responded well to ADT and whose response duration was more than 12 months.[24] CaP that recurred earlier or failed to respond to ADT had no AR gene amplification. Median survival after CaP recurrence was twice as long for patients with AR gene amplification as for those with no amplification ($P = .03$). A subsequent report from the same group that examined prostatic tissues from a larger cohort of CRCaP

patients failed to detect an association between AR gene amplification and survival.[25]

Our group detected AR gene amplification in 33% of CRCaP specimens obtained from the primary site, which was associated with increased AR protein expression.[26] However, no association was found between AR gene amplification and duration of survival after ADT. More recently, AR gene amplification was detected in 50% to 85% of circulating tumor cells in patients with CRCaP.[27,28] These differences in reported rates of AR overexpression could be attributed to study cohort differences, tumor heterogeneity, and technical improvements.

Holzbeierlein and colleagues[29] performed a genome-wide analysis and identified gene expression changes that occur during ADT and in CRCaP. Many AR-regulated genes that were suppressed when patients were started on ADT were reexpressed in CRCaP, specifically AR and steroid-synthesis enzymes, which suggests that CRCaP tumors have increased sensitivity to, and endogenously synthesize androgens (intracrine androgen synthesis; see later discussion). Chen and colleagues[30] selected 7 CaP xenografts for castration resistance by passing tumors in castrated mice. The AR gene was the only overexpressed gene common to all CRCaP xenografts when the expression profiles of all 7 pairs were compared. In addition, AR overexpression converted bicalutamide, flutamide, and cyproterone acetate from AR antagonists to agonists, which suggests that AR overexpression can cause, at least in part, the antiandrogen withdrawal syndrome. Abundance of AR increases the total AR content of the tumor that is available for ligand binding and allows seemingly androgen-independent cancer cells to proliferate in an androgen-depleted environment.

Palmberg and colleagues[25] suggested better response to antiandrogen therapy addition to gonadotropin-releasing hormone analogues in CRCaP patients whose AR was amplified compared with patients without it, which suggested continued dependence of CRCaP on residual androgens. One mechanism of increasing AR expression is through endothelin-1 (ET-1). ET-1 is highly expressed by CaP cell lines and tumor specimens, and elevated plasma levels of ET-1 are present in men with CRCaP.[31,32] ET-1 binds endothelin A receptor, which activates Src/phosphatidylinositol 3-kinase (PI3K) signaling pathways (see section on the outlaw pathway) and augments AR expression via c-Myc.[33] ET-1 also stimulates osteoblasts and plays a role in osteoblastic bone metastasis.[32]

Increased AR Sensitivity to Androgens

The authors' group was the first to demonstrate increased stability of AR in the "absence of androgens" when androgen-sensitive LNCaP cells were compared with androgen-independent LNCaP-C4-2 and CWR-R1 cells, and castration-recurrent CWR22 xenograft tumors.[34] AR in LNCaP cells was unstable, with a degradation half-time ($t_{1/2}$) of 3 hours. By contrast, AR was more stable in androgen-independent CWR-R1 ($t_{1/2} = 6$ hours) and LNCaP-C4-2 cell lines ($t_{1/2} = 7$ hours), and castration-recurrent CWR22 tumors ($t_{1/2} > 12$ hours). The concentration of dihydrotestosterone (DHT) required for growth stimulation of androgen-independent cells (CWR-R1 and LNCaP-C4-2) was 4 orders of magnitude lower than that required for LNCaP cells. The increased sensitivity to androgens was not associated with major differences in AR expression, AR binding affinity to androgens, or AR-androgen dissociation times. These results suggested that increased AR stability may increase AR nuclear retention time, which could result in an increased biological response at lower DHT levels

with little change in AR levels or affinity. The authors' group provided a molecular mechanism to explain increased AR sensitivity to low androgen levels in CRCaP; the AR coactivator profile changed from SRC1 to TIF2 in castration-recurrent CWR22 xenografts and CRCaP clinical samples.[35] Other common mechanisms that hypersensitize AR to low androgen levels in CRCaP include growth factor and/or cytokine-induced AR phosphorylation via signal transduction pathways, for example, AR tyrosine phosphorylation at Y534 by Src kinase,[36] and Y267 and Y363 by Ack1 kinase (see section on the outlaw pathway).[37]

INTRACRINE SYNTHESIS OF ANDROGENS BY CRCaP TISSUE

CRCaP increases the availability of testicular androgen to AR by de novo synthesis of testicular androgens from ubiquitous substrates.

Testosterone (T) is the main circulating testicular androgen, whereas DHT is the main intracellular testicular androgen. DHT is the preferred AR ligand because DHT has higher affinity for AR than T owing to slower off time,[38] and 10-fold higher potency of inducing AR signaling than T.[39] T is converted to DHT by the enzyme 5α-reductase (5α-R). Whereas the DHT:T ratio in benign prostate and ASCaP tissues is 2.5:1 to 20:1, DHT levels drop significantly in CRCaP tissues and the ratio becomes 0.25:1 to 0.5:1.[40,41] This change in ratios is likely a consequence of changes in 5α-R isozyme tissue expression during CaP progression. The authors' group and others reported relative increases in 5α-R isozymes 1 and 3, and a relative decrease in isozyme 2 in CRCaP, versus ASCaP.[42,43] The total 5α-reducing capability in CRCaP versus ASCaP is probably decreased because isozyme 2 is the most efficient 5α-reducing enzyme at physiologic (intracellular) pH.[44] Despite the significant reduction in DHT levels in CRCaP tissues, AR signaling remains active. Comparing levels of T and DHT between benign prostatic and ASCaP tissues on one hand, with CRCaP tissues reveals persistent and even elevated androgen levels in CRCaP tissues, well within the range that is capable of activating wild-type and mutated ARs.[40,41]

The authors' group compared prostatic tissue levels of T and DHT between androgen-stimulated benign prostate and CRCaP. T levels were similar and DHT levels were 80% to 90% lower.[40,45] Mean DHT levels were 8.13 pmol/g versus 1.45 pmol/g tissue using mass spectrometry (MS), and 13.7 pmol/g versus 1.25 pmol/g tissue using radioimmunoassay (RIA), levels sufficient to activate even a molecularly "normal" AR (wild-type unphosphorylated AR with normal coregulator profile). Continued AR activation in CRCaP was suggested by continued expression of PSA. These results were confirmed by others.[41] T level was 3-fold higher, whereas DHT level was 11-fold lower (mean 0.25 ng/g tissue), in metastatic CRCaP lesions compared with prostatic tissue from eugonadal patients with ASCaP.[41] Expression of AR and PSA proteins was higher and similar, respectively, between metastatic CRCaP (bone metastasis) and ASCaP tissues, again indicating continued AR signaling in CRCaP.

Tissue levels of androgens are difficult to measure using either MS or RIA because of problems with tissue procurement, low tissue androgen levels, and assay sensitivity. However, tissue androgen levels appear similar when measured by different groups using different methods to assay different types of tissues (Table 2). In CWR-R1 and LNCaP-C4-2 cell lines (both exhibiting mutated ARs), a DHT level as low as 10^{-14} M (2.92×10^{-6} ng/g tissue) was sufficient for growth stimulation.[34,46]

Substrates for de novo androgen synthesis in CRCaP cells include cholesterol, cholesterol precursors (eg, acetic acid), and adrenal androgens.[46–48] Furthermore, all enzymes necessary for DHT synthesis from cholesterol are expressed, and most are upregulated (3–30 fold) in CRCaP tissue.[29,41]

Two closely intertwined pathways exist that ultimately lead to DHT synthesis from cholesterol: the front-door pathway (via the adrenal androgens dehydroepiandrosterone [DHEA] and androstenedione [ASD]) and the back-door pathway (via pregnanedione and androstanediol) (Fig. 2).[49] In the classic pathway, C21 steroids such as pregnenolone and progesterone are first converted to the C19 adrenal androgens DHEA and ASD via sequential 17α-hydroxylase and 17,20-lyase activities of CYP17A, followed by the activities of 17β-hydroxysteroid dehydrogenase (17βHSD) and 5α-R. In the back-door pathway, the order of steps is reversed whereby C21 steroids are first 5α-reduced, followed by sequential CYP17A and 17βHSD actions.[49] Androstanediol is the major degradation product of DHT from the reductive 3α-hydroxysteroid dehydrogenase (HSD) activity of 3α-HSD aldo-keto reductases 1C (AKR1C). The authors' group demonstrated AR transactivation by androstanediol in benign and malignant prostate-derived cell lines via oxidation of androstanediol into DHT.[50] Administration of androstanediol to castration-recurrent CWR22 tumor xenografts resulted in a 28-fold increase in intratumoral DHT levels.

Clinical indicators of the significance of residual prostatic tissue androgens in CRCaP include the benefits of secondary or tertiary hormonal therapies in CRCaP patients. Ketoconazole administration in CRCaP is associated a PSA response ($\geq 50\%$ decrease in PSA from baseline) in 50% to 60% of patients.[51] 5α-Reductase inhibitors (5α-RI) used

Table 2
Comparison of prostatic tissue testicular androgen levels measured by different groups

Mass Spectrometry			Radioimmunoassay		
	T	DHT		T	DHT
Titus et al,[45] 2005			Mohler et al,[40] 2004		
ASBP (n = 18)	2.75	13.7	ASBP (n = 30)	3.26	8.13
CRCaP (n = 18)	3.75	1.25	CRCaP (n = 15)	2.78	1.45
Montgomery et al,[41] 2008			Geller et al,[135] 1979		
ASBP (n = 6)	0.04	1.92	ASBP (n = 17)	NM	17.6
ASCaP (n = 4)	0.23	2.75	CaP orch ± DES (n = 9)	NM	4.47
CR-Met CaP (n = 8)	0.74	0.25	CaP DES 1 mg (n = 6)	NM	12.4
			Labrie et al,[136] 1989		
			Human CaP (n = NS)	NM	18.6
			Orch (n = 5, 2–12 mo)	NM	9.29
			Orch + FL (n = 4, 2 mo)	NM	ND

Abbreviations: ASBP, androgen-stimulated benign prostate; CRCaP, castration-recurrent prostate cancer; CR-Met CaP, metastatic castration-recurrent prostate cancer; DES, diethylstilbestrol; DHT, dihydrotestosterone; FL, flutamide; mo, months; n, number of subjects; ND, not detected; NM, not measured; NS, not specified; orch, orchiectomy; T, testosterone.

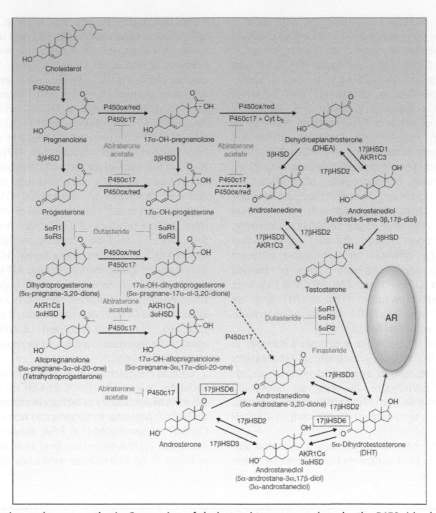

Fig. 2. Intracrine androgen synthesis. Conversion of cholesterol to pregnenolone by the P450 side-chain cleavage enzyme (P450ssc) is the first committed step in steroid biosynthesis. The 17α-hydroxylase/17,20-lyase (P450c17) catalyzes multiple 17α-hydroxylase and 17,20-lyase reactions in the steroidogenic pathway that require P450 oxidoreductase (P450ox/red) electron transfer. P450c17, coded by the CYP17A1 gene, is the target for inhibition by abiraterone acetate. Progesterone, 17α-hydroxyprogesterone (17α-OH-progesterone), and T are substrates for 5α-reductase types 1 to 3 (5αR1, 2, or 3). Finasteride is a 5αR2,3 inhibitor. Dutasteride is an inhibitor of 5αR types 1 to 3. Isozymes of 3β-hydroxysteroid dehydrogenase (3βHSD), 17β-hydroxysteroid dehydrogenase (17βHSD), and aldo-keto reductase (AKR1C3) are often reversible enzymes with oxidative and reductive activities that require nicotinamide adenine dinucleotide cofactors. T and DHT are the 2 biologically active androgens that activate AR. T is the major circulating active androgen formed in the testis. DHT is formed from T in the testis, and can be synthesized in a so-called back-door pathway (green) from progesterone and androsterone precursors, independent of DHEA, androstenedione, or T intermediates. The back-door pathway of DHT synthesis involves the conversion of androstanediol to DHT by 17β-HSD6. (*Reproduced from* Mohler JL, Titus MA, Wilson EM. Potential prostate cancer drug target: bioactivation of androstanediol by conversion to dihydrotestosterone. Clin Cancer Res 2011;17(18):5844–9.)

singly or in combination with an antiandrogen or ketoconazole and hydrocortisone resulted in PSA decreases of variable magnitudes and durations in more than half of the patients with CRCaP.[52,53] Abiraterone, a CYP17A inhibitor of adrenal and testicular androgen synthesis, prolongs overall survival in post-docetaxel CRCaP patients by nearly 4 months.[54] Abiraterone also decreases "castrate" serum T level in CRCaP patients from less than 50 ng/dL to less than 1 ng/dL.[55]

These results strongly support that CRCaP tissue is capable of intracrine testicular androgen synthesis from ubiquitous substrates. Therapeutic strategies designed to more effectively ablate tumor androgens are needed and are likely to improve CRCaP outcomes.

THE PROMISCUOUS PATHWAY

AR specificity is broadened such that AR could be activated by nonandrogenic steroids or even anti-androgens. The broadened specificity might be achieved either through mutations in the LBD or through alterations in the coregulator profile.

AR Mutations

The AR gene is not necessary for survival, as is evident by the germline loss-of-function mutations that lead to androgen insensitivity syndrome.[56] CRCaP that acquires somatic gain-of-function mutations in the LBD of the AR gene have broad-ened ligand specificity, which allows AR activation by nontesticular androgens and antiandrogens.[57] AR mutations seen in androgen insensitivity syndrome and CRCaP involve different parts of the AR gene. AR mutations can explain the antian-drogen withdrawal syndrome observed on discon-tinuation of antiandrogens (flutamide, nilutamide,[58] bicalutamide,[59] and cyproterone acetate[60]).

The first such AR mutation was identified in LNCaP cells, which were activated by testicular and adrenal androgens, progesterone, estradiol, and flutamide, but not bicalutamide.[61] Sequencing the AR gene from LNCaP cells revealed a missense mutation in amino acid 877, located in the LBD. This mutation caused the substitution of alanine for threonine (T877A). CaP cells possessing this mutation were able to be clonally selected to grow in a castrate environment, leading to CRCaP.

The frequency of AR mutations reported in the literature varies widely (0%–50%). AR mutations were initially reported in 50% (5 of 10) of patients with CRCaP from whom specimens were obtained from metastatic lesions (bone marrow, skin, and pleural fluid) using a cloning-based method whereby polymerase chain reaction integrity may have been problematic.[62] Subsequent reports from the same group identified AR mutations at lower frequencies. AR mutations were reported in 10% to 30% of CRCaP patients who were treated for long periods of time with castration and antiandrogens, and specimens were obtained from bone marrow metastases.[57,63] Work by the authors' group using different methods suggested similar frequency of AR mutations in CRCaP. The T877A mutation was detected in 10% of 25 pros-tatectomy specimens from CRCaP patients using denaturing gradient gel electrophoresis (DGGE) of exons B to H, and direct sequencing of exon A

and any possible mutations suggested by DGGE.[64] Factors that make it difficult to determine the true in vivo frequency of AR mutations include patient selection, tumor heterogeneity, tissue source (prostate gland vs metastases), method of tissue preservation, duration of antiandrogen therapy, and molecular methods.[63]

The human CaP xenograft CWR22 cells have an H874Y (substitution of tyrosine for histidine) mutant AR that is activated by testicular and adrenal androgens, estradiol, progesterone, and flutamide. The H874Y mutation occurs in the LBD and broadens AR specificity by changing co-activator binding to AR. Passage of these cells in castrate nude mice gives rise to castration-recurrent CWR22 cells, also known as CWR-R1 cells, which exhibit the same AR mutation.[34,65]

MDA PCa 2a and 2b cell lines were established from bone metastasis in a CRCaP patient. These cell lines harbor a promiscuous AR that has reduced affinity for androgens.[66] Two distinct missense mutations in the AR LBD were detected in these cell lines: the T877A mutation and the leucine-to-histidine substitution at amino acid 701 (L701H). The L701H mutation alone decreases AR affinity for DHT and increases affinity to cortisol. The T877A mutation broadens AR speci-ficity to include progesterone and estradiol, and provides a synergistic effect by increasing AR affinity for cortisol 3-fold more than the L701H mutation alone. Cortisol was associated with the highest transactivation response in L701H-T877A transfected cells.[67] The frequency of this mutation in CRCaP remains unknown.

Recent work that reported AR transactivation by androstanediol[50] demonstrated the ability of CRCaP cells to convert a weak androgen into DHT. Other weak AR ligands may be converted to testicular androgens by CRCaP cells instead of transactivating a promiscuous AR directly. This new concept questions the significance of AR mutations and must cause a reexamination of publications describing broadened specificity of any steroid receptor for its ligands.

Many other mutations in the AR gene have been identified and are cataloged in the Androgen Receptor Gene Mutations Database (http://andro gendb.mcgill.ca/), but it is unclear how many other mutations use the promiscuous receptor mechanism.

Altered Coregulator Profiles

Several proteins modulate the function of AR and act as either coactivators or corepressors of DNA transcription. More than 170 AR coregulator proteins have been reported.[68] Each coregulator either interacts directly with AR or is found in a transcriptional complex that includes AR.[69] Alterations in AR coregulator levels and function may contribute to the development of CRCaP. In addition, overexpression of some coregulators in CaP clinical specimens was associated with unfavorable clinical outcomes.[70]

Increase in coactivator proteins

Several AR coactivators, such as TIF2, SRC1, Tip60, and CARM1, are overexpressed in CRCaP.[34,71,72] Proposed mechanisms for AR coactivator–induced growth stimulation in CRCaP include increased AR sensitivity to ligands and/or through broadened AR specificity.

Clinical samples of androgen-stimulated benign prostate, ASCaP, CRCaP, and androgen-stimulated and castration-recurrent CWR22 tumor xenografts were used to detect overexpression of AR and 2 AR coactivators; TIF2 and SRC1, in CRCaP samples.[35] TIF2 was more overexpressed than SRC1 so that the transcriptional complex had a predominance of TIF2. Overexpression of TIF2 in cotransfection assays increased AR transcriptional activity in the presence of physiologic concentrations of adrenal androgens. Furthermore, overexpressed TIF2 increased the transcriptional activity of the mutant ARs (T877A in LNCaP) and (H874Y in CWR22) in the presence of unchanged levels of testicular and adrenal androgens, progesterone, estradiol, and hydroxyflutamide. These results show that overexpression of TIF2 and/or SRC1 in CRCaP increases AR transactivation in wild-type and mutant ARs in response to low and physiologic concentrations of testicular and adrenal androgens, and other steroids with affinity for AR. Agoulnik and colleagues[73] found that reducing SRC1 expression decreased cell growth and PSA synthesis in the AR-dependent LNCaP and LNCaP-C4-2 cell lines, whereas proliferation was unaffected in the AR-negative PC-3 and DU145 cell lines, suggesting that the effects of SRC1 are AR-dependent. Unlike SRC1, the effects of TIF2 seem to be a combination of AR-dependent and AR-independent mechanisms, because reducing the expression of TIF2 negatively affected the growth of both LNCaP and PC-3 cells.[74]

Yeh and colleagues[75,76] transfected DU145 CaP cells with AR and found that overexpression of the AR coactivator (ARA70) enhanced AR transactivation 10-fold in the presence of DHT or T, and greater than 30-fold in the presence of estradiol.

Halkidou and colleagues[71] studied the expression and subcellular localization of the AR coactivator Tip60 in CaP cell lines, and in benign and malignant prostate clinical samples. On androgen withdrawal, Tip60 expression was upregulated and shifted to the nucleus in LNCaP cell culture and in CWR22 xenografts. Androgen exposure decreased the expression of Tip60 and increased its cytoplasmic distribution. In clinical samples, Tip60 had a diffuse cellular distribution in benign prostatic and ASCaP tissues, whereas in CRCaP, localization was mainly nuclear.

The AR coactivator CARM1 is overexpressed in CRCaP but not in ASCaP. Reducing CARM1 expression decreased PSA expression and CaP cell growth, and induced apoptosis.[72] Many other coactivators have been identified, but their contributions to AR action have not been characterized fully.

Decrease in corepressor proteins

Corepressors reduce AR activity through a variety of mechanisms such as prevention of nuclear localization and DNA binding, recruiting histone deacetylases that deacetylate chromatin and other proteins required for transcriptional activity, competing with coactivators for binding to AR, reducing NTD/LBD interactions required for optimal transcriptional activation of AR, and functioning as scaffolds for other AR coregulators.[77] Examples include NCoR1, SMRT/NCoR2, DAX-1, cyclin D1a (an estrogen-receptor coactivator), histone deacetylases, and the less well characterized proteins Hey1 and FoxH1.[78–83] Recruitment of NCoR1 and SMRT by agonist-bound AR has been shown to suppress agonist-induced activation of androgen-regulated genes such as PSA, TSC22, NKX3.1 and B2M.[84,85] Recruitment of corepressors is believed to be a key mediator of antagonist-mediated inhibition of steroid receptors including AR, which suggests that loss of expression of corepressors could facilitate tumor growth in the presence of AR antagonists used in conjunction with castration.[86–88] The large number of AR coregulators and their inherent redundancy make AR coregulators challenging targets for drug development.

THE OUTLAW PATHWAY

AR activation by nonsteroid molecules, such as growth factors and cytokines, has been referred to as the outlaw pathway. This method of activation occurs in the absence of androgens or other steroid ligands, but is dependent on AR. Growth factors, including insulin-like growth factor 1 (IGF-1), keratinocyte growth factor (KGF), and epidermal growth factor (EGF), and cytokines such as interleukin (IL)-6, are capable of activating AR via signal transduction pathways.[89,90] In addition, IL-6 is capable of increasing AR sensitivity to low androgen levels[90] and plays a role in CaP bone metastasis (see section on the role of inflammation). IGF-1, EGF, and IL-6 can each activate AR in the presumed absence of ligands,[89–92] and all were reported to be upregulated in CRCaP.[93–95]

Signal transduction pathways are a complex network of membrane-bound and intracellular kinases, capable of activating AR by phosphorylating either AR coactivators (eg, TIF2 and SRC1)[91,92] or AR itself, at several amino acid residues.[36,37,91,92,96,97] In addition, some of these kinases, such as AKT (protein kinase B), are capable of inhibiting apoptosis.[98] AR phosphorylation could occur at several serine or threonine residues by mitogen-activated protein kinase (MAPK), PI3K/AKT, protein kinase A, and protein kinase C.[91,92,96,97] AR also could be phosphorylated and activated by tyrosine kinases such as Src and Ack1 kinases.[36,37]

Culig and colleagues[89] reported androgen-independent AR transactivation by IGF-1, KGF, or EGF in AR-cotransfected DU145 CaP cells. IGF-1 was the most potent. All 3 growth factors had no stimulatory effects in DU145 cells that lacked AR. Combining IGF-1 with the synthetic androgen methyltrienolone (R1881) did not have any additive or synergistic effects on AR transactivation. Bicalutamide completely inhibited the AR-stimulatory effects of all 3 growth factors. These results provide evidence that IGF-I, KGF, and EGF are capable of directly activating AR in the absence of androgens, via the LBD.

AR-cotransfected DU145 and LNCaP cells were used to prove the existence of cross-talk between IL-6 and AR transactivation.[90] IL-6 upregulated AR activity in a ligand-independent manner, as well as synergistically, with very low doses of R1881. The maximal induction of reporter gene activity by IL-6 alone was 67% of the maximal induction stimulated by 1 nM R1881. The concentration of the androgen required to achieve maximal AR transactivation was reduced 100-fold in the presence of IL-6. IL-6 did not induce reporter gene activity when the AR expression vector was replaced with an empty vector. Bicalutamide inhibited AR transactivation by IL-6 alone, and in combination with R1881. Inhibitors of the protein kinase A, protein kinase C, and MAPK pathways abolished AR transactivation induced by IL-6 but had minimal or no effect on AR transactivation induced by R1881. In LNCaP cells, IL-6 induced AR-regulated PSA mRNA and protein synthesis that was antagonized by bicalutamide, and by inhibitors of the protein kinase A or MAPK signaling pathways. These experiments support the ability of IL-6 to stimulate, in an androgen-independent manner, AR transactivation via the LBD through

signal transduction pathways. In addition, IL-6 hypersensitizes AR to low androgen levels, which raises the specter of intracrine metabolism of DHT from media components, such as cholesterol. Investigators must consider and control for problems previously not considered, such as steroid hormone contaminants in the pores of plastic ware.

Receptor HER-2/neu is another mechanism of outlaw activation of AR. HER-2/neu, also known as ErbB-2, is a member of the EGF receptor family of plasma membrane-bound receptor tyrosine kinases. Unlike the other family members, HER-2/neu has no known ligands and is therefore considered an orphan receptor. HER-2/neu was found to be overexpressed in LAPC-4-cell lines generated from xenografts implanted in castrated mice.[99] Forced overexpression of HER-2/neu in androgen-sensitive CaP cells was sufficient to confer androgen-independent growth in vitro and accelerate growth in castrated mice.[99] HER-2/neu activated AR signaling in the absence of ligands and enhanced the magnitude of AR transactivation in the presence of low levels of androgens, but not in the absence of AR. Unlike IGF-1, KGF, EGF, and IL-6, bicalutamide did not inhibit AR transactivation mediated by HER-2/neu, which suggests that HER-2/neu affects AR signaling through a mechanism independent of the AR LBD.[99] Several signal transduction pathways mediate the effects of HER-2/neu, such as MAPK, PI3K/AKT, phospholipase C, and protein kinase C.[100]

AR SPLICE VARIANTS

Variants of the wild-type (full-length) AR protein lacking the LBD are synthesized using either somatic nonsense mutations or posttranslational proteolysis. Splice variants have been demonstrated to be constitutively active in the absence of androgens.[101,102] Hu and colleagues[103] detected 7 AR splice variants (AR-V1 to AR-V7) in clinical samples of ASCaP (n = 82), CRCaP (n = 25), and CWR22Rv1. These AR variants were encoded by AR transcripts with "intronic" insertions (ie, cryptic exons) downstream of the coding sequence for the AR DBD. The premature stop codons present in the cryptic exons caused the translated AR proteins to be truncated. Only the NTD, DBD, and a short variant-specific peptide were retained. The 2 most abundantly expressed variants, AR-V1 and AR-V7, showed an average 20-fold higher expression in CRCaP compared with ASCaP at the mRNA level. At the protein level, AR-V1 was detected in at least 67% of CRCaP versus 11% in ASCaP samples. Among ASCaP

Table 3
Agents targeting CRCaP

Agent	Mechanism	Pathway
Abiraterone TAK-700	Inhibit CYP17	Inhibit adrenal and intracrine androgen synthesis
MDV-3100 AZD-3514 ARN-509 BMS-641988	Pure AR antagonists	Inhibit ligand-dependent AR activation
TOK-001	Dual CYP17 inhibitor and AR antagonist	Inhibits adrenal and intracrine androgen synthesis and ligand-dependent AR activation
Dutasteride Finasteride	5α-Reductase inhibitors	Decrease DHT synthesis and interfere with intracrine androgen production
EPI-001	Inhibits AR NTD	Inhibits AR-dependent mechanisms
Geldanamycin Tanespimycin (17-AAG) Alvespimycin (17-DMAG)	Inhibit HSP90	Inhibit AR chaperones and increase AR degradation
OGX-427	Inhibits HSP27	Inhibits AR chaperones and increases AR degradation
Romidepsin Suberoylanilide hydroxamic acid (SAHA) LBH-589 Trichostatin A Depsipeptide	Inhibit histone deacetylases	Inhibit transcription of AR target genes
Erlotinib Gefitinib	Inhibit EGFR-TK activity	Target the outlaw pathway
Lapatinib	Inhibits EGFR-TK and HER2/neu-TK activity	Targets the outlaw pathway
Imantinib	Multireceptor TKI including PDGFR	Targets the outlaw pathway
Trastuzumab Pertuzumab	Monoclonal antibodies against HER2/neu	Target the outlaw pathway
Dasatinib AZD-0530	Inhibit Src-TK activities	Targets the outlaw pathway
CP-751,871 IMC-A12	Monoclonal antibodies against IGF-1 receptor	Inhibit the outlaw pathway
Atrasentan ZD-4054	ER-A blockers	Target AR overexpression and inhibit osteoblastic bone metastasis
Denosumab	Monoclonal antibody against RANKL	Inhibits osteoclast activation and lytic bone metastasis
Zoledronic acid	Bisphosphonate	Binds hydroxyapatite of damaged bone and inhibits osteoclasts
Strontium Samarium	Radioisotopes	Bind hydroxyapatite of damaged bone and deliver radiation to the entire tumor microenvironment in bone
Bevacizumab	Monoclonal antibody against VEGF	Inhibits angiogenesis

(continued on next page)

Agent	Mechanism	Pathway
Table 3 *(continued)*		
Aflibercept	Inhibits VEGF	Inhibits angiogenesis
Sunitinib	Multireceptor TKI including VEGFR	Inhibits angiogenesis
Gossypol G-3139 (Oblimersen)	Inhibit Bcl-2	Inhibit the bypass pathway by stimulating apoptosis
AT-101	Inhibits multiple antiapoptotic BCL-2 family members (BCL-2, BCL-XL, BCL-W, MCL-1)	Inhibit the bypass pathway by stimulating apoptosis
OGX-011	Inhibits Clusterin	Inhibits the bypass pathway by stimulating apoptosis
Docetaxel Cabazitaxel	Stabilize microtubules and inhibit their disassembly	Inhibit mitosis
Provenge	Stimulates T cells against PAP-positive cells	Cancer vaccine
GVAX	Stimulates the immune system against multiple CaP antigens (irradiated LNCaP and PC-3 cells)	Cancer vaccine
Ipilimumab	Monoclonal antibody against CTLA-4	Enhances and maintains tumor-specific T-cell activity

Abbreviations: EGFR, epidermal growth factor receptor; ER-A, endothelin receptor A; HSP, heat-shock protein; IGF-1, insulin-like growth factor-1; NTD, N-terminus domain; PAP, prostate acid phosphatase; PDGFR, platelet-derived growth factor receptor; RANKL, receptor activator of nuclear factor κB ligand; TK, tyrosine kinase; TKI, tyrosine kinase inhibitor; VEGF, vascular endothelial growth factor; VEGFR, vascular endothelial growth factor receptor.

samples, higher expression of AR-V7 was associated with biochemical failure after radical prostatectomy ($P = .012$), unlike the expression of wild-type AR and AR-V1. AR-V7 was localized in the nuclei of cultured CaP cells under androgen-depleted conditions, and was constitutively active in inducing the expression of androgen-responsive genes.

Guo and colleagues[104] detected 3 AR splice variants (AR3, AR4, AR5) in several CaP cell lines, where higher expression of all 3 was noted in androgen-independent versus androgen-sensitive cell lines. AR3, AR4, and AR5 are identical to the respective splice variants AR-V7, AR-V1, and AR-V4 described by Hu and colleagues.[103] AR3 was the most abundantly expressed and the most active of the 3 AR splice variants. AR3 activity was not enhanced by the addition of DHT and was unaffected by bicalutamide. AR3 overexpression enhanced the growth of androgen-sensitive LNCaP cells in androgen-depleted cell-culture conditions and in castrated mice. AR3 knockdown in the androgen-independent CaP cell lines CWR-R1 and 22Rv1 attenuated their growth in androgen-depleted conditions. Using tissue microarrays constructed from androgen-stimulated benign

prostate, ASCaP, and CRCaP clinical samples, AR3 protein was found to be significantly overexpressed in CaP in comparison with benign prostate, and to be redistributed from the cytoplasm to the nucleus in CRCaP in comparison with ASCaP. AR3 overexpression was independently associated with a 2.5-fold increased risk of biochemical failure after radical prostatectomy, which was higher than risks posed by Gleason score, preoperative PSA, or positive surgical margin. Thus AR splice variants allow ligand-independent AR transactivation, could be present before castration, and would serve as a biomarker of the lethal phenotype.

ROLE OF INFLAMMATION

Approximately 20% of human cancers are caused by chronic inflammation.[105] Inflammation plays a role in progression to CRCaP through a combination of mechanisms, which include the bypass and outlaw pathways, and contributes to CaP bone metastasis. IL-6 is a proinflammatory agent that is involved in the regulation of various cellular functions, including proliferation, differentiation, apoptosis, angiogenesis, and regulation of immune response. IL-6 is expressed in benign and malignant prostate tissue, and the levels of this cytokine and its receptor increase during prostate carcinogenesis.[106] Binding of IL-6 to the IL-6 receptor complex leads to phosphorylation and activation of Janus kinase (JAK). JAK activates several intracellular signal transduction pathways, such as Signal Transducer and Activator of Transcription (STAT), MAPK, and PI3K/AKT pathways.[107] STAT3 leads to increased receptor activator of nuclear factor κB ligand (RANKL) expression, which activates osteoclasts and plays an important role in CaP bone metastasis.[108] STAT3 also increases expression of NF-κB2/p52, which has antiapoptotic effects and is capable of ligand-independent AR activation.[109–111] Cyclooxygenase-2 (COX-2) is a proinflammatory enzyme necessary for prostaglandin synthesis. Inhibition of the COX-2 pathway downregulates several important targets of CRCaP, such as AR, EGFR, AKT, and cyclin D.[112] Analysis of data from the Radiation Therapy Oncology Group (RTOG 92-02) trial concluded that increased COX-2 expression was significantly associated with biochemical failure, distant metastasis, and treatment failure.[113]

THE BYPASS PATHWAY

CaP cells seem capable of survival independent of AR transactivation. Blocking apoptosis is one way that allows the bypassing of AR signaling because androgens stimulate CaP cell proliferation and ADT leads to apoptosis. CRCaP cells have been shown to upregulate the antiapoptotic protein, B-cell lymphoma 2 (Bcl-2).[114] Liu and colleagues[115] detected Bcl-2 expression in CaP cells that initially did not express it by selecting for growth of CaP xenografts in castrated mice. Blocking Bcl-2 with antisense oligonucleotides delayed the emergence of CRCaP in the LNCaP xenograft model.[116] Another bypass pathway mechanism is by inactivating the proapoptotic tumor suppressor gene Phosphatase and Tensin Homologue (PTEN). PTEN dephosphorylates phosphatidylinositol 3,4,5-triphosphate, a second messenger that activates the AKT protein kinase pathway.[117,118] The AKT pathway phosphorylates and activates AR in the absence of ligands, that is, in response to growth factors, cytokines, or HER-2/neu. The AKT pathway also phosphorylates and inactivates several proapoptotic proteins, which include BAD and procaspase 9.[98] Increased AKT activity was reported in androgen-independent LNAI cells compared with parental androgen-sensitive LNCaP cells.[119] Overexpressing AKT in LNCaP xenograft tumors accelerated tumor growth 6-fold and downregulated the expression of the cell-cycle inhibitor, p27.[119]

AR bypass can also be achieved via neuroendocrine differentiation of CaP cells. Neuroendocrine cells have a low rate of proliferation that allows them to survive treatment with androgen deprivation, chemotherapy, and radiation.[120] Neuroendocrine cells are more prevalent in CRCaP than in ASCaP, and are present in 40% to 100% of patients with CRCaP.[120] Neuroendocrine cells secrete neuropeptides, such as serotonin and bombesin, which can increase the proliferation of neighboring CaP cells, allowing progression in an androgen-deprived environment.[121,122]

Estrogen receptors (ER) have been suggested as another bypass mechanism in CRCaP based on the profound changes in their expression in CRCaP tissues.[123] In benign prostate, ERα is expressed mainly in stromal and basal epithelial cells and ERβ is expressed predominantly in luminal epithelial cells. ERα mediate epithelial proliferation, whereas ERβ stimulate epithelial differentiation and apoptosis. CaP development and progression was associated with increased expression of ERα and the ERα-regulated progesterone receptor,[124,125] and decreased expression of ERβ.[126] In addition, the expression of the TMPRSS2:ERG gene fusion, a molecular marker for aggressive CaP, was increased by ERα agonists and decreased by ERβ agonists.[127] Whether and how ER bypasses AR in CRCaP remain to be determined. One possibility is through ER-regulated expression of growth factors such as IGF-1, which in turn activate AR (ie, a combination of bypass and outlaw pathways).[128]

THE STEM-CELL PATHWAY

Approximately 1% of prostate basal epithelial cells are putative stem cells that express CD44/α2β1/CD133 but not PSA.[129] These stem cells are androgen-independent and capable of generating differentiated epithelium that expresses AR and PSA. In the stem-cell pathway, a small clone of prostate epithelial stem cells is tumorigenic, and proliferates under the selective pressure of ADT, which leads to regeneration of the phenotypically mixed population of CaP cells.[130] CaP stem cells occur at a frequency of 0.1% of cells in any CaP tumor and express the phenotype CD44/α2β1/CD133. These cells are capable of self-renewal and are multidrug-resistant.[130,131]

FUTURE TARGETS FOR THE PREVENTION AND TREATMENT OF CRCaP

Several agents targeting various pathways implicated in CRCaP development have been or are being tested in clinical trials, and have been reviewed by others (see **Fig. 2**; **Table 3**).[132–134]

One caveat of these trials is that each trial usually targets a single pathway. CaP cells are capable of bypassing blocked pathways by using other pathways for continued growth. Trials of multiple agents with different mechanisms of action used simultaneously are eagerly awaited, because targeting as many CRCaP pathways as possible in one setting may induce more complete responses and/or longer-lasting remissions.

SUMMARY

ADT is only palliative for advanced and metastatic CaP. CRCaP continues to grow, using several mechanisms that depend on AR signaling in most cases. These mechanisms include the hypersensitive, intracrine metabolism, promiscuous, outlaw, bypass, and stem-cell pathways. In the hypersensitive pathway, CRCaP increases its sensitivity to castrate androgen levels by amplifying AR or increasing its sensitivity. CRCaP may synthesize testicular androgens, the most potent AR ligands, from weak adrenal androgens, cholesterol, or even acetate. In the promiscuous pathway, CRCaP broadens its ligand specificity so that it is activated by adrenal androgens, estradiol, progesterone, cortisol, or antiandrogens. In the outlaw pathway, CRCaP acquires the ability to become activated by growth factors and cytokines, in a ligand-independent but AR-dependent mechanism. Inhibition of apoptosis and/or entry into the cell cycle, neuroendocrine differentiation, and the use of estrogen-receptor signaling are other mechanisms used by CRCaP to bypass AR, and are collectively referred to as the bypass pathway. In the stem-cell pathway, a small population of prostate epithelial stem cells is tumorigenic and survives castration to regenerate a drug-resistant, phenotypically mixed tumor. Several pathways use similar molecular processes, such as upregulation of AR coactivators, and increased synthesis of IL-6, which can sensitize AR to AR ligands, activate AR in a ligand-independent fashion, and inhibit apoptosis.

Men with CRCaP have new agents approved by the Food and Drug Administration for the treatment of CRCaP: abiraterone acetate, sipuleucel-T, docetaxel, and cabazitaxel. More promising agents are in clinical trials. Simultaneous multitargeted attacks on CRCaP growth mechanisms may induce longer-lasting remissions and even cure some men with advanced disease.

REFERENCES

1. Huggins C, Hodges CV. Studies on prostatic cancer. I. The effect of castration, of estrogen and of androgen injection on serum phosphatases in metastatic carcinoma of the prostate. 1941. J Urol 2002;167(2 Pt 2):948–51.
2. Chen Y, Clegg NJ, Scher HI. Anti-androgens and androgen-depleting therapies in prostate cancer: new agents for an established target. Lancet Oncol 2009;10(10):981–91.
3. Gelmann EP. Molecular biology of the androgen receptor. J Clin Oncol 2002;20(13):3001–15.
4. Simental JA, Sar M, Lane MV, et al. Transcriptional activation and nuclear targeting signals of the human androgen receptor. J Biol Chem 1991; 266(1):510–8.
5. Jenster G, van der Korput HA, Trapman J, et al. Identification of two transcription activation units in the N-terminal domain of the human androgen receptor. J Biol Chem 1995;270:7341–6.
6. Platz EA, Rimm EB, Willett WC, et al. Racial variation in prostate cancer incidence and in hormonal system markers among male health professionals. J Natl Cancer Inst 2000;92(24):2009–17.
7. Stanford JL, Just JJ, Gibbs M, et al. Polymorphic repeats in the androgen receptor gene: molecular markers of prostate cancer risk. Cancer Res 1997;57(6):1194–8.
8. Zeegers MP, Kiemeney LA, Nieder AM, et al. How strong is the association between CAG and GGN repeat length polymorphisms in the androgen receptor gene and prostate cancer risk? Cancer Epidemiol Biomarkers Prev 2004;13(11 Pt 1): 1765–71.
9. Bratt O, Borg A, Kristoffersson U, et al. CAG repeat length in the androgen receptor gene is related to age at diagnosis of prostate cancer and response to endocrine therapy, but not to prostate cancer risk. Br J Cancer 1999;81(4):672–6.
10. Correa-Cerro L, Wohr G, Haussler J, et al. (CAG) nCAA and GGN repeats in the human androgen receptor gene are not associated with prostate cancer in a French-German population. Eur J Hum Genet 1999;7(3):357–62.
11. Walcott JL, Merry DE. Trinucleotide repeat disease. The androgen receptor in spinal and bulbar muscular atrophy. Vitam Horm 2002;65:127–47.
12. Hard T, Kellenbach E, Boelens R, et al. Solution structure of the glucocorticoid receptor DNA-binding domain. Science 1990;249:157–60.
13. Schoenmakers E, Alen P, Verrijdt G, et al. Differential DNA binding by the androgen and glucocorticoid receptors involves the second Zn-finger and a C-terminal extension of the DNA-binding domains. Biochem J 1999;341(Part 3):515–21.
14. Gioeli D, Ficarro SB, Kwiek JJ, et al. Androgen receptor phosphorylation. Regulation and identification of the phosphorylation sites. J Biol Chem 2002;277:29304–14.
15. Fu M, Rao M, Wang C, et al. Acetylation of androgen receptor enhances coactivator binding

and promotes prostate cancer cell growth. Mol Cell Biol 2003;23:8563–75.

16. Zhou ZX, Kemppainen JA, Wilson EM. Identification of three proline-directed phosphorylation sites in the human androgen receptor. Mol Endocrinol 1995;9(5):605–15.

17. Sack JS, Kish KF, Wang C, et al. Crystallographic structures of the ligand-binding domains of the androgen receptor and its T877A mutant complexed with the natural agonist dihydrotestosterone. Proc Natl Acad Sci U S A 2001;98:4904–9.

18. Bourguet W, Ruff M, Chambon P, et al. Crystal structure of the ligand-binding domain of the human nuclear receptor RXR-a. Nature 1995;375:377–82.

19. Pratt WB, Toft DO. Steroid receptor interactions with heat shock protein and immunophilin chaperones. Endocr Rev 1997;18:306–60.

20. Prescott J, Coetzee GA. Molecular chaperones throughout the life cycle of the androgen receptor. Cancer Lett 2006;231:12–9.

21. Li J, Al-Azzawi F. Mechanism of androgen receptor action. Maturitas 2009;63(2):142–8.

22. Heinlein CA, Chang C. Androgen receptor (AR) coregulators: an overview. Endocr Rev 2002; 23(2):175–200.

23. Visakorpi T, Hyytinen E, Koivisto P, et al. In vivo amplification of the androgen receptor gene and progression of human prostate cancer. Nat Genet 1995;9(4):401–6.

24. Koivisto P, Kononen J, Palmberg C, et al. Androgen receptor gene amplification: a possible molecular mechanism for androgen deprivation therapy failure in prostate cancer. Cancer Res 1997;57(2): 314–9.

25. Palmberg C, Koivisto P, Kakkola L, et al. Androgen receptor gene amplification at primary progression predicts response to combined androgen blockade as second line therapy for advanced prostate cancer. J Urol 2000;164(6):1992–5.

26. Ford OH 3rd, Gregory CW, Kim D, et al. Androgen receptor gene amplification and protein expression in recurrent prostate cancer. J Urol 2003;170(5): 1817–21.

27. Attard G, Swennenhuis JF, Olmos D, et al. Characterization of ERG, AR and PTEN gene status in circulating tumor cells from patients with castration-resistant prostate cancer. Cancer Res 2009;69(7): 2912–8.

28. Leversha MA, Han J, Asgari Z, et al. Fluorescence in situ hybridization analysis of circulating tumor cells in metastatic prostate cancer. Clin Cancer Res 2009;15(6):2091–7.

29. Holzbeierlein J, Lal P, LaTulippe E, et al. Gene expression analysis of human prostate carcinoma during hormonal therapy identifies androgen-responsive genes and mechanisms of therapy resistance. Am J Pathol 2004;164(1):217–27.

30. Chen CD, Welsbie DS, Tran C, et al. Molecular determinants of resistance to antiandrogen therapy. Nat Med 2004;10(1):33–9.

31. Nelson JB, Chan-Tack K, Hedican SP, et al. Endothelin-1 production and decreased endothelin B receptor expression in advanced prostate cancer. Cancer Res 1996;56:663–8.

32. Nelson JB, Hedican SP, George DJ, et al. Identification of endothelin-1 in the pathophysiology of metastatic adenocarcinoma of the prostate. Nat Med 1995;1:944–9.

33. Lee JG, Zheng R, McCafferty-Cepero JM, et al. Endothelin-1 enhances the expression of the androgen receptor via activation of the c-myc pathway in prostate cancer cells. Mol Carcinog 2009;48(2):141–9.

34. Gregory CW, Johnson RT Jr, Mohler JL, et al. Androgen receptor stabilization in recurrent prostate cancer is associated with hypersensitivity to low androgen. Cancer Res 2001;61(7):2892–8.

35. Gregory C, He B, Johnson R, et al. A mechanism for androgen receptor-mediated prostate cancer recurrence after androgen deprivation therapy. Cancer Res 2001;61:4315–9.

36. Guo Z, Dai B, Jiang T, et al. Regulation of androgen receptor activity by tyrosine phosphorylation. Cancer Cell 2006;10:309–19.

37. Mahajan NP, Liu Y, Majumder S, et al. Activated Cdc42-associated kinase Ack1 promotes prostate cancer progression via androgen receptor tyrosine phosphorylation. Proc Natl Acad Sci U S A 2007; 104:8438–43.

38. Askew EB, Gampe RT Jr, Stanley TB, et al. Modulation of androgen receptor activation function 2 by testosterone and dihydrotestosterone. J Biol Chem 2007;282(35):25801–16.

39. Deslypere JP, Young M, Wilson JD, et al. Testosterone and 5 alpha-dihydrotestosterone interact differently with the androgen receptor to enhance transcription of the MMTV-CAT reporter gene. Mol Cell Endocrinol 1992;88(1–3):15–22.

40. Mohler JL, Gregory CW, Ford OH 3rd, et al. The androgen axis in recurrent prostate cancer. Clin Cancer Res 2004;10(2):440–8.

41. Montgomery RB, Mostaghel EA, Vessella R, et al. Maintenance of intratumoral androgens in metastatic prostate cancer: a mechanism for castration-resistant tumor growth. Cancer Res 2008;68(11): 4447–54.

42. Thomas L, Lazier C, Gupta R, et al. Differential alterations in 5α-reductase type 1 and type 2 levels during development and progression of prostate cancer. Prostate 2005;63:231–9.

43. Godoy A, Kawinski E, Li Y, et al. 5α-Reductase 3 expression in human benign and malignant tissues: a comparative analysis during prostate cancer progression. Prostate 2011;71(10):1033–46.

44. Russell DW, Wilson JD. Steroid 5a-reductase: two genes/two enzymes. Annu Rev Biochem 1994;63:25–61.

45. Titus MA, Schell MJ, Lih FB, et al. Testosterone and dihydrotestosterone tissue levels in recurrent prostate cancer. Clin Cancer Res 2005;11(13):4653–7.

46. Leon C, Locke J, Adomat H, et al. Alterations in cholesterol regulation contribute to the production of intratumoral androgens during progression to castration-resistant prostate cancer in a mouse xenograft model. Prostate 2010;70:390–400.

47. Locke J, Guns E, Lubik A, et al. Androgen levels increase by intratumoral de novo steroidogenesis during progression of castration-resistant prostate cancer. Cancer Res 2008;68(15):6407–15.

48. Harper ME, Pike A, Peeling WB, et al. Steroids of adrenal origin metabolized by human prostatic tissue both in vivo and in vitro. J Endocrinol 1974;60(1):117–25.

49. Mohler JL, Titus MA, Wilson EM. Potential prostate cancer drug target: bioactivation of androstanediol by conversion to dihydrotestosterone. Clin Cancer Res 2011;17(18):5844–9.

50. Mohler JL, Titus MA, Bai S, et al. Activation of the androgen receptor by intratumoral bioconversion of androstanediol to dihydrotestosterone in prostate cancer. Cancer Res 2011;71(4):1486–96.

51. Small EJ, Ryan CJ. The case for secondary hormonal therapies in the chemotherapy age. J Urol 2006;176(6 Pt 2):S66–71.

52. Shah S, Trump D, Sartor O, et al. Phase II study of dutasteride in recurrent prostate cancer during androgen-deprivation therapy. J Urol 2009;181:621–6.

53. Azzouni F, Mohler J. Role of 5α-reductase inhibitors in prostate cancer prevention and treatment. Urology 2012;79(6):1197–205 [Epub 2012 Mar 23].

54. de Bono JS, Logothetis CJ, Molina A, et al. Abiraterone and increased survival in metastatic prostate cancer. N Engl J Med 2011;364(21):1995–2005.

55. Ryan CJ, Smith MR, Fong L, et al. Phase I clinical trial of the CYP17 inhibitor abiraterone acetate demonstrating clinical activity in patients with castration-resistant prostate cancer who received prior ketoconazole therapy. J Clin Oncol 2010;28(9):1481–8.

56. Feldman B, Feldman D. The development of androgen-independent prostate cancer. Nat Rev Cancer 2001;1(1):34–45.

57. Taplin ME, Bubley GJ, Ko YJ, et al. Selection for androgen receptor mutations in prostate cancers treated with androgen antagonist. Cancer Res 1999;59(11):2511–5.

58. Fenton MA, Shuster TD, Fertig AM, et al. Functional characterization of mutant androgen receptors from androgen-independent prostate cancer. Clin Cancer Res 1997;3(8):1383–8.

59. Terakawa T, Miyake H, Kumano M, et al. The antiandrogen bicalutamide activates the androgen receptor (AR) with a mutation in codon 741 through the mitogen activated protein kinase (MARK) pathway in human prostate cancer PC3 cells. Oncol Rep 2010;24(5):1395–9.

60. Veldscholte J, Ris-Stalpers C, Kuiper GG, et al. A mutation in the ligand binding domain of the androgen receptor of human LNCaP cells affects steroid binding characteristics and response to anti-androgens. Biochem Biophys Res Commun 1990;173(2):534–40.

61. Veldscholte J, Berrevoets CA, Ris-Stalpers C, et al. The androgen receptor in LNCaP cells contains a mutation in the ligand binding domain which affects steroid binding characteristics and response to antiandrogens. J Steroid Biochem Mol Biol 1992;41(3–8):665–9.

62. Taplin ME, Bubley GJ, Shuster TD, et al. Mutation of the androgen-receptor gene in metastatic androgen-independent prostate cancer. N Engl J Med 1995;332(21):1393–8.

63. Taplin ME, Rajeshkumar B, Halabi S, et al. Androgen receptor mutations in androgen-independent prostate cancer: Cancer and Leukemia Group B Study 9663. J Clin Oncol 2003;21(14):2673–8.

64. Greene SL, Stockton P, Kozyreva OG, et al. Molecular analysis of the androgen receptor using laser capture microdissection and direct sequencing. In: Terrian DM, editor. Cancer cell signalling: methods and protocols. Totowa (NJ): Humana Press, Inc; 2003. p. 287–302.

65. McDonald S, Brive L, Agus DB, et al. Ligand responsiveness in human prostate cancer: structural analysis of mutant androgen receptors from LNCaP and CWR22 tumors. Cancer Res 2000;60(9):2317–22.

66. Zhao XY, Boyle B, Krishnan AV, et al. Two mutations identified in the androgen receptor of the new human prostate cancer cell line MDA PCa 2a. J Urol 1999;162(6):2192–9.

67. Zhao XY, Malloy PJ, Krishnan AV, et al. Glucocorticoids can promote androgen-independent growth of prostate cancer cells through a mutated androgen receptor. Nat Med 2000;6(6):703–6.

68. Hu R, Denmeade SR, Luo J. Molecular processes leading to aberrant androgen receptor signaling and castration resistance in prostate cancer. Expert Rev Endocrinol Metab 2010;5(5):753–64.

69. Agoulnik IU, Weigel NL. Androgen receptor coactivators and prostate cancer. Adv Exp Med Biol 2008;617:245–55.

70. Chmelar R, Buchanan G, Need EF, et al. Androgen receptor coregulators and their involvement in the development and progression of prostate cancer. Int J Cancer 2007;120(4):719–33.

71. Halkidou K, Gnanapragasam VJ, Mehta PB, et al. Expression of Tip60, an androgen receptor coactivator, and its role in prostate cancer development. Oncogene 2003;22(16):2466–77.

72. Majumder S, Liu Y, Ford OH, et al. Involvement of arginine methyltransferase CARM1 in androgen receptor function and prostate cancer cell viability. Prostate 2006;66:1292–301.

73. Agoulnik IU, Vaid A, Bingman WE 3rd, et al. Role of SRC-1 in the promotion of prostate cancer cell growth and tumor progression. Cancer Res 2005; 65(17):7959–67.

74. Agoulnik IU, Vaid A, Nakka M, et al. Androgens modulate expression of TIF2, an androgen receptor coactivator whose expression level correlates with early biochemical recurrence in prostate cancer. Cancer Res 2006;66:10594–602.

75. Yeh S, Chang C. Cloning and characterization of a specific coactivator, ARA70, for the androgen receptor in human prostate cells. Proc Natl Acad Sci U S A 1996;93(11):5517–21.

76. Yeh S-H, Miyamoto H, Shima H, et al. From estrogen to androgen receptor: a new pathway for sex hormones in prostate. Proc Natl Acad Sci U S A 1998;95(10):5527–32.

77. Wang L, Hsu CL, Chang C. Androgen receptor corepressors: an overview. Prostate 2005;63: 117–30.

78. Agoulnik IU, Krause WC, Bingman WEI, et al. Repressors of androgen and progesterone receptor action. J Biol Chem 2003;278:31136–48.

79. Burd CJ, Petre CE, Morey LM, et al. Cyclin D1b variant influences prostate cancer growth through aberrant androgen receptor regulation. Proc Natl Acad Sci U S A 2006;103:2190–5.

80. Martinez ED, Danielsen M. Loss of androgen receptor transcriptional activity at the G(1)/S transition. J Biol Chem 2002;277:29719–29.

81. Karvonen U, Janne OA, Palvimo JJ, et al. Androgen receptor regulates nuclear trafficking and nuclear domain residency of corepressor HDAC7 in a ligand-dependent fashion. Exp Cell Res 2006; 312(16):3165–83.

82. Chen G, Nomura M, Morinago H, et al. Modulation of androgen receptor transactivation by FoxH1. A newly identified androgen receptor corepressor. J Biol Chem 2005;280:36355–63.

83. Belandia B, Powell SM, Garcia-Pedrero JM, et al. Hey1, a mediator of notch signaling, is an androgen receptor corepressor. Mol Cell Biol 2005;25:1425–36.

84. Yoon HG, Wong J. The corepressors SMRT and N-CoR are involved in agonist- and antagonist-regulated transcription by androgen receptor. Mol Endocrinol 2006;20:1048–60.

85. Berrevoets CA, Umar A, Trapman J, et al. Differential modulation of androgen receptor transcriptional activity by the nuclear receptor co-repressor (N-CoR). Biochem J 2004;379(Part 3):731–8.

86. Jackson TA, Richer JK, Bain DL, et al. The partial agonist activity of antagonist-occupied steroid receptors is controlled by a novel hinge domain-binding coactivator L7/SPA and the corepressors N-CoR or SMRT. Mol Endocrinol 1997;11:693–705.

87. Liao G, Chen LY, Zhang A, et al. Regulation of androgen receptor activity by the nuclear receptor corepressor SMRT. J Biol Chem 2003;278:5052–61.

88. Miyamoto H, Rahman MM, Chang C. Molecular basis for the antiandrogens withdrawal syndrome. J Cell Biochem 2004;91:3–12.

89. Culig Z, Hobisch A, Cronauer MV, et al. Androgen receptor activation in prostatic tumor cell lines by insulin-like growth factor-I, keratinocyte growth factor, and epidermal growth factor. Cancer Res 1994;54(20):5474–8.

90. Hobisch A, Eder IE, Putz T, et al. Interleukin-6 regulates prostate-specific protein expression in prostate carcinoma cells by activation of the androgen receptor. Cancer Res 1998;58(20):4640–5.

91. Gregory CW, Fei X, Ponguta LA, et al. Epidermal growth factor increases coactivation of the androgen receptor in recurrent prostate cancer. J Biol Chem 2004;279(8):7119–30.

92. Ueda T, Mawji NR, Bruchovsky N, et al. Ligand-independent activation of the androgen receptor by interleukin-6 and the role of steroid receptor coactivator-1 in prostate cancer cells. J Biol Chem 2002;277(41):38087–94.

93. Krueckl SL, Sikes RA, Edlund NM, et al. Increased insulin-like growth factor I receptor expression and signaling are components of androgen-independent progression in a lineage-derived prostate cancer progression model. Cancer Res 2004;64(23):8620–9.

94. George DJ, Halabi S, Shepard TF, et al. The prognostic significance of plasma interleukin-6 levels in patients with metastatic hormone-refractory prostate cancer: results from cancer and leukemia group B 9480. Clin Cancer Res 2005;11(5):1815–20.

95. Di Lorenzo G, Tortora G, D'Armiento FP, et al. Expression of epidermal growth factor receptor correlates with disease relapse and progression to androgen-independence in human prostate cancer. Clin Cancer Res 2002;8(11):3438–44.

96. Lin HK, Yeh S, Kang HY, et al. AKT suppresses androgen-induced apoptosis by phosphorylating and inhibiting androgen receptor. Proc Natl Acad Sci U S A 2001;98(13):7200–5.

97. Yeh S, Lin H, Kang H, et al. From HER2/Neu signal cascade to androgen receptor and its coactivators: a novel pathway by induction of androgen target genes through MAP kinase in prostate cancer cells. Proc Natl Acad Sci U S A 1999;96(10): 5458–63.

98. Zhou H, Li X, Meinkoth J, et al. AKT regulates cell survival and apoptosis at a post-mitochondrial level. J Cell Biol 2000;151:483–94.

99. Craft N, Shostak Y, Carey M, et al. A mechanism for hormone-independent prostate cancer through modulation of androgen receptor signaling by the HER-2/neu tyrosine kinase. Nat Med 1999;5(3):280–5.

100. Roy V, Perez EA. Beyond trastuzumab: small molecule tyrosine kinase inhibitors in HER-2-positive breast cancer. Oncologist 2009;14(11):1061–9.

101. Ceraline J, Cruchant MD, Erdmann E, et al. Constitutive activation of the androgen receptor by a point mutation in the hinge region: a new mechanism for androgen-independent growth in prostate cancer. Int J Cancer 2004;108:152.

102. Libertini SJ, Tepper CG, Rodriguez V, et al. Evidence for calpain-mediated androgen receptor cleavage as a mechanism for androgen independence. Cancer Res 2007;67:9001–5.

103. Hu R, Dunn TA, Wei S, et al. Ligand-independent androgen receptor variants derived from splicing of cryptic exons signify hormone-refractory prostate cancer. Cancer Res 2009;69(1):16–22.

104. Guo Z, Yang X, Sun F, et al. A novel androgen receptor splice variant is up-regulated during prostate cancer progression and promotes androgen depletion-resistant growth. Cancer Res 2009;69(6):2305–13.

105. De Marzo AM, Platz EA, Sutcliffe S, et al. Inflammation in prostate carcinogenesis. Nat Rev Cancer 2007;7(4):256–69.

106. Drachenberg DE, Elgamal AA, Rowbotham R, et al. Circulating levels of interleukin-6 in patients with hormone refractory prostate cancer. Prostate 1999;41:127–33.

107. Rose-John S. Coordination of interleukin-6 biology by membrane bound and soluble receptors. Adv Exp Med Biol 2001;495:145–51.

108. Azevedo A, Cunha V, Teixeira AL, et al. IL-6/IL-6R as a potential key signaling pathway in prostate cancer development. World J Clin Oncol 2011;2(12):384–96.

109. Nadiminty N, Lou W, Lee SO, et al. Stat3 activation of NF-κB p100 processing involves CBP/p300-mediated acetylation. Proc Natl Acad Sci U S A 2006;103:7264–9.

110. Nadiminty N, Chun JY, Lou W, et al. NF-κB2/p52 enhances androgen-independent growth of human LNCaP cells via protection from apoptotic cell death and cell cycle arrest induced by androgen deprivation. Prostate 2008;68:1725–33.

111. Nadiminty N, Lou W, Sun M, et al. Aberrant activation of the androgen receptor by NF-κB2/p52 in prostate cancer cells. Cancer Res 2010;70(8):3309–19.

112. Narayanan BA, Reddy BS, Bosland MC, et al. Exisulind in combination with celecoxib modulates epidermal growth factor receptor, cyclooxygenase-2, and cyclin D1 against prostate carcinogenesis: In vivo evidence. Clin Cancer Res 2007;13:5965–73.

113. Khor LY, Bae K, Pollack A, et al. COX-2 expression predicts prostate-cancer outcome: analysis of data from the RTOG 92–02 trial. Lancet Oncol 2007;8(10):912–20.

114. Colombel M, Symmans F, Gil S, et al. Detection of the apoptosis-suppressing oncoprotein bc1-2 in hormone-refractory human prostate cancers. Am J Pathol 1993;143(2):390–400.

115. Liu A, Corey E, Bladou F, et al. Prostatic cell lineage markers: emergence of Bcl2+ cells of human prostate cancer xenograft LuCaP 23 following castration. Int J Cancer 1996;65(1):85–9.

116. Gleave M, Tolcher A, Miyake H, et al. Progression to androgen independence is delayed by adjuvant treatment with antisense Bcl-2 oligodeoxynucleotides after castration in the LNCaP prostate tumor model. Clin Cancer Res 1999;5(10):2891–8.

117. Datta S, Brunet A, Greenberg M. Cellular survival: a play in three AKTs. Genes Dev 1999;13(22):2905–27.

118. Stambolic V, Suzuki A, de la Pompa JL, et al. Negative regulation of PKB/AKT dependent cell survival by the tumor suppressor PTEN. Cell 1998;95(1):29–39.

119. Graff JR, Konicek BW, McNulty AM, et al. Increased AKT activity contributes to prostate cancer progression by dramatically accelerating prostate tumor growth and diminishing p27Kip1 expression. J Biol Chem 2000;275(32):24500–5.

120. Debes JD, Tindall DJ. Mechanisms of androgen-refractory prostate cancer. N Engl J Med 2004;351(15):1488–90.

121. Fixemer T, Remberger K, Bonkhoff H. Apoptosis resistance of neuroendocrine phenotypes in prostatic adenocarcinoma. Prostate 2002;53(2):118–23.

122. Bonkhoff H. Neuroendocrine differentiation in human prostate cancer. Morphogenesis, proliferation and androgen receptor status. Ann Oncol 2001;12(Suppl 2):S141–4.

123. Bonkhoff H, Berges R. The evolving role of oestrogens and their receptors in the development and progression of prostate cancer. Eur Urol 2009;55:533–42.

124. Bonkhoff H, Fixemer T, Hunsicker I, et al. Estrogen receptor expression in prostate cancer and premalignant prostatic lesions. Am J Pathol 1999;155:641–7.

125. Bonkhoff H, Fixemer T, Hunsicker I, et al. Progesterone receptor expression in human prostate cancer: correlation with tumor progression. Prostate 2001;48:285–91.

126. Fixemer T, Remberger K, Bonkhoff H. Differential expression of the estrogen receptor beta (ER beta) in human prostate tissue, premalignant changes, and in primary, metastatic, and recurrent prostatic adenocarcinoma. Prostate 2003;54:79–87.

127. Setlur SR, Mertz KD, Hoshida Y, et al. Estrogen-dependent signaling in a molecularly distinct subclass of aggressive prostate cancer. J Natl Cancer Inst 2008;100:815–25.

128. Ricke W, Wang Y, Cunha G. Steroid hormones and carcinogenesis of the prostate: the role of estrogens. Differentiation 2007;75:871–82.

129. Collins AT, Habib FK, Maitland NJ, et al. Identification and isolation of human prostate epithelial stem cells based on α2β1-integrin expression. J Cell Sci 2001;114:3865–72.

130. Collins AT, Berry PA, Hyde C, et al. Prospective identification of tumorigenic prostate cancer stem cells. Cancer Res 2005;65(23):10946–51.

131. Leong KG, Wang BE, Johnson L, et al. Generation of a prostate from a single adult stem cell. Nature 2008;456(7223):804–8.

132. Pienta K, Bradley D. Mechanisms underlying the development of androgen-independent prostate cancer. Clin Cancer Res 2006;12(6): 1665–71.

133. Chi KN, Bjartell A, Dearnaley D, et al. Castration-resistant prostate cancer: from new pathophysiology to new treatment targets. Eur Urol 2009; 56(4):594–605.

134. Attard G, Richards J, de Bono JS. New strategies in metastatic prostate cancer: targeting the androgen receptor signaling pathway. Clin Cancer Res 2011;17(7):1649–57.

135. Geller J, Albert J, Nachtsheim D, et al. Steroid levels in cancer of the prostate—markers of tumor differentiation and adequacy of anti-androgen therapy. Prog Clin Biol Res 1979;33:103–11.

136. Labrie F, Dupont A, Bélanger A, et al. Anti-hormone treatment for prostate cancer relapsing after treatment with flutamide and castration. Addition of aminoglutethimide and low dose hydrocortisone to combination therapy. Br J Urol 1989;63(6):634–8.

Targeting the Androgen Receptor

Terence W. Friedlander, MD*, Charles J. Ryan, MD

KEYWORDS

- Castration-resistant prostate cancer • Androgen receptor • Abiraterone acetate • Orteronel
- Galeterone • MDV3100 • ARN-509 • EPI-001

KEY POINTS

- Androgen receptor (AR)-mediated signaling is critical to the growth and survival of prostate cancer.
- Recent work exploring the molecular structure and evolution of the AR in response to hormonal therapies has revealed novel mechanisms of progression and yielded new targets for drug development.
- The vast majority of castration-resistant tumors still rely on AR activity.

INTRODUCTION

Prostate cancer is the most common cancer in men and is unique in that its growth is largely dependent on androgen signaling. This dependence was first recognized more than 70 years ago when Huggins and Hodges[1,2] observed striking regressions of metastatic prostate cancer in men who underwent either surgical or medical castration. Indeed, in men with metastatic prostate cancer, androgen deprivation improves bone pain, lessens lower urinary tract symptoms, and increases overall quality of life.

Despite the impressive clinical improvements observed with androgen deprivation therapy (ADT), androgen suppression is not curative, and all men eventually develop disease growth despite castrate levels of testosterone. Tumor growth in the castrate environment is lethal and accounts for close to 30,000 deaths annually in the United States.[3] The median survival for a man with castrate-resistant disease is between 2 and 3 years from the time of diagnosis of castration resistance.[4]

Until recently, the terms androgen-independent prostate cancer (AIPC) or hormone refractory prostate cancer (HRPC) were used in the literature to describe this clinical state, implying largely that tumor growth occurred through pathways completely independent of the androgen signaling. Work in recent years, however, has dispelled this misconception and has clearly demonstrated that signaling through the androgen receptor (AR) remains crucial to tumor growth in the castrate tumor environment. With this understanding, the term castration-resistant prostate cancer (CRPC) has gradually emerged to describe this clinical state. The term "CRPC" is especially useful in that it connotes only the clinical state of disease growth despite castrate levels of serum testosterone, while not indicating the potential, one way or another, for response to further androgen manipulation.

As we shall see in this review, castration resistance can develop in many ways, including through the development of AR mutations, through AR amplification, through the production of androgens within tumors (intracrine androgen synthesis), through the

Authors' disclosures of potential conflicts of interest: The authors declare no potential conflict of interest.
Division of Genitourinary Medical Oncology, Helen Diller Family Comprehensive Cancer Center, 1600 Divisadero Street, Box 1711, University of California, San Francisco, CA 94143, USA
* Corresponding author.
E-mail address: terence.friedlander@ucsf.edu

Urol Clin N Am 39 (2012) 453–464
http://dx.doi.org/10.1016/j.ucl.2012.07.003

emergence of truncated AR proteins (splice variants) capable of ligand-independent signaling, and through other mechanisms. Understanding these mechanisms has led the way for the development of multiple novel agents that target the AR itself. Indeed, enzalutamide, a novel antiandrogen that directly inhibits AR function, and abiraterone acetate (Zytiga), an inhibitor of androgen synthesis that lowers circulating ligand, have both been shown to improve overall survival in well-powered randomized Phase III studies and are discussed later in this article. Additionally, a number of new agents are in clinical development, including agents that directly target the AR, such as ARN-509 and EPI-001, as well as those, like abiraterone acetate, that indirectly target the AR, such as orteronel (TAK-700), galeterone (TOK-001), and others.

To understand the clinical development of these agents, we first review our current understanding of the structure and function of the AR, then explore how castration resistance emerges, focusing specifically on mechanisms that lead to persistent AR signaling in a low testosterone environment. We then review the clinical development of agents that target the AR, focusing on recently approved agents and those currently in clinical development.

AR STRUCTURE AND FUNCTION

The AR gene is located on chromosome Xq11-12 and is a member of the steroid hormone receptor family that includes, among others, the estrogen receptor, progesterone receptor, and the glucocorticoid receptor. All share a similar structure. Histologically, the AR is present in benign prostate epithelial cells as well as in all stages and grades of primary and metastatic prostate cancer.[5,6] Functionally, the AR is a 110-kDa ligand-activated transcription factor consisting of 917 amino acids that contain 3 important distinct domains (**Fig. 1**A): a carboxy-terminal ligand-binding domain (LBD), which binds androgens, a DNA-binding domain (DBD), and a regulatory N-terminal domain (NTD).[7] Within the N-terminal domain lies the activation function 1 (AF-1) and AF-5 domains, which contain binding sites for transcriptional coregulators and are essential for AR activity.[8,9]

Under normal conditions, inactive AR is found in the cytoplasm of prostate cancer cells and is stabilized there by various heat-shock proteins (HSPs), which expose the LBD to surrounding proteins and allow for androgen binding. Once bound to androgenic ligands, a conformational change occurs in the AR, causing dissociation of HSPs, AR receptor dimerization, and AR migration to the nucleus (see **Fig. 1**B).[10] Once inside the

nucleus, the AR DBD binds to specific androgen response elements (AREs) on the promoter or enhancer regions of androgen-regulated genes. Transcription of genes necessary for prostate cancer growth and survival can then be initiated, and is enhanced by the binding of transcription coregulators to the AF-1 binding site in the AR-NTD.[11] Among the many genes under AR transcriptional control is prostate-specific antigen (PSA), and hence serum PSA measurement serves as a clinically useful biomarker for AR transcriptional activity and, by extension, disease growth.

EVOLUTION OF AR STRUCTURE AND FUNCTION IN PROSTATE CANCER

Depletion of circulating testicular androgens through either orchiectomy or luteinizing hormone–releasing hormone (LHRH) therapy drastically decreases androgenic ligand levels, reduces AR signaling, lowers PSA, and results in regression of disease the vast majority of cases. Both the rate of PSA decline and the nadir PSA on therapy are predictive of overall response to initial ADT, with higher nadir PSA values and shorter times to PSA nadir associated with poor survival.[12] This observation further highlights the role that AR-mediated signaling has on disease progression and disease aggressiveness.

Antiandrogens, such as bicalutamide (Casodex), nilutamide (Nilandron), and flutamide (Eulexin), have been in clinical use for decades, and observations about their use illustrate one of the first clinically relevant, identifiable steps in AR evolution. It was first noted in the early 1990s that disease progression, despite the combination of an LHRH agonist and an antiandrogen, could be stopped and reversed simply through discontinuation of the antiandrogen.[13] This antiandrogen withdrawal effect (AAWD) was best characterized in a study by Small and colleagues[14] who observed that discontinuation of an antiandrogen in men with a rising PSA leads to sustained PSA declines of more than 75% in more than 10% of men. Further work demonstrated that mutations in the AR can cause AR inhibitors, such as bicalutamide that bind to the LBD, to paradoxically stimulate AR and result in disease growth.[15] Although this mechanism remains incompletely understood, this observation illustrates the point that genomic changes occur or arise in the AR in response to therapy and can have important functional and clinical implications. Whether these genomic changes are present in a subpopulation of cells at baseline, or whether they are acquired in response to the selective pressure of AR-targeted therapy, is still unknown.

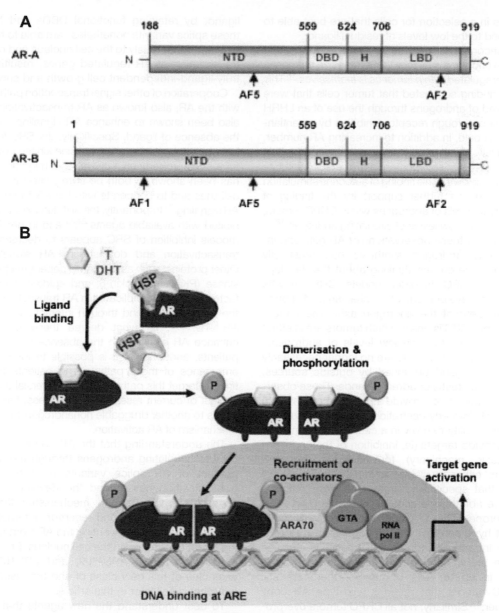

Fig. 1. (*A*) Structural domains of 2 isoforms of the androgen receptor (AR-A and AR-B). Numbers above the bars refer to the amino acid residues that separate the domains starting from the N-terminus (*left*) to C-terminus (*right*). (*B*) The presence of testosterone (T) or dihydrotestosterone (DHT) causes dissociation of HSP, dimerization, and phosphorylation (P) of the AR and translocation to the nucleus where the AR binds to an ARE, causing recruitment of DNA transcriptional machinery and gene transcription. (*Adapted from* Li J, Al-Azzawi F. Mechanism of androgen receptor action. Maturitas 2009;63:142–8; with permission.)

Further observation about the state of the AR as tumors transition from castration-sensitive to castration-resistant have had important function implications and have helped guide the development of new therapies. In a landmark study, Stanbrough and colleagues[16] profiled the expression signatures of primary and metastatic prostate tumors, including both castration-sensitive and castration-resistant tumors, and found significantly higher levels of AR mRNA in castrate-resistant tumors compared with castration-sensitive tumors. Subsequent studies of metastatic CRPC tumors obtained at autopsy showed that the genomic segment of chromosome X encoding the AR is itself amplified, up to 60-fold in some cases, and other studies has shown that the AR protein is overexpressed in metastatic CRPC tumors.[17] These observations suggest that depletion of circulating androgens results in a selection for cells that are best able to respond to the low levels of residual ligand.

A second critical laboratory observation is that mRNA encoding enzymes that synthesize hormones are upregulated *within tumor cells themselves*.[16] This novel finding suggested that tumor cells that were deprived of androgens through the use of an LHRH agonist or through receptor inhibition by an antiandrogen could, in addition to increasing AR number, potentially synthesize their own androgens within the local tumor environment and thereby stimulate their own growth. This finding of autocrine stimulation has been lent further support by the finding of increased levels of androgens within CRPC tumors, even despite low levels of circulating androgen.[18]

Coupling these observations of AR gain and intratumoral androgen synthesis has drastically changed the current thinking about the development of CRPC. In older models, CRPC results from the development of mechanisms of growth independent of the androgen axis. The current model of CRPC is one in which tumors are in effect *hypersensitive* to even low levels of androgens, and one in which tumors are no longer necessarily reliant on ligand produced by outside sources, such as the testis or adrenal glands. These observations, therefore, provide a plausible mechanism by which formerly castration-sensitive tumors regain the ability to grow in a castrate environment, and provide targets (ie, inhibition of the androgen synthesis machinery) for drug development. Agents either available or in late-stage clinical trials that specifically target androgen synthesis include abiraterone acetate, orteronel (TAK-700), galeterone (TOK-001), and ketoconazole (Nizoral).

Yet hypersensitivity to androgens and upregulated intracrine androgen synthesis is not the whole story. Although AR amplification can be seen in up to 70% of tumors, there are still CRPC tumors that retain a wild-type AR copy number.[17] Similarly, not all CRPC tumors overproduce androgens at a local level. Thus, recent work has explored other mechanisms of autonomous AR activation in men with castrate levels of serum testosterone. Perhaps the most intriguing of these observations is that aberrations can occur in the post-transcriptional splicing of AR mRNA, leading to various forms of a truncated AR protein. Although many forms of these splice-variants are maladaptive and lead to a nonfunctioning AR protein, multiple studies have found the presence, in CRPC tumors, of AR proteins that no longer contains an LBD, but retains the DBD and NTD.[19,20] Lacking a binding site for ligand, these AR splice-variant mutants can thereby be rendered insensitive to manipulation of circulating or local hormone levels. Despite their insensitivity to

ligand, by retaining functional DBDs and NTDs these splice variants nonetheless are able to translocate autonomously to the cell nucleus and cause transcription of AR regulated genes, resulting in truly ligand-independent cell growth and survival.

Cooperation of other signal transduction pathways with the AR, also known as AR transactivation, has also been shown to enhance AR signaling even in the absence of ligand. Specifically, the SRC kinase is a ubiquitous nonreceptor tyrosine kinase involved tumor cell proliferation, survival, and migration, and has been shown to both be upregulated in CRPC cell lines and to cooperate with the AR to enhance AR signaling.[21] Importantly, the SRC kinase can be inhibited with available agents,[22,23] and in preclinical models inhibition of SRC appears to decrease AR transactivation and downstream AR signaling.[24] Other proteins, such as the cAMP dependent protein kinase (PKA), interleukin-6, and epidermal growth factor, have been implicated in AR transactivation in the absence of ligand through interaction with the AR-NTD.[25–27] To what degree these pathways enhance AR signaling in the absence of ligand in patients, and whether it is possible to identify the emergence of these pathways in patients in real time to target this pathway, is controversial and the subject of current research. Nonetheless, this work points to another druggable nonandrogen-mediated mechanism of AR activation.

The understanding that the AR can lose sensitivity to circulating androgens through the development of AR splice variants or through AR transactivation has guided the development of novel AR inhibitors with mechanisms that go beyond impairing ligand-receptor interactions, but rather focus on preventing the AR from reaching target sequences in the cell nucleus. Enzalutamide (MDV-3100), ARN-509, and EPI-100 are examples of this new class of and are discussed in further detail later in this article.

To best understand the new agents that have been recently approved or are in clinical development, it is best to think about these agents as a class. This review, therefore, first explores agents that "indirectly" target the AR by inhibiting androgenic ligand production, then focuses on agents that "directly" inhibit interactions between ligand and the AR LBD, and last focuses on agents that impair the interaction of the AR with target sequences in the DNA.

INDIRECTLY TARGETING THE AR: INHIBITORS OF ANDROGEN SYNTHESIS
Androgen Deprivation Therapy

ADT can be accomplished either through bilateral orchiectomy or medically through the use of gonadotropin-releasing hormone (GnRH) therapy. The GnRH agonists leuprolide (Lupron), goserelin (Zoladex), and triptorelin (Trelstar) are synthetic GnRH analogs that are more than 100 times more potent than natural GnRH and less susceptible to enzymatic degradation.[28] Binding of these agents to receptors in the pituitary gland causes a burst of LHRH release and an initial rise in testosterone production by testicular Leydig cells. Persistent GnRH stimulation over time, however, leads to a downregulation in pituitary GnRH receptors, leading to declines in LHRH secretion and compensatory falls in testicular testosterone production to castrate levels.

Because GnRH agonists cause an initial serum testosterone flare, novel GnRH antagonists, which avoid raising serum testosterone levels, have been developed. Degarelix (Firmagon) was approved by the Food and Drug Administration (FDA) in 2008 and works by inhibiting the interaction of endogenous GnRH with receptors on pituitary gonadotropin-producing cells. Although useful for patients with newly diagnosed widespread metastatic disease in whom a testosterone flare should be avoided, the higher incidence of local injection site reactions (40% vs <1% for men receiving leuprolide) and the need for monthly injections make long-term treatment with this agent less desirable for most practictioners.[29]

Regardless of the method, ADT to achieve a serum testosterone level lower than 50 ng/dL is the mainstay of the treatment of metastatic prostate cancer, and is beneficial when combined with radiation therapy for patients with high-risk localized disease.[30–32] Recent work has shown that the degree of AR suppression achieved by initial ADT, as measured by serum PSA production, is significantly correlated with the duration of response to hormone therapy. In a study of men receiving ADT for metastatic disease, a time to nadir PSA of less than 6 months was associated with shorter overall survival on univariate analysis.[12] Similarly, the median survival for men with a PSA nadir of 0.2 ng/mL or less was 75 months, compared with 44 months for men with a nadir PSA between 0.2 to 4.0 ng/mL, and only 13 months for men who never nadired below 4.0 ng/mL. These findings support the notion that incomplete suppression of AR signaling leads to AR-mediated disease growth and faster disease progression.

Ketoconazole

Ketoconazole is a synthetic oral imidazole antifungal designed to disrupt fungal cell membranes through inhibition of ergosterol synthesis. Because of the homology between specific fungal and human enzymes, ketoconazole also impairs androgen synthesis in humans, specifically though inhibition of CYP51A, CYP11A1, CYP11B1, CYP11B2, CYP17, and CYP19.[33] Because it also suppresses mineralocorticoid and glucocorticoid synthesis, ketoconazole is given with a replacement dose of corticosteroid, usually oral hydrocortisone. In the largest randomized study to date, ketoconazole was given to men with CRPC at the time of AAWD.[14] PSA responses were observed in 32% of patients taking ketoconazole compared with 10% of men undergoing AAWD alone ($P<.001$), with twice as many patients having objective responses in the ketoconazole arm. Although crossover of patients randomized to AAWD alone to ketoconazole likely obscured any overall survival benefit, 2 important observations to come out of this study were that patients who had a more than 50% PSA decline had a 41-month survival, compared with 13 months in those who did not ($P<.001$), and that patients with high baseline circulating androstenedione levels were more likely to benefit from therapy than those with low circulating levels.[34] Both of these observations suggest that androgens remain important even after the development of castration-resistance, and show that decreasing the levels of other androgenic ligands in tumors still reliant on ligand-receptor stimulation can greatly slow the growth of the CRPC. Whether baseline circulating androgen levels can be used to identify a population of patients with CRPC more likely to benefit from ketoconazole is still the subject of debate.

Abiraterone Acetate

The recognition that inhibition of androgen synthesis by ketoconazole could result in both PSA and sustained objective responses led the way for the search for better inhibitors of androgen synthesis. Abiraterone acetate is the prodrug of abiraterone, a potent and selective inhibitor of CYP17 (17alpha-hydroxylase/C17,20-lyase), an enzyme that catalyzes key steps in the synthetic pathway of androgens (**Figs. 2** and **3**). Abiraterone acetate plus prednisone was tested against placebo plus prednisone in a randomized Phase III study of 1195 men with metastatic CRPC who had previously received docetaxel. After a median follow-up of 12.8 months, a statistically significant survival benefit was observed in the abiraterone/prednisone arm with median survival of 14.8 months in this arm, compared with 10.9 months in the placebo/prednisone arm (hazard ratio, 0.65; $P<.001$).[35] This study was the first ever to show an

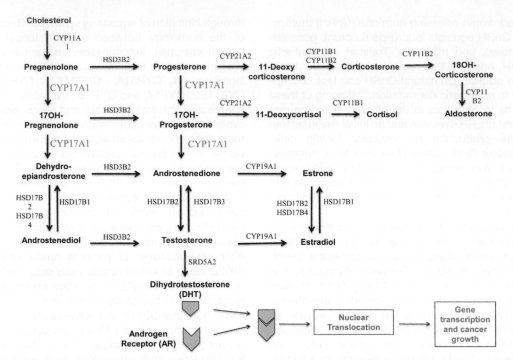

Fig. 2. Androgen synthesis cascade. CYP17A1 is inhibited by abiraterone, orteronel, and galeterone. Blockade of downstream synthesis is hypothesized to deprive tumors of androgenic ligand and thereby impair tumor growth.

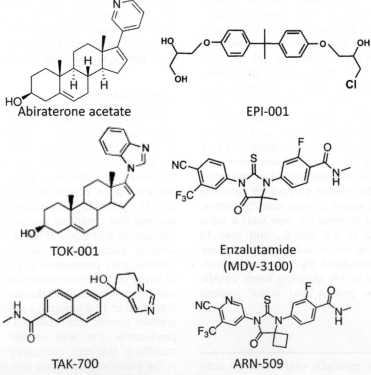

Fig. 3. Molecular structure of 6 novel agents that target the AR.

overall survival benefit to a "secondary" hormonal therapy, as well as the first ever to show a survival benefit for patients with docetaxel-treated CRPC. With the results of this study, abiraterone acetate received FDA approval in 2011 and has become a standard of care for men with docetaxel-treated CRPC.

A second randomized, placebo-controlled Phase III study of abiraterone acetate in men with docetaxel-naïve CRPC with coprimary end points of radiographic progression-free survival (rPFS) and overall survival (OS) was unblinded in March 2011 after the second of 3 pre-planned interim analyses performed after 43% of events revealed a statistically significant improvement in rPFS. rPFS for patients treated with placebo plus prednisone was 8.3 months, compared with an approximate doubling for patients treated with abiraterone plus prednisone. Additionally, a trend to improvement in overall survival was observed.[36] Based on these data, it is possible that abiraterone will become an option for all men with metastatic CRPC, regardless of prior docetaxel use.

Inhibition of CYP17 blocks androgen and cortisol production; however, does not impair mineralocorticoid synthesis. Reductions in cortisol levels are sensed by the pituitary, which responds by increasing serum adrenocorticotropic hormone (ACTH) levels; as abiraterone blocks further cortisol and androgen synthesis, the net effect of increased ACTH is to increase mineralocorticoid synthesis. Thus, most side effects of abiraterone are a result of mineralocorticoid excess, with any grade of hypertension, hyperkalemia, and fluid retention observed in 10%, 17%, and 31% of patients, respectively, treated on the post-docetaxel study. Data from early-phase testing showed that the addition of prednisone, 5 mg twice a day, can abrogate many of these effects, and therefore prednisone should be given concurrently with abiraterone therapy. Although rare, Grade 3 and 4 elevations in liver enzymes have also been observed, and frequent liver function test monitoring, especially at the initiation of therapy, is recommended.

Work is under way to better understand which patients are likely to respond to abiraterone. In accordance with the mechanism of action of abiraterone, higher baseline tumor CYP17 expression and higher baseline circulating androgen levels both correlate with response to therapy.[37] This finding reinforces the idea that patients harboring tumors that still depend on AR signaling stand to benefit from ligand-targeted therapy. Similarly, how resistance to abiraterone develops is still unknown; whether resistance is due to upregulation of androgen synthesis by the host adrenal gland, upregulation of intracrine androgen synthesis within tumors, impairment of abiraterone transport within cancer cells, or evolution of the AR to a ligand-independent state will need to be addressed in future studies.

Orteronel (TAK-700)

Similar to abiraterone acetate, orteronel is a rationally designed inhibitor of CYP17 with increased selectivity for inhibition of the 17,20-lyase activity over the 17-hydroxylase activity of the enzyme (see **Figs. 2** and **3**). The differential selectivity has been hypothesized to result in less overall mineralocorticoid toxicity and has allowed for the omission of concurrent replacement steroids in early clinical trials. Doses above 300 mg twice daily, however, do appear to suppress cortisol synthesis and therefore concomitant prednisone has been incorporated in the ongoing studies.

In a phase I/II study, 26 patients received orteronel in dosages ranging between 200 and 600 mg twice daily with or without concurrent prednisone, and an additional 65 received 400 mg twice a day in the dose-expansion portion.[38] All patients who received more than 300 mg twice a day in the Phase I study had PSA declines, including 12 patients with a more than 50% PSA decline and 4 patients with a greater than 90% decline. Efficacy was similar in the Phase II portion, with 54% of patients achieving a more than 50% PSA response by week 12. The most common treatment-related adverse events were fatigue, nausea, constipation, headache, and diarrhea, and although Grade 3 hypokalemia, hyponatremia, and hyperglycemia was seen in 2 patients each, there were no dose-limiting toxicities. Consistent with preclinical data, both testosterone and dehydroepiandrostenedione sulfate (DHEA-S) decreased dramatically, and blunted responses to ACTH stimulation were observed in patients receiving more than 300 mg twice a day dosing, indicative of impaired cortisol synthesis in patients not receiving concurrent prednisone.

Based on these results, 2 concurrent Phase III studies are under way exploring the efficacy of orteronel plus prednisone versus prednisone alone in men with either chemotherapy-naïve or docetaxel-treated metastatic CRPC. The primary end point of these studies is overall survival, with a co-primary end point of rPFS in the chemotherapy-naïve study. If positive, orteronel plus prednisone would represent an alternative to abiraterone or ketoconazole to impair androgen synthesis for men with metastatic CRPC. Although there are data to suggest that abiraterone is effective in some men who have previously received ketoconazole,[39] it is unknown if patients who have developed disease progression while on ketoconazole or abiraterone will respond to orteronel.

Galeterone (TOK-001)

Galeterone is another inhibitor of CYP17. In preclinical testing, it was shown to have a higher specificity for CYP17 inhibition, with a half-maximal inhibitory concentration (IC_{50}) of 300 nM compared with 800 nM for abiraterone (see **Figs. 2** and **3**).[40] In addition to its activity against CYP17, it also competitively blocks androgen binding at the AR and downregulates AR expression in cell lines, thus functioning in some respects as both an indirect and a direct inhibitor of the AR.[40] Importantly, galeterone retains activity in cell lines resistant to bicalutamide expressing higher levels of AR.[41]

In the phase I ARMOR-1 study, 49 patients with chemotherapy-naïve nonmetastatic CRPC received single or split daily dosages ranging from 650 mg to 2600 mg for a minimum of 12 weeks without concurrent prednisone.[42] PSA reductions of 30% or greater were seen in 49% of patients, with 22% of patients having a 50% or greater decline in PSA. The most common side effects were fatigue, liver function test (LFT) abnormalities, pruritis, nausea, and diarrhea. Although Grades 2 and 3 LFT abnormalities were observed, most were asymptomatic and resolved with discontinuation of the drug. Six of 7 patients holding drug for LFT abnormalities were successfully rechallenged with galeterone without recurrent grade 3 LFT elevations. One case of grade 4 rhabdomyolysis was observed in a patient taking concurrent simvastatin; however, no maximum tolerated dose was reached. A Phase II study is expected to open in late 2012.

DIRECTLY TARGETING THE AR: INHIBITORS OF THE AR LIGAND BINDING DOMAIN
Bicalutamide, Flutamide, Nilutamide

The nonsteroidal antiandrogens bicalutamide, flutamide, and nilutamide block androgen-mediated signaling by binding to the AR LBD. Addition of an antiandrogen at the time of CRPC in men treated with androgen deprivation alone can lower PSA by 50% or more in more than a third of patients, and response to an antiandrogen in this setting has been associated with improved cause-specific survival.[43] Although several studies of high-dose bicalutamide monotherapy have been performed in men with CRPC, PSA declines of 50% or more occur in only approximately one-quarter of patients,[44–46] and in light of a number of new therapies, this strategy is not commonly

used. There are no data supporting the superiority of one antiandrogen over another; however, bicalutamide has an increased affinity for both the wild-type and mutated AR,[47] and therefore may work in cases in which AR antagonism with flutamide have failed. Similarly nilutamide has been shown to induce PSA declines in men who have developed resistance to AR inhibition with flutamide or bicalutamide.[48]

Long-term treatment with any of the nonsteroidal antiandrogens may select for cells with AR mutations that allow for paradoxic stimulation of the AR by the antiandrogen. Stopping the antiandrogen in men with a rising PSA, termed AAWD, can result in PSA declines in between 10% and 20% of men.[14,49] Withdrawal responses should be seen within 4 weeks following discontinuation of flutamide or nilutamide, and up to 6 weeks following discontinuation of bicalutamide.

DIRECTLY TARGETING THE AR: BEYOND THE LIGAND-BINDING DOMAIN
Enzalutamide (MDV-3100)

The recognition that persistent AR signaling is still important at the time of castration resistance led to the search for more potent inhibitors of the AR, including the search for compounds that could inhibit binding of the AR to nuclear response elements (NREs) and thereby act independently of the LBD. One of the most significant findings came from the identification of enzalutamide, a compound that has a more than fivefold greater affinity for the AR than bicalutamide (see **Fig. 3**).[50] Enzalutamide was subsequently shown to both impair AR nuclear translocation and induce a conformational change in the AR that impairs DNA binding and cofactor recruitment. Promising results from Phase I and II studies led the way for the Phase III study, a double-blinded randomized study of 1199 men with CRPC previously treated with docetaxel. Patients were randomized 2:1 to receive enzalutamide or placebo, and continuation of corticosteroids was allowed but not required. The study was unblinded after a pre-planned interim analysis after 520 deaths showed a significant overall survival benefit ($P<.001$; hazard ratio 0.631), with median overall survival of 18.4 months in the enzalutamide arm compared with 13.6 months in the placebo.[21] Secondary end points, including rPFS, soft tissue response rate, and time to PSA progression, all favored enzalutamide. Impressively, 54% of patients treated experienced a more than 50% PSA decline compared with 1.5% of placebo-treated patients and 25% of patients treated experienced a more than 90% PSA decline compared with 1% of placebo-treated patients. Improvement in quality of life was significantly higher as assessed by the Functional Assessment of Cancer Therapy – Prostate (FACT-P) questionnaire in enzalutamide-treated patients compared with those treated with placebo (43.2% vs 18.3%, P<.0001). Common side effects included fatigue, diarrhea, and hot flashes. Seizures, which had been a concern in the early-phase testing were reported in 5 patients (<1%) treated with enzalutamide.

Enzalutamide is currently being evaluated in a Phase III study of men with chemotherapy-naïve metastatic CRPC. This study has enrolled 1680 patients and has co-primary end points of overall survival and progression-free survival. Results of this study and a decision regarding FDA approval of enzalutamide are expected in late 2012 or early 2013.

ARN-509

ARN-509 is a structural analog of enzalutamide, which has been shown to have similar in vitro activity, but greater in vivo activity (see **Fig. 3**).[51] ARN-509 binds the AR with a 7- to 10-fold greater affinity than bicalutamide and specifically inhibits the growth of cells overexpressing the androgen receptor. Similar to enzalutamide, ARN-509 impairs AR nuclear localization and binding to NREs, and unlike bicalutamide has no intrinsic AR-agonist activity. ARN-509 showed improved efficacy in preclinical models at lower steady-state plasma concentrations than enzalutamide, implying potentially a higher therapeutic index. ARN-509 is currently being evaluated in Phase I and Phase II studies in multiple different CRPC populations, including in men with nonmetastatic CRPC, as well as in men previously treated with chemotherapy and/or abiraterone acetate.

EPI-001

The clinical efficacy of enzalutamide supports the hypothesis that inhibition of interaction between the AR and AREs in the nucleus can reduce PSA and slow disease growth in men with CRPC. Similarly, there is increasing evidence that AR-splice variants and transactivated ARs still rely on intact AR DBDs and AR NTDs for function in the absence of ligand. Therefore, it is hypothesized that pure inhibitors of the DBD or NTD should be able to block interaction of the AR with nuclear response elements regardless of the presence of ligand.

This hypothesis led to the identification of the molecule EPI-001 though a screen of extracts from marine sponges looking specifically for molecules that could block the AR-NTD. EPI-001 was found to inhibit AR activity in vitro regardless of the presence of ligand, both in cells bearing wild-type AR as well as in those with a constitutively active AR splice variant lacking an AR LBD (see **Fig. 3**).[52] EPI-001 blocks the expression of TMPRSS2, PSA, and other AR-mediated mRNAs though inhibition of binding of the AR to nuclear response elements in the promoters of these genes. EPI-001 is specific for the AR and does not inhibit the progesterone or glucocorticoid receptors. Importantly, EPI-001 does not inhibit ligand binding and is thought to work exclusively through inhibition of the AR-NTD. In mouse models, EPI-001 decreases tumor growth and reduces PSA expression without significant toxicity, including in castrated mice bearing castration-resistant LNCaP xenografts. Phase I–II clinical trials with EPI-001 are currently in planning, including combinatorial approaches with androgen synthesis inhibitors and other novel AR inhibitors.

SUMMARY

Much has been learned about the pivotal role of the AR in the 70+ years since androgens were first identified as the major drivers of prostate cancer. Recent work has shown that the vast majority of castration-resistant tumors still rely on AR activity and recent clinical trials using agents that either directly or indirectly target the AR have shown clear efficacy. Understanding of the molecular structure and function of the AR has allowed for the development of therapies that block necessary and specific receptor domains.

Given the clinical efficacy of abiraterone acetate, orteronel, and galeterone, it seems likely that inhibition of AR ligand production is sufficient in most tumors to slow AR signaling through deprivation of ligand. None of these therapies are curative, however, and more work will need to be performed to understand the exact mechanisms of resistance to these agents. It is possible that multiple different mechanisms may be at work, including but not limited to selection for cells capable of further AR amplification, the emergence of cells bearing constitutively active AR splice variants, and selection for cells capable of ligand-independent AR transactivation.

Enzalutamide, ARN-509, and EPI-001 represent an exciting new class of agents that are capable of targeting the AR regardless of the presence of ligand, and are able to impair downstream AR functions through inhibition of interactions between the AR and nuclear response elements.

Beyond establishing efficacy and safety of each of these agents, further research will be needed to better understand the optimal sequence of use of these novel agents and to better evaluate whether combinatorial approaches will be more effective at suppressing AR-mediated cell growth than sequential therapy. Will sequential use of the novel androgen synthesis inhibitors have clinical benefit, or will resistance to one predict resistance to the entire class? Similarly, will agents like abiraterone have efficacy in cells resistant to direct AR inhibitors, such as enzalutamide? Finally, will resistance to AR-targeted therapy involve the emergence of pathways that are completely independent of the AR, and if so, will we be able to identify and target these mechanisms? We eagerly await the answers to these questions.

REFERENCES

1. Huggins C, Hodges CV. Studies on prostatic cancer. I. The effect of castration, of estrogen and androgen injection on serum phosphatases in metastatic carcinoma of the prostate. CA Cancer J Clin 1972; 22:232–40.

2. Huggins C. HCV: studies on prostatic cancer II: the effects of castration on advanced carcinoma of the prostate gland. Arch Surg 1941;43:209–23.

3. Siegel R, Naishadham D, Jemal A. Cancer statistics, 2012. CA Cancer J Clin 2012;62:10–29.

4. Halabi S, Small EJ, Kantoff PW, et al. Prognostic model for predicting survival in men with hormone-refractory metastatic prostate cancer. J Clin Oncol 2003;21:1232–7.

5. Ruizeveld de Winter JA, Trapman J, Vermey M, et al. Androgen receptor expression in human tissues: an immunohistochemical study. J Histochem Cytochem 1991;39:927–36.

6. Ekman P, Brolin J. Steroid receptor profile in human prostate cancer metastases as compared with primary prostatic carcinoma. Prostate 1991;18: 147–53.

7. Li J, Al-Azzawi F. Mechanism of androgen receptor action. Maturitas 2009;63:142–8.

8. Jenster G, van der Korput HA, van Vroonhoven C, et al. Domains of the human androgen receptor involved in steroid binding, transcriptional activation, and subcellular localization. Mol Endocrinol 1991;5:1396–404.

9. Rundlett SE, Wu XP, Miesfeld RL. Functional characterizations of the androgen receptor confirm that the molecular basis of androgen action is transcriptional regulation. Mol Endocrinol 1990;4:708–14.

10. Heemers HV, Tindall DJ. Androgen receptor (AR) coregulators: a diversity of functions converging on and regulating the AR transcriptional complex. Endocr Rev 2007;28:778–808.

11. Bevan CL, Hoare S, Claessens F, et al. The AF1 and AF2 domains of the androgen receptor interact with distinct regions of SRC1. Mol Cell Biol 1999;19: 8383–92.

12. Choueiri TK, Xie W, D'Amico AV, et al. Time to prostate-specific antigen nadir independently predicts overall survival in patients who have metastatic hormone-sensitive prostate cancer treated with androgen-deprivation therapy. Cancer 2009;115: 981–7.

13. Kelly WK, Scher HI. Prostate specific antigen decline after antiandrogen withdrawal: the flutamide withdrawal syndrome. J Urol 1993;149:607–9.

14. Small EJ, Halabi S, Dawson NA, et al. Antiandrogen withdrawal alone or in combination with ketoconazole in androgen-independent prostate cancer patients: a phase III trial (CALGB 9583). J Clin Oncol 2004; 22:1025–33.

15. Fenton MA, Shuster TD, Fertig AM, et al. Functional characterization of mutant androgen receptors from androgen-independent prostate cancer. Clin Cancer Res 1997;3:1383–8.

16. Stanbrough M, Bubley GJ, Ross K, et al. Increased expression of genes converting adrenal androgens to testosterone in androgen-independent prostate cancer. Cancer Res 2006;66:2815–25.

17. Friedlander TW, Roy R, Tomlins SA, et al. Common structural and epigenetic changes in the genome of castration-resistant prostate cancer. Cancer Res 2012;72:616–25.

18. Montgomery RB, Mostaghel EA, Vessella R, et al. Maintenance of intratumoral androgens in metastatic prostate cancer: a mechanism for castration-resistant tumor growth. Cancer Res 2008;68:4447–54.

19. Dehm SM, Schmidt LJ, Heemers HV, et al. Splicing of a novel androgen receptor exon generates a constitutively active androgen receptor that mediates prostate cancer therapy resistance. Cancer Res 2008;68:5469–77.

20. Li Y, Alsagabi M, Fan D, et al. Intragenic rearrangement and altered RNA splicing of the androgen receptor in a cell-based model of prostate cancer progression. Cancer Res 2011;71:2108–17.

21. De Bono JS, Saad F, Taplin ME, et al. Primary, secondary, and quality-of-life endpoint results from the phase III AFFIRM study of MDV3100, an androgen receptor signalling inhibitor. American Society of Clinical Oncology Annual Meeting. Chicago, June 2, 2012.

22. Summy JM, Trevino JG, Lesslie DP, et al. AP23846, a novel and highly potent Src family kinase inhibitor, reduces vascular endothelial growth factor and interleukin-8 expression in human solid tumor cell lines and abrogates downstream angiogenic processes. Mol Cancer Ther 2005;4:1900–11.

23. Mendiratta P, Mostaghel E, Guinney J, et al. Genomic strategy for targeting therapy in castration-resistant prostate cancer. J Clin Oncol 2009;27:2022–9.

24. Asim M, Siddiqui IA, Hafeez BB, et al. Src kinase potentiates androgen receptor transactivation function and invasion of androgen-independent prostate cancer C4-2 cells. Oncogene 2008;27:3596–604.

25. Ueda T, Bruchovsky N, Sadar MD. Activation of the androgen receptor N-terminal domain by interleukin-6 via MAPK and STAT3 signal transduction pathways. J Biol Chem 2002;277:7076–85.

26. Culig Z, Hobisch A, Cronauer MV, et al. Androgen receptor activation in prostatic tumor cell lines by insulin-like growth factor-I, keratinocyte growth factor, and epidermal growth factor. Cancer Res 1994;54:5474–8.

27. Nazareth LV, Weigel NL. Activation of the human androgen receptor through a protein kinase A signaling pathway. J Biol Chem 1996;271:19900–7.

28. Schally AV, Coy DH, Arimura A. LH-RH agonists and antagonists. Int J Gynaecol Obstet 1980;18:318–24.

29. Klotz L, Boccon-Gibod L, Shore ND, et al. The efficacy and safety of degarelix: a 12-month, comparative, randomized, open-label, parallel-group phase III study in patients with prostate cancer. BJU Int 2008;102:1531–8.

30. Roach M 3rd, Bae K, Speight J, et al. Short-term neoadjuvant androgen deprivation therapy and external-beam radiotherapy for locally advanced prostate cancer: long-term results of RTOG 8610. J Clin Oncol 2008;26:585–91.

31. Bolla M, Van Tienhoven G, Warde P, et al. External irradiation with or without long-term androgen suppression for prostate cancer with high metastatic risk: 10-year results of an EORTC randomised study. Lancet Oncol 2010;11:1066–73.

32. Pilepich MV, Winter K, Lawton CA, et al. Androgen suppression adjuvant to definitive radiotherapy in prostate carcinoma—long-term results of phase III RTOG 85–31. Int J Radiat Oncol Biol Phys 2005;61:1285–90.

33. Lamberts SW, Bons EG, Bruining HA, et al. Differential effects of the imidazole derivatives etomidate, ketoconazole and miconazole and of metyrapone on the secretion of cortisol and its precursors by human adrenocortical cells. J Pharmacol Exp Ther 1987;240:259–64.

34. Ryan CJ, Halabi S, Ou SS, et al. Adrenal androgen levels as predictors of outcome in prostate cancer patients treated with ketoconazole plus antiandrogen withdrawal: results from a cancer and leukemia group B study. Clin Cancer Res 2007;13:2030–7.

35. De Bono JS, Scher HI, Montgomery RB, et al. Circulating tumor cells predict survival benefit from treatment in metastatic castration-resistant prostate cancer. Clin Cancer Res 2008;14:6302–9.

36. Ryan CJ. Interim analysis (IA) results of COU-AA-302, a randomized, Phase III study of abiraterone acetate (AA) in chemotherapy-naive patients (pts) with metastatic castration-resistant prostate cancer (mCRPC), American Society of Clinical Oncology Annual Meeting. Chicago, June 2, 2012.

37. Ryan C, Li J, Kheoh T, et al. Baseline serum adrenal androgens are prognostic and predictive of overall survival (OS) in patients (pts) with metastatic castrate-resistant prostate cancer (mCRPC): results of the COU-AA-301 phase 3 randomized trial. American Association of Cancer Researchers Annual Meeting. Chicago, April 3, 2012.

38. Dreicer R, Agus DB, MacVicar GR, et al. Safety, pharmacokinetics, and efficacy of TAK-700 in castration-resistant, metastatic prostate cancer: a phase I/II, open-label study. American Society of Clinical Oncology Genitourinary Symposium. San Francisco, March 5, 2010.

39. Ryan CJ. Abiraterone acetate (AA) in patients with metastatic castration-resistant prostate cancer (mCRPC) and prior therapy with ketoconazole: a prostate cancer clinical trials consortium study. American Society of Clinical Oncology Annual Meeting. Chicago, June 4, 2011.

40. Vasaitis TS, Bruno RD, Njar VC. CYP17 inhibitors for prostate cancer therapy. J Steroid Biochem Mol Biol 2011;125(1–2):23–31.

41. Schayowitz A, Sabnis G, Njar VC, et al. Synergistic effect of a novel antiandrogen, VN/124–1, and signal transduction inhibitors in prostate cancer progression to hormone independence in vitro. Mol Cancer Ther 2008;7:121–32.

42. Taplin M, Franklin C, Morrison JP, et al. ARMOR1: Safety of galeterone (TOK-001) in a Phase 1 clinical trial in chemotherapy naïve patients with castration resistant prostate cancer (CRPC), American Association of Clinical Researchers Annual Meeting. Chicago, April 3, 2012.

43. Suzuki H, Okihara K, Miyake H, et al. Alternative nonsteroidal antiandrogen therapy for advanced prostate cancer that relapsed after initial maximum androgen blockade. J Urol 2008;180:921–7.

44. Scher HI, Liebertz C, Kelly WK, et al. Bicalutamide for advanced prostate cancer: the natural versus treated history of disease. J Clin Oncol 1997;15:2928–38.

45. Joyce R, Fenton MA, Rode P, et al. High dose bicalutamide for androgen independent prostate cancer: effect of prior hormonal therapy. J Urol 1998;159:149–53.

46. Kucuk O, Fisher E, Moinpour CM, et al. Phase II trial of bicalutamide in patients with advanced prostate cancer in whom conventional hormonal therapy failed: a Southwest Oncology Group study (SWOG 9235). Urology 2001;58:53–8.

47. Danila DC, Morris MJ, de Bono JS, et al. Phase II multicenter study of abiraterone acetate plus prednisone therapy in patients with docetaxel-treated castration-resistant prostate cancer. J Clin Oncol 2010;28:1496–501.

48. Kassouf W, Tanguay S, Aprikian AG. Nilutamide as second line hormone therapy for prostate cancer after androgen ablation fails. J Urol 2003;169:1742–4.

49. de Bono JS, Oudard S, Ozguroglu M, et al. Prednisone plus cabazitaxel or mitoxantrone for metastatic castration-resistant prostate cancer progressing after docetaxel treatment: a randomised open-label trial. Lancet 2010;376:1147–54.

50. Tran C, Ouk S, Clegg NJ, et al. Development of a second-generation antiandrogen for treatment of advanced prostate cancer. Science 2009;324:787–90.

51. Clegg NJ, Wongvipat J, Joseph JD, et al. ARN-509: a novel antiandrogen for prostate cancer treatment. Cancer Res 2012;72:1494–503.

52. Andersen RJ, Mawji NR, Wang J, et al. Regression of castrate-recurrent prostate cancer by a small-molecule inhibitor of the amino-terminus domain of the androgen receptor. Cancer Cell 2010;17: 535–46.

Immunotherapy for Castration-Resistant Prostate Cancer

Guru Sonpavde, MD[a], Philip W. Kantoff, MD[b],*

KEYWORDS

- Immunotherapy • Castration-resistant • Prostate cancer • Sipuleucel-T, CTLA-4
- PROSTVAC-VF TRICOM • Immune response • Overall survival

KEY POINTS

- Sipuleucel-T is approved for the therapy of asymptomatic or minimally symptomatic men with metastatic castration-resistant prostate cancer.
- Immunotherapy seems to be a valid strategy and further vigorous development of other promising modalities is ongoing (eg, T-cell checkpoint inhibitor, ipilimumab, and the poxvirus-based agent, PROSTVAC-VF TRICOM).
- Rational development of immunotherapy needs to focus on biomarkers predictive of benefit.
- Immunotherapy seems to generally yield survival benefits with little evidence for early clinical benefits.
- Clinical trials evaluating immunotherapy in early-disease and low-disease burden settings should be vigorously supported because this strategy may yield the greatest benefits.

INTRODUCTION

Prostate cancer is well suited for developing immunotherapy owing to early detection, relatively indolent pace of progression, and the expression of organ-specific antigens in a nonessential organ. The rationale for immunotherapy, for malignancies in general, is predicated on overcoming the evasion of the immune system owing to defective tumor antigen processing and presentation by APCs to T lymphocytes, presumably the primary drivers of the host antitumor immune response. The defective presentation may be partly due to downregulation of major histocompatibility complex (MHC) class I molecules.[1–3] Malignancies also promote an immunosuppressive microenvironment resulting from immunosuppressive cytokines (interleukin [IL]-4, IL-6, IL-10, transforming growth factor-beta, vascular endothelial growth factor, tumor necrosis factor), arachidonic acid metabolites, and depletion of tryptophan (due to overexpressed indoleamine 2, 3-dioxygenase). These inhibitory pathways occur in conjunction with the increased activity of immunosuppressive cells. These include tolerogenic APCs, myeloid-derived suppressive cells, T_{REG} cells, T-cell receptor (TCR) dysfunction, and upregulation of checkpoint pathways that inhibit T-cell response (eg, cytotoxic T lymphocyte-associated antigen 4 [CTLA-4] and programmed cell death 1 [PD-1]).[2,4–13] Thus, enhanced presentation of the tumor antigen to the immune system and inhibiting pathways that suppress the immune response may both be anticipated to confer antitumor activity.

The success of sipuleucel-T (Provenge, APC8015, Dendreon Corp, WA, USA) in men with metastatic castration-resistant prostate cancer (CRPC) provides the impetus to further develop

Relevant disclosures. Guru Sonpavde: Research funding to institution from Bellicum Pharmaceuticals and BMS; speaker for Dendreon. Philip W. Kantoff: Paid consultant to Bellicum Pharmaceuticals, Dendreon, and BN-IT.
[a] Department of Medicine, Section of Medical Oncology, University of Alabama at Birmingham (UAB) Comprehensive Cancer Center, 1802 6th Avenue South, WTI-520A, Birmingham, AL 35294, USA; [b] Lank Center for Genitourinary Oncology, Dana-Farber Cancer Institute, Harvard Medical School, 450 Brookline Avenue, Boston, MA 02215, USA
* Corresponding author.
E-mail address: philip_kantoff@dfci.harvard.edu

immunotherapy to treat this disease (**Table 1**).[14] Multiple novel immunotherapeutic platforms are emerging. In addition to novel APC-based agents, promising immunotherapeutic approaches are undergoing vigorous investigation. These include T-lymphocyte checkpoint blockade, poxvirus-based immunotherapy, radioimmunoconjugates (RICs), as well as designer T lymphocytes, allogeneic-cell line-based, adenovirus-based, peptide-based, DNA-based, and *Listeria*-based approaches (**Fig. 1**). This article reviews current immunotherapy with sipuleucel-T and some of

Table 1
Reported randomized trials of immunotherapy for CRPC

Trial (First Author)	Target Antigen	Phase of Trial	N	Standard Regimen	Experimental Regimen	Clinical Outcomes
Kantoff et al,[14] 2010	PAP	III	512	Autologous APCs not pulsed with antigen	Autologous APCs pulsed with PAP-GM-CSF fusion protein (sipuleucel-T)	Extended median OS (25.8 vs 21.7 mo, HR = 0.77; P = .02) and 3-y OS (31.7% vs 23.0%)
Small et al,[15] 2006	PAP	II	127	Autologous APCs not pulsed with antigen	Autologous APCs pulsed with PAP-GM-CSF fusion protein (sipuleucel-T)	Extended median OS (25.8 vs 21.4 mo; P = .01
Kantoff et al,[16] 2010	PSA	II	125	Empty poxvirus vector + placebo	PROSTVAC-TRICOM + GM-CSF	Extended median OS (25.1 vs 16.6 mo, P = .006) and 3-y OS (30% vs 17%)
Kaufman et al,[17] 2004	PSA	II	64	PROSTVAC-TRICOM rF-PSA × 4	PROSTVAC-TRICOM rF-PSA × 3 → rV-PSA or rV-PSA × 1 → rF-PSA × 3	Trend for PSA progression favoring priming dose of rV-PSA.
Gulley et al,[18] 2010	PSA	II	32	PROSTVAC-TRICOM	PROSTVAC-TRICOM + GM-CSF (multiple doses)	13 of 28 evaluable subjects had >twofold increases in PSA-specific T-cell responses by ELISPOT; 4 of 5 high responders survived >40 mo and others had a median OS of 20 mo
Arlen et al,[19] 2006	PSA	II	28	PROSTVAC-TRICOM → Docetaxel-dexamethasone	PROSTVAC-TRICOM Plus docetaxel-dexamethasone	Median PFS on docetaxel was 6.1 mo after receiving vaccine vs 3.7 mo in historical controls
Noguchi et al,[20] 2010	PPV[a]	II	57	EMP	EMP plus PPV	PPV plus EMP was associated with improvement in PSA-PFS compared with EMP (8.5 vs 2.8 mo)
Higano et al,[21] 2009	Multiple prostate antigens	III	626	Docetaxel-prednisone	GVAX	<30% chance of improvement in OS led to early termination
Small et al,[22] 2009	Multiple prostate antigens	III	408	Docetaxel-prednisone	Docetaxel plus GVAX	Shorter median OS (12.2 vs 14.1 mo, P = .0076) for GVAX-docetaxel

Abbreviations: EMP, estramustine phosphate; GM-CSF, granulocyte-macrophage colony-stimulating factor; HR, hazard ratio; OS, overall survival; PAP, prostatic acid phosphatase; PPV, personalized peptide vaccine; PSA, prostate-specific antigen; rF, recombinant fowlpox; rV, recombinant vaccinia.
[a] Personalized peptide vaccine for HLA-A2 or A24+ men.

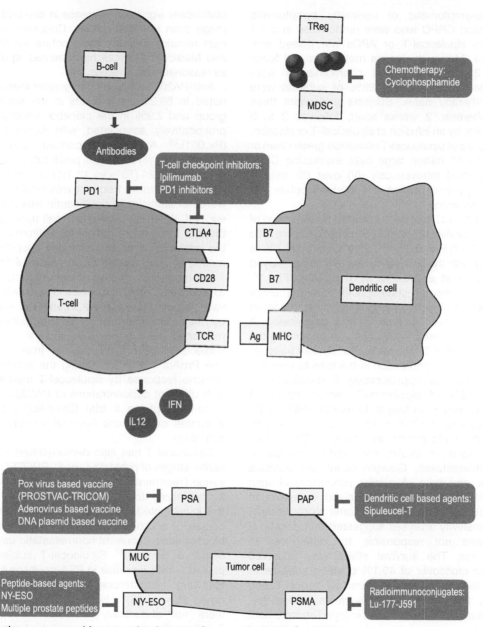

Fig. 1. Pathways targeted by emerging immunotherapeutic agents for CRPC.

the most promising emerging immunotherapeutic approaches for CRPC.

AUTOLOGOUS APC-BASED IMMUNOTHERAPY
Sipuleucel-T

Sipuleucel-T was designed for targeted induction of the immune system to recognize and specifically eradicate prostate tumor cells. In the laboratory, the APCs are exposed to a prostate antigen-containing fusion protein followed by infusion,

which is predicated to train the immune system to generate prostate-specific T cells. Sipuleucel-T is based on a platform of CD54+ APCs collected by leukapheresis and pulsed with PA2024, which is a prostatic acid phosphatase (PAP)–granulocyte-macrophage colony-stimulating factor (GM-CSF) fusion construct. A consistent extension in survival in two smaller randomized trials totaling 225 men (n = 127 and n = 98, respectively), followed by the pivotal immunotherapy for prostate adeno-carcinoma treatment (IMPACT) phase III trial (n = 512).[14,15,23] The IMPACT trial included men with asymptomatic or minimally symptomatic metastatic CRPC who were randomized in a 2:1 ratio to sipuleucel-T or APCs not pulsed with PA2024. Men with visceral metastasis and fewer than 3 months beyond chemotherapy were excluded. Approximately 85% of subjects were chemotherapy naïve. Subjects underwent three leukapheresis, 2 weeks apart, followed 2 to 3 days later by an infusion of sipuleucel-T or placebo. Each dose of sipuleucel-T contained greater than or equal to 40 million large cells expressing CD54 administered intravenously (IV) over 60 minutes following premedication with acetaminophen and an antihistamine.

The IMPACT trial demonstrated an extension of median survival (25.8 vs 21.7 months, hazard ratio [HR] = 0.77; P = .02) and 3-year survival (31.7% vs 23.0%), with the survival curves exhibiting delayed separation at approximately 6 months (**Fig. 2**). However, few prostate-specific antigen (PSA) declines or objective responses occurred and no delay was seen in time to first progression. A subsequent retrospective analysis integrating the results of IMPACT and the earlier, smaller trials detected delayed separation in the time to disease-related pain at approximately 6 months, such that 39.3% of sipuleucel-T versus 18.9% of controls were pain-free at 12 months (HR = 0.84 [95% CI: 0.64, 1.12]; P = .24).[24] There was no preferential benefit based on baseline PSA, lactate dehydrogenase, alkaline phosphatase, number of bone metastases, Gleason score, performance status, and pain. A similar proportion of men (~55%) in both groups received docetaxel at a median of 12 to 13 months after study therapy, but sensitivity analyses suggested that docetaxel use was not responsible for differences in outcomes. The survival effect was observed despite crossover of 49.1% placebo subjects to initial salvage frozen and stored sipuleucel-T, and at any time, in 63.7% of subjects. Intriguingly, crossover subjects (n = 109) enjoyed an increment in postprogression survival relative to untreated controls (n = 62) with a median survival of 23.8 versus 11.6 months (HR = 0.52 [95% CI: 0.37, 0.73]; P = .0001). Because such an analysis may be confounded by more favorable subjects who are crossing over from placebo to sipuleucel-T, an additional analysis was undertaken by invoking the rank-preserving structural failure time model.[25] This analysis also suggested an extension of survival in the crossover subjects.

The toxicity profile was excellent with manageable infusional adverse events including fever (22.5%) and chills (51.2%). The ongoing PROCEED registry study (NCT01306890) is collecting toxicity data to allay concerns regarding a possible non–

statistically significant increase in cerebral hemorrhage seen in initial studies. Concerns regarding cost remain, although the Centers for Medicare and Medicaid Services has deemed sipuleucel-T as reasonable and necessary.

Anti-PA2024 antibody titer greater than 400 was noted in 66.2% of subjects in the sipuleucel-T group and 2.9% in the placebo group and was provocatively associated with survival benefit (P<.001).[26] Antibody responses against PAP (28.5% vs 1.4%) and T-cell proliferation responses to both PA2024 (73% vs 12.1%) and PAP (27.3% vs 8%) were more frequent with sipuleucel-T but were not statistically significantly associated with survival. Whereas cytotoxic T-cell upregulation is thought to be more critical for antitumor activity, the association of the antibody response with outcomes may merely be a surrogate for better T-cell responses or may reflect imprecise assays to measure T-cell responses. The quality of the vaccine product may predict benefit as suggested by the association of CD54 upregulation and nucleated cell counts with survival in placebo subjects who crossed over to frozen product. The ProAct trial is evaluating the differences in immune response by sipuleucel-T manufactured with different concentrations of PA2024. Another open-label phase II trial (OpenAct) extensively evaluates cellular and humoral immune system activation.

Sipuleucel-T has also demonstrated activity in earlier stages of prostate cancer. PROTECT (PROvenge Treatment and Early Cancer Treatment) was a randomized double-blind phase III trial (n = 176) that investigated sipuleucel-T after a 3- to 4-month course of androgen deprivation therapy (ADT) in biochemically recurrent nonmetastatic castration-sensitive disease.[27] Sipuleucel-T subjects displayed a 48% increase in PSA-doubling time (DT) following testosterone recovery (155 vs 105 days, P = .038). However, clinical outcomes were not statistically different.[28] Remarkably, T-cell proliferative and enzyme-linked immunosorbent spot (ELISPOT) responses to PA2024 were observed at a median of 22.6 months and up to 67.3 months. In another trial, sipuleucel-T favorably modified PSA kinetics and produced immune responses when combined with bevacizumab in hormone-naïve prostate cancer.[29] A recent report demonstrated the biologic activity of neoadjuvant sipuleucel-T preceding radical prostatectomy.[30] Greater than twofold increases in $CD3^+$ and $CD4^+$ T cells were observed at the tumor rim where benign and malignant glands interface, compared with the pretreatment biopsy.

An ongoing phase III international trial (P-10-4) is investigating the efficacy of combining ADT with

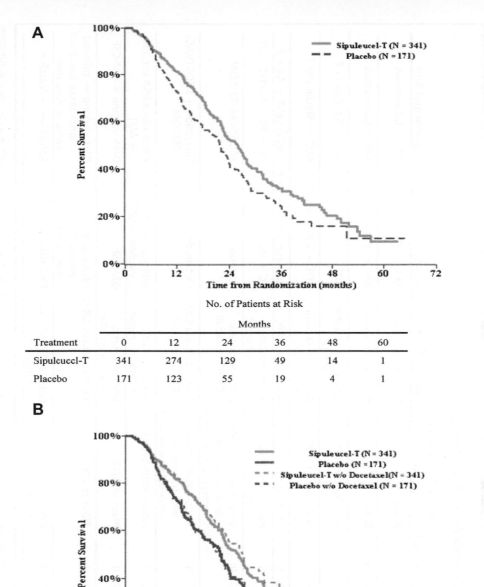

Fig. 2. Survival for sipuleucel-T compared with placebo: IMPACT trial. (*A*) The primary survival analysis and (*B*) analysis with and without censoring at the time of posttrial docetaxel therapy, which showed a consistent treatment effect with sipuleucel-T. (*Reprinted from* Kantoff PW, Higano CS, Shore ND, et al. Sipuleucel-T immunotherapy for castration-resistant prostate cancer. N Engl J Med 2010;363:411–22; with permission.)

sipuleucel-T in metastatic castration-sensitive prostate cancer (**Table 2**). Other randomized phase II trials use immune response–based primary endpoints to evaluate the sequencing of sipuleucel-T and hormonal agents (see **Table 2**).

In one study, sipuleucel-T is administered 2 weeks before or 12 weeks into a 12-month course of ADT for hormone-sensitive metastatic disease. Another trial randomizes men with metastatic CRPC to receive sipuleucel-T followed by abiraterone

Table 2
Ongoing randomized trials of immunotherapeutic agents for prostate cancer

Molecular Target	Institution	Trial Identifier	Phase of Trial	Class of Therapeutic Agent	Line of Therapy	Standard Arm	Experimental Arm
CTLA-4	International	NCT01057810	III	MAb	First, metastatic CRPC	XRT → Placebo	XRT → Ipilimumab
CTLA-4	International	NCT00861614	III	MAb	Second, metastatic CRPC	XRT → Placebo	XRT → Ipilimumab
PAP	International	P-10-4	III	Autologous APC	Castration-sensitive, metastatic	ADT	ADT + Sipuleucel-T
PAP	Multicenter	NCT01431391	II	Autologous APC	Castration-sensitive, metastatic	ADT + Sipuleucel-T	ADT → Sipuleucel-T
PAP	Multicenter	NCT01487863	II	Autologous APC	Metastatic CRPC	Sipuleucel-T → AA+ P	Sipuleucel-T + AA+ P
PSMA	Cornell-led multicenter	NCT00859781	II	Radioisotope Lu-177 tagged MAb	Nonmetastatic CRPC, phase II	KC + HC	KC + HC + Lu-177-J591
PSA	Multicenter	NCT01322490	III	Virus-based antigen and costimulatory molecule expression	First, metastatic CRPC, phase III	Placebo	PROSTVAC-TRICOM
PSA	NIH, USA	NCT00450463	II	Virus-based antigen and costimulatory molecule expression	First, nonmetastatic CRPC, phase II	Flutamide	Flutamide + PROSTVAC-TRICOM
PSA	University of Iowa	NCT00583752	II	Adenovirus-based	Nonmetastatic, hormone naïve	Adenovirus-PSA vaccine→ ADT	Adenovirus-PSA vaccine + ADT
PAP	University of Wisconsin	NCT01341652	II	Plasmid DNA	Nonmetastatic, hormone naïve	GM-CSF	DNA vaccine + GM-CSF
PAP	University of Wisconsin	NCT00849121	II	Plasmid DNA	Nonmetastatic CRPC	DNA vaccine Induction → maintenance	DNA vaccine → tailored maintenance based on immune response
Gene-mediated immunotherapy	Multicenter	NCT01436968	III	AdV-HSV-tk + valacyclovir	Localized high-risk untreated	Radiation	Radiation → Vaccine

Abbreviations: AA, abiraterone acetate; ADT, androgen deprivation therapy; HC, hydrocortisone; KC, ketoconazole; LU-177, lutetium 177; MAb, monoclonal antibody; P, prednisone; PSMA, prostate-specific membrane antigen; XRT, radiation.

acetate (in combination with prednisone), or to concurrent therapy with both of these agents.

Emerging Autologous APC-Based Agents

APCs engineered to express drug-inducible D40 receptors using an adenovirus vector were preclinically shown to engage CD4+ T-helper cells within the lymph node paracortex to augment cytotoxic lymphocyte activation.[31,32] The CD40 receptor was then activated in vivo by a dimerizer (AP1903) in a temporally controlled manner, which was expected to prolong the activated state of APCs.[33] A phase I-II clinical trial enrolled 18 men with metastatic CRPC and reported feasibility and promising activity for this approach when targeting prostate-specific membrane antigen (PSMA).[34]

POXVIRUS-BASED IMMUNOTHERAPY

Viral vaccines display high immunogenicity, do not require patient-specific manufacture, and are capable of carrying a large payload of genetic material.[35,36] Poxviruses engineered to carry a tumor antigen can infect host cells and replicate within the cytoplasm. The tumor antigen may then generate neutralizing antibodies to the encoded antigen (eg, PSA) and may also be taken up by APCs and presented to T cells. Thus, in addition to an immune response against the poxvirus, a tumor antigen-specific immune response may be anticipated. The critical barrier is the induction of antibodies against the poxvirus-based vector, which may neutralize the immunogenicity of a booster dose. To overcome this problem, a different poxvirus or avipoxvirus vector has been used as the booster.[36,37] The poxvirus agent in trials, PROSTVAC-VF TRICOM (Bavarian Nordic, Washington, DC, USA), consists of an initial priming dose of recombinant vaccinia (rV) followed by a booster dose of recombinant fowlpox (rF) subcutaneously. Each of these vectors was engineered to express PSA and TRICOM consisting of the costimulatory molecules intercellular adhesion molecule 1 (ICAM-1 [CD54]), B7.1 (CD80), and leukocyte function-associated antigen 3 (CD58).

An initial randomized phase II trial evaluated different schedules of this prime-boost approach.[17] This trial randomized 64 subjects with PSA progression after local therapy to receive rF-PSA × 4, rF-PSA × 3 → rV-PSA, or rV-PSA × 1→ rF-PSA × 3. Among eligible subjects, 45.3% were free of PSA progression at 19.1 months and 78.1% demonstrated clinical progression-free survival (PFS). There was a trend for PSA progression favoring the group that received a priming dose of rV-PSA. Although no significant increases in anti-

PSA antibody titers were detected, 46% of subjects demonstrated an increase in PSA-reactive T cells.

Subsequently, a double-blind randomized phase II trial enrolled 122 subjects with chemotherapy-naïve, minimally symptomatic metastatic CRPC, Gleason score less than or equal to 7 and no visceral metastasis (see **Table 1**).[16] Therapy was administered subcutaneously on days 1, 14, 28, 56, 84, 112, and 140 and consisted of one priming dose and 6 booster doses. The PROSTVAC arm subjects received priming with rV-PSA-TRICOM followed by boosts using rF-PSA-TRICOM. GM-CSF was administered within 5 mm of vaccination as an adjuvant on the day of and for 3 consecutive days thereafter. The control arm received priming immunization with empty vaccinia vector and boosts with empty fowlpox vector, in conjunction with placebo saline injections instead of GM-CSF. Nineteen of the 40 subjects in the control arm, crossed over to PROSTVAC-VF. PFS was similar in the two groups (P = .56). However, with mature follow-up, PROSTVAC-VF TRICOM conferred a significant extension of median survival (25.1 vs 16.6 months, P = .006) and 3-year survival (30% vs 17%), again characterized by a delayed separation in survival curves (**Fig. 3**).

There was a slight imbalance in favor of the PROSTVAC arm in PSA, hemoglobin, lactate dehydrogenase, and alkaline phosphatase, which was not considered significant. Another limitation was the lack of posttrial-treatment data (eg, docetaxel administration). Estimating predicted survival by a nomogram revealed a 1-month mean and 2-month median difference in predicted survival (mean and median of 20.4 months for controls vs mean of 21.4 months and median of 22.5 months for PROSTVAC), whereas the median survival difference of 8.5 months exceeded the nomogram-predicted survival. Hence, an imbalance in docetaxel administration, which yields a median survival extension of approximately 3 months, was thought unlikely to yield the magnitude of extension in this trial. Finally, the role of GM-CSF as an adjuvant is unclear. Most adverse events were injection site reactions with manageable fatigue, fevers, and nausea.

Subjects did not mount antibody responses to PSA, although robust antibody responses were observed to the vaccinia vector and all but one also generated antibody responses to fowlpox vector. There was no correlation of antivector antibody responses with overall survival (OS), and T-cell responses were not evaluated. Another trial in metastatic CRPC investigated the combination of GM-CSF and PROSTVAC-VF TRICOM and did demonstrate T-cell responses.[18] In this trial, 13 of 28 evaluable subjects had less than twofold

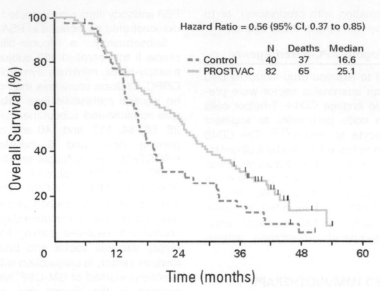

Fig. 3. Survival for PROSTVAC-VF-TRICOM compared with placebo. (*Reprinted from* Kantoff PW, Schuetz TJ, Blumenstein BA, et al. Overall survival analysis of a phase II randomized controlled trial of a Poxviral-based PSA-targeted immunotherapy in metastatic castration-resistant prostate cancer. J Clin Oncol 2010;28:1099; with permission from American Society of Clinical Oncology.)

increases in PSA-specific T-cell immune responses by ELISPOT assay (interferon gamma [IFN-γ] secretion in response to PSA), and four of five high responders (>sixfold increase) survived less than 40 months, while low or nonresponders exhibited a median OS of 20 months. Subjects with a predicted survival greater than or equal to 18 months seemed to preferentially benefit, suggesting that those with more indolent disease may preferentially benefit.[18] Those with less than 18-months predicted survival (actual median predicted was 12.3 months) exhibited an actual median OS of 14.6 mo, while those with baseline predicted median OS greater than or equal to 18 months (actual median predicted survival was 20.9 months) exhibited an actual median OS of greater than or equal to 37.3 months.

Trials investigating PROSTVAC have also provided data that may inform optimal sequencing and combinations. One trial (n = 28) suggested that concurrent weekly docetaxel and dexamethasone does not have a deleterious effect on immune response compared with vaccine alone.[19,38] The median increase in T-cell precursors to PSA was 3.33-fold in both arms following 3 months of therapy. Median PFS on docetaxel was 6.1 months after prior vaccine compared with 3.7 months in historical controls. Two subjects who crossed over to docetaxel after vaccine exhibited additional increases in T-cell responses over 308 and 427 days, respectively. In other preclinical studies, cyclophosphamide

chemotherapy has been shown to deplete T_{REG} cells and enhance the activity of vaccination. Conversely, a favorable vaccination may be associated with an augmented response to subsequent chemotherapy.[39–41] Immune responses to multiple other tumor-associated antigens (TAAs) not found in the vaccine (epitope spreading) was evaluated by testing for T cells directed against known HLA-A2 epitopes of three additional prostate cancer–associated antigens. Indeed, all three subjects tested developed T-cell responses to at least one of these additional TAAs including PSMA, PAP, and/or Mucin 1, cell surface associated antigen (MUC-1). Additionally, the sequence of immunotherapy preceding ADT seemed optimal in a clinical trial enrolling nonmetastatic CRPC.[42,43] In this trial, 42 subjects received either nilutamide or PROSTVAC-VF TRICOM and were crossed over on progression. Twelve subjects receiving vaccine had nilutamide added at the time of PSA progression and exhibited a longer median time to treatment failure from initiation of therapy (25.9 months) compared with the reverse sequence in 8 subjects (15.9 months).

Confirmation of the activity of PROSTVAC-VF TRICOM is ongoing in a phase III trial enrolling minimally symptomatic or asymptomatic men with metastatic CRPC (see **Table 2**). Novel combinations are also undergoing evaluation as in a Phase I trial that combined ipilimumab and PROSTVAC-VF TRICOM vaccine in metastatic CRPC.[44] Interestingly, only one of six subjects previously exposed to chemotherapy displayed a PSA decline, whereas 14 of 24 chemotherapy-naïve subjects (58%) had PSA declines, of which six were greater than 50%. Toxicities were attributable to ipilimumab. An ongoing randomized trial is comparing flutamide alone or with PROSTVAC-VF TRICOM in subjects progressing on ADT alone. A phase II trial randomizes chemotherapy-naïve men with metastatic CRPC to either five doses of ProstVac-VF followed by docetaxel or to initial docetaxel alone (see **Table 2**). Another poxvirus-based agent, TG4010, a recombinant, attenuated modified vaccinia virus Ankara expressing both the MUC1 antigen (a glycoprotein amplified in epithelial malignancies) and IL2 has been evaluated in a small randomized phase II trial (n = 40).[45] Two schedules were explored in men with PSA progression alone after local therapy. Thirteen of 40 subjects exhibited less than twofold slowing of PSA-DT, which was associated with MUC1-specific T-cell responses.

T-LYMPHOCYTE CHECKPOINT INHIBITORS
CTLA-4 Inhibitors

Optimal antigen presentation by the MHC class I molecule on APCs to TCRs on cytotoxic CD8+ T cells requires complementary signals.[46] CD28 on T cells interacts with B7 receptors on APCs to augment cytotoxic T-cell response. Conversely, CTLA-4 and PD-1 on T cells downregulate the immune response and maintain tolerance for self antigens.[36,47–40] The CTLA-4–inhibiting IgG1 human monoclonal antibody, ipilimumab, has extended survival in advanced melanoma.[50] Early phase I clinical trials of ipilimumab, administered IV, have yielded clinical and PSA responses in advanced CRPC.[51,52] A phase I-II trial (n = 45) used ipilimumab 10 mg/kg every 3 weeks for 4 weeks with or without prior priming by single fraction of radiation to a metastatic bony site.[53] The rationale for prior radiation was based on its potential augmenting role when preceding immunotherapy.[54–57] Radiation has been shown to alter tumor-cell phenotype and upregulate TAAs, MHC class I, Fas, and TLR4 agonists.[54,56,58,59] Seventeen men (38%) experienced immune-related adverse events including diarrhea and/or colitis, rash and/or pruritus, hepatitis, and endocrinopathy attributable to nonspecific systemic upregulation of the immune system. Eleven subjects (24%) experienced greater than or equal to grade 3 gastrointestinal or hepatic immune-related adverse events, which resolved with immunosuppression. Addition of radiation was well tolerated. Ten subjects (22%; 95% CI 10%–34%) exhibited confirmed PSA declines greater than or equal to 50.

These encouraging data led to two phase III clinical trials in men with metastatic CRPC who are either chemotherapy naïve or following prior chemotherapy (see **Table 2**). Both of these trials are placebo-controlled and a metastatic bone site was irradiated before therapy. The combination of ipilimumab with other immunotherapeutic modalities (PROSTVAC-VF TRICOM or GVAX [Cell GeneSys, South San Francisco, CA]) is also feasible (see later discussion).[44,60]

PD-1 Inhibitors

Another coinhibitory signaling pathway, PD-L1/PD-1 is also upregulated in prostate cancer tumor infiltrating immune cells.[5,61] Unlike early lethality in CTLA-4 knockout mice, PD-1–deficient animals develop a mild form of late onset strain-specific autoimmunity.[62] Early evidence of clinical activity and feasibility has been demonstrated for IV administered PD-1 targeting monoclonal antibodies and advanced solid tumors with higher baseline B7-H1 (PD-L1) expressions seeming to derive a preferential benefit.[63–65] Subjects with colorectal cancer, melanoma, renal carcinoma, and non–small-cell lung cancer demonstrated clinical benefits, including durable responses and stable disease. Responses were not reported in subjects with advanced prostate cancer, although this finding may reflect the difficulties of determining benefit from immunotherapy (which may be aggravated by poorly measurable disease in CRPC) or the small number of subjects. Most encouragingly, the toxicity profile seemed highly favorable and grade 3 or 4 toxic effects considered related to treatment occurred in only 9% of subjects.[64] Further investigation is planned.

MONOCLONAL ANTIBODIES AND THEIR CONJUGATES

The naked anti-PSMA antibody, J591, was engineered as a therapeutic agent and is rapidly internalized upon binding to PSMA. The naked antibody was feasible and demonstrated dose-dependent antibody-dependent cell mediated cytotoxicity but yielded marginal antitumor activity.[66] However, a risk of hepatotoxicity and marrow toxicity from immunoconjugates was anticipated due to increased uptake in these organ sites. Hepatic uptake diminished as antibody mass increased, suggesting that the uptake was related to antibody binding. The PSMA antibody may also have antiangiogenic activity owing to expression of this antigen in neovasculature.[67] In one phase I trial, 27 subjects with a variety of advanced solid tumors known to express PSMA in their vasculature received J591. Twenty (74%)

of 27 subjects had at least one site of metastatic disease targeted by indium 111–labeled J591.[3] Seven of 10 subject tumor specimens available for immunohistochemical assessment demonstrated PSMA staining in neovasculature. Although, no objective tumor regressions were noted, one subject with metastatic colon cancer had a 53% decline in carcinoembryonic antigen and two subjects had stable disease. One subject with metastatic rectal cancer and another with bladder cancer experienced pain relief. One small trial enrolling heterogeneous subjects with prostate cancer (n = 17) administered continuous low-dose subcutaneous IL-2 daily for 8 weeks with weekly intravenous infusions of J591 during weeks 4 to 6, which demonstrated a trend for NK cell expansion in those without progression.[68]

Unlike the naked antibody, the immunoconjugate of the PSMA antibody designed to deliver the maytansinoid antimicrotubule agent, DM-1, yielded PSA responses in two (22%) of nine subjects treated at 264 or 343 mg/m^2 accompanied by one measurable tumor regression.[69] However, neuropathy occurred in 8 (35%) of 23 subjects, including five of six subjects treated at 343 mg/m^2, suggesting the need for a more optimal linker between J591 and DM-1 (a potentially neurotoxic agent). Similarly, RICs of J591 and radiopharmaceuticals or toxins have demonstrated more promising activity.[69–71] Two phase II trials investigating yttrium 90 [(90)Y]-J591 were conducted in subjects with metastatic CRPC. In the first trial (n = 29), dose-limiting toxicity was thrombocytopenia with non–life-threatening bleeding.[71] Nonhematologic toxicity was not dose limiting. Targeting of known sites of bone and soft tissue metastases was seen in most subjects and no immunogenicity was seen. Two subjects experienced 85% and 70% declines in PSA lasting 8 and 8.6 months, respectively, which were accompanied by objective responses. In the second phase II trial of (90)Y-J591 (n = 35), four subjects experienced greater than or equal to 50% PSA declines.[70]

Subsequently, phase I and II trials established the safety of lutetium 177 (Lu-177)–tagged J591.[72,73] Unlike (90)Y, this radiopharmaceutical emits both β and γ radiation, which allows concurrent imaging. In the phase II trial, 28 men with metastatic CRPC received two fractionated doses 2 weeks apart, which seemed to allow higher cumulative doses of Lu-177–tagged J591 with less toxicity. Additionally, a suggestion of dose response was observed with targeting of metastatic sites. An ongoing phase II trial is evaluating Lu-177–tagged J591 in nonmetastatic CRPC with rapidly rising PSA (PSA-DT <8 months and PSA ≥2 ng/mL) and/or PSA ≥20 ng/mL to target microscopic metastatic disease (see **Table 2**). Another phase I trial in metastatic CRPC is evaluating Lu-177–tagged J591 in combination with docetaxel.

DNA-BASED IMMUNOTHERAPY

Phase I and II clinical trials have evaluated DNA plasmids encoding PSA or PAP.[74,75] In a phase I trial of eight subjects with CRPC receiving GM-CSF and IL-2 in combination with a DNA vaccine bearing the PSA gene, a PSA-specific cellular immune response, and humoral response were detected in two of three subjects in the highest dose cohort.[75] In another larger phase I-II trial, 22 subjects with castration-sensitive prostate cancer and biochemical recurrence received an intradermally plasmid DNA–expressing PAP in combination with GM-CSF.[74] Three subjects (14%) developed ELISPOT responses (ie, PAP-specific IFN-γ– secreting CD8+ T cells), and nine subjects (41%) developed PAP-specific CD4+ and/or CD8+ T-cell proliferative responses. The vaccine seemed moderately immunogenic coupled with somewhat delayed immune responses, although the toxicity profile was excellent. Antibody responses against PAP were not identified.

There was a suggestion of antitumor activity with the median PSA-DT increasing from 6.5 months at baseline to 8.5 months during treatment (P = .033) and 9.3 months in the post-treatment year (P = .054). PAP-specific interferon-γ–secreting T-cell responses (ELISPOT) were detectable in six of eight men with prolongation of PSA-doubling time (DT) greater than or equal to 200%, but in only 1 of 14 subjects without a change in PSA-DT (P = .001).[76] Moreover, HLA-A2–expressing individuals seemed to derive greater benefit. A phase II trial accruing nonmetastatic CRPC randomized subjects to six doses every 2 weeks followed by every 3 months boosting or to six initial doses followed by a tailored booster schedule based on T-cell immune responses (biweekly, monthly, or 3 monthly) (see **Table 2**). Another phase II trial compares this vaccine against GM-CSF (see **Table 2**).

ALLOGENEIC CELL LINE–BASED IMMUNOTHERAPY

The allogeneic cell based agent, GVAX is also an off-the-shelf product with convenient intradermal administration. It has completed extensive phase III evaluation but has reported disappointing results.[77,78] GVAX consists of a platform of irradiated hormone sensitive (LnCaP) and hormone resistant (PC-3) prostate cancer cell lines transduced with a replication-defective retrovirus bearing GM-CSF. Theoretically, this approach was designed to incite an immune response against a broad panel of prostate tumor antigens expressed by both cell lines. Early trials seemed promising with generation of immune responses as well as potential antitumor activity in terms of favorable modulation of PSA kinetics and extension of survival compared with historical data.

A phase 3 trial (VITAL-1) randomized 600 relatively asymptomatic metastatic CRPC subjects to GVAX or docetaxel-prednisone, and the second phase III trial (VITAL-2) randomized symptomatic subjects to GVAX plus docetaxel or docetaxel-prednisone (see **Table 1**). Unfortunately, VITAL-2 (n = 408) demonstrated an excess of deaths (67 vs 47) and shorter median survival (12.2 vs 14.1 months, $P = .0076$) for GVAX-docetaxel.[22] These data prompted an unplanned analysis of VITAL-1 trial (n = 626), which suggested a less than 30% chance of improvement in survival and a decision was made for early termination.[21,79] It is unclear whether these negative results reflect a flaw in the design of these trials or real lack of clinical efficacy of GVAX.

A recent paper reported the feasibility and activity of combination GVAX and ipilimumab.[60] An earlier trial accrued 60 subjects with CRPC and investigated another allogeneic cell line–based vaccine manufactured from three of four selected cell lines in combination with *Mycobacterium vaccae* as an adjuvant.[80] Each of four groups received a different combination of four cell lines. The vaccine was safe and well-tolerated with no major side-effects, although PSA declines could not be attributed solely to the vaccine. Immune responses were seen as reflected by cytokine production, antibody response, and T-cell proliferation.

PEPTIDE-BASED IMMUNOTHERAPY

Peptide-based immunotherapy requires a specific HLA allele to enable recognition by host T lymphocytes. This barrier may be addressed by using a cocktail of peptides. One randomized phase II trial compared low-dose estramustine phosphate (EMP) alone or with a subcutaneously administered personalized peptide vaccine (PPV) in 57 HLA-A2–positive or HLA-A24–positive metastatic CRPC subjects.[20] The peptides were derived from PSA, PAP, PSMA, multidrug-resistant protein, and other epithelial tumor antigens. PPV plus low-dose EMP was also associated with an improvement in PSA-progression–based PFS compared with EMP alone (8.5 vs 2.8 months, $P = .0012$). The HR for OS was 0.3 in favor of the vaccine plus EMP group despite

crossover. The peptide plus EMP combination was well tolerated and demonstrated IgG and cytotoxic-T cell responses. In another retrospective study of a broad spectrum of tumor-receiving personalized peptide-based immunotherapy, IgG response was found to be superior to cytotoxic T-cell response as a predictive biomarker for survival.[81] Intriguingly, this study also demonstrated an association between baseline lymphocyte count and survival.

The NY-ESO-1 and LAGE-1 antigens are amplified in multiple malignancies, including prostate cancer.[82] These peptides have induced immune responses and yielded antitumor activity in preclinical systems.[83,84] Early trials are ongoing to tailor therapy based on subject HLA subtypes and gene expression profiling.[85] Peptide vaccines may be prepared readily and cheaply and hence warrant further evaluation given the preliminary evidence for activity and feasibility.

ADENOVIRAL VECTOR–BASED IMMUNOTHERAPY

Adenoviruses carrying the PSA gene induced anti-PSA T-cell responses and antitumor activity in a preclinical mouse model of prostate cancer.[86,87] These data led to a phase I clinical trial in which 32 subjects with metastatic CRPC received a single subcutaneous injection.[88] Anti-PSA antibodies were observed in 34% and T-cell responses were seen in 68% of subjects. Also, subjects receiving an aqueous suspension of the vaccine developed anti-PSA antibodies more frequently than those receiving the vaccine in collagen matrix did. Conversely, T-cell responses were more frequent in subjects receiving the collagen matrix–based vaccine. PSA-DT increases were noted in 48%, and longer than nomogram-predicted survival was observed in 55%. Antibody responses correlated better with increases in PSA-DT than did T-cell responses; whereas increased survival correlated better with T-cell responses The toxicity profile was excellent.

A phase II trial is ongoing to evaluate the Ad5-PSA vaccine either alone or in combination with androgen deprivation in those with PSA recurrence (see **Table 2**). This study is evaluating immune responses with or without androgen deprivation and may shed light on the potential synergism between immunotherapy and androgen deprivation. Prior data have demonstrated the induction of an immune response against the prostate (T-cell infiltration of the prostate) and thymic regeneration after androgen deprivation.[89–93] Another phase II trial is also evaluating the impact of the vaccine in CRPC. Preclinically, adenovirus vaccines in combination with intratumoral CpG ODN, a TLR-9 agonist seemed to yield a more potent immune response compared with the vaccine alone.[94]

LISTERIA-BASED IMMUNOTHERAPY

Attenuated strains of Listeria monocytogenes, an intracellular bacterial antigen, have been used to carry a payload of tumor antigens and induce tumor regressions and antigen-specific immune responses in murine models. L monocytogenes can access to both phagosomal and cytosolic compartments and thus antigens delivered by L monocytogenes can presumably be presented by infected APCs to T cells in the context of both MHC I and II molecules, resulting in antigen-specific cellular immune responses.[95] Conjugation with a truncated form of listeriolysin O (LLO) increased the immunogenicity of antigens expressed by L monocytogenes. Immunization with L monocytogenes-LLO-PSA downregulated the number of tumor-infiltrating T-regulatory cells and induced complete regression of over 80% of prostate tumors in a preclinical system.[96] Additionally, better humoral and cytotoxic immune responses were also observed when using L monocytogenes-LLO-PSA when compared with PSA-based plasmid DNA and vaccinia vaccines.

The first phase I study of this modality evaluated a live-attenuated L monocytogenes expressing the HPV-E16 E7 antigen fused to LLO in previously treated cervical carcinoma.[97] Subjects received 1 of 3 dose levels of L monocytogenes-LLO-E7 as an intravenous infusion, followed by a second dose 3 weeks later. All subjects experienced a flu-like syndrome that was manageable. These adverse events were acute and transient in most subjects, although dose-limiting diastolic hypotension was observed. Stable disease was reported in seven subjects and an unconfirmed partial tumor response was seen in one subject. Immune response was not comprehensively evaluated in this trial.

Another phase I clinical trial evaluated a live attenuated L monocytogenes vaccine expressing mesothelin in a variety of solid tumors and demonstrated antigen-specific T-cell immune responses.[98] In this recently reported trial, a single intravenous injection of ANZ-100, a live-attenuated L monocytogenes strain, engineered to express human mesothelin (CRS-207), was evaluated in a dose escalation study in subjects with liver metastases. Both a single infusion of ANZ-100 and multiple infusions of CRS-207 were well tolerated. Dose-dependent immune activation was observed for both ANZ-100 and CRS-207 as measured by serum cytokine-chemokine levels and NK cell activation. In the CRS-207 cohort, LLO and mesothelin-specific

T-cell responses were detected. Toxicities included transient laboratory abnormalities and symptoms mediated by cytokine release.

CLINICAL ENDPOINTS FOR THE DEVELOPMENT OF IMMUNOTHERAPY

A pattern of delayed responses occasionally coupled with early progression (possibly from immune response in tumor stroma) and prolonged survival has been observed with immunotherapy across the spectrum of agents. Early tumor regressions, PSA responses, or extension of PFS have not been observed with immunotherapy and this phenomenon is exacerbated by the difficulty of objectively assessing tumor burden in prostate cancer.[99] Potentially, the slowing of PSA-DT may provide an early signal of antitumor activity, although this endpoint has yet to be validated and correlated with meaningful clinical endpoints.[100] Circulating tumor cell alterations seem useful in the setting of chemotherapy and abiraterone but require validation in the context of immunotherapy.[101] Therefore, until intermediate endpoints can be validated, OS remains the most reliable and objective endpoint.

One important advance in the arena of objective response assessment in the context of immunotherapy is the recent formulation of immune-related response criteria.[102] These criteria attempt to capture four distinct response patterns: immediate response, durable stable disease, response after tumor burden increase, and response in the presence of new lesions.[102,103] The recommendations advocate the assessment of tumor burden as a continuous variable considering index as well as new lesions (ie, the appearance of new lesions alone does not constitute immune-related–PD if tumor burden does not increase greater than or equal to 25%).[103] Statistical models describing HR as a function of time, recognizing differences before and after separation of survival curves, were advocated.

DEVELOPMENT OF PREDICTIVE BIOMARKERS FOR THE EFFICACY OF IMMUNOTHERAPY

Biomarkers to predict benefit from immunotherapy require extensive study and validation and may vary between agents and individuals. Potentially, the baseline immune state of the host (ie, host genomics), tumor tissue and/or stroma genomics, and quality of the immunotherapeutic product may impact on the immune response and subsequent outcomes. Gene expression profiling in peripheral blood mononuclear cells seemed informative for prognosticating in men with CRPC receiving personalized peptide vaccines.[85]

Early immune response may serve as a pharmacodynamic marker to signal continued benefit from extending therapy and may also help develop rational regimens. However, the optimal measure of immune response (ie, T cell, humoral, or cytokine responses) is unclear. An antibody response measured by ELISA is a robust and extensively used assay and has significant advantages of reproducibility, although it is unclear whether it captures the mechanism of antitumor activity or is merely a surrogate for cytotoxic T-cell response. The ELISpot assay measures cytokine (eg, IFN-γ) release from T cells in response to specific peptides but has been less extensively studied and refined. Variability and reproducibility are still barriers in its interpretation and validation is, therefore, warranted.[104–106] T-cell response may also be measured by proliferative capacity, cytolytic activity, and markers of activation. An additional caveat in measuring immune responses only to the targeted antigen is that epitope spreading may lead to the immune response targeting other tumor antigens, which may be responsible antitumor activity.[107]

SUMMARY

Immunotherapy has substantially advanced the prevention of malignancies (eg, immunization against hepatitis B and human papillomavirus [HPV] are established for the prevention of hepatocellular carcinoma and cervical cancer).[108,109] Now, immunotherapy has been validated as a therapeutic modality for advanced malignancies, with the approvals of ipilimumab for melanoma and sipuleucel-T for CRPC.[14,50] Fortunately, the toxicity profile is also excellent with most emerging agents, although T-cell checkpoint inhibitors are not designed to be antigen specific and are characterized by systemic immune phenomena. However, the median extension of survival may still be characterized as modest. Given the cost issues, a focus on developing predictive biomarkers to select subjects likely to derive the most durable benefits is warranted. For example, the finding that sipuleucel-T extends 3-year survival to 31.7% compared with 23.0% with controls implies that only an additional absolute 8.7% of subjects derive durable extensions of survival. Hence, biomarkers to identify the subset of subjects destined to enjoy the most durable benefits may yield higher cost-effectiveness. The identification of such biomarkers is likely to be challenging and expensive, but the economic issues facing society demand that investigators

develop agents rationally from the early stages of clinical trials.

Reducing the cost of manufacture by evaluating off the shelf agents may also be prudent, given the financial barriers. The emerging data suggestive of synergism between other therapeutic modalities (radiation, androgen deprivation, chemotherapy) and immunotherapy needs further exploration of both concurrent novel combinations and sequences. Rational and safe combinations of immunotherapeutic agents also warrant exploration. Given the delayed benefits, intermediate endpoints to capture signals of activity are a significant unmet need. Concurrently, immune-related response criteria require validation in CRPC. Moreover, the application of immunotherapy to early-disease and-low disease burden settings, especially in the adjuvant setting may likely yield the greatest benefits. In this context, intraprostatic injection of deleted tumor suppressor genes have yielded systemic immune responses and suicide gene therapy in undergoing phase III evaluation in the adjuvant setting (see **Table 2**).[110]

REFERENCES

1. Blades RA, Keating PJ, McWilliam LJ, et al. Loss of HLA class I expression in prostate cancer: implications for immunotherapy. Urology 1995;46:681.
2. Miller AM, Pisa P. Tumor escape mechanisms in prostate cancer. Cancer Immunol Immunother 2007;56:81.
3. Zhang H, Melamed J, Wei P, et al. Concordant down-regulation of proto-oncogene PML and major histocompatibility antigen HLA class I expression in high-grade prostate cancer. Cancer Immun 2003;3:2.
4. Badawi AF. The role of prostaglandin synthesis in prostate cancer. BJU Int 2000;85:451.
5. Barach YS, Lee JS, Zang X. T cell coinhibition in prostate cancer: new immune evasion pathways and emerging therapeutics. Trends Mol Med 2010. [Epub ahead of print].
6. Elsasser-Beile U, Gierschner D, Jantscheff P, et al. Different basal expression of type T1 and T2 cytokines in peripheral lymphocytes of patients with adenocarcinomas and benign hyperplasia of the prostate. Anticancer Res 2003;23:4027.
7. Filella X, Alcover J, Zarco MA, et al. Analysis of type T1 and T2 cytokines in patients with prostate cancer. Prostate 2000;44:271.
8. Katz JB, Muller AJ, Prendergast GC. Indoleamine 2,3-dioxygenase in T-cell tolerance and tumoral immune escape. Immunol Rev 2008;222:206.
9. Kusmartsev S, Vieweg J. Enhancing the efficacy of cancer vaccines in urologic oncology: new directions. Nat Rev Urol 2009;6:540.

10. Mantovani A, Allavena P, Sica A, et al. Cancer-related inflammation. Nature 2008;454:436.

11. Murdoch C, Muthana M, Coffelt SB, et al. The role of myeloid cells in the promotion of tumour angiogenesis. Nat Rev Cancer 2008;8:618.

12. Sanda MG, Restifo NP, Walsh JC, et al. Molecular characterization of defective antigen processing in human prostate cancer. J Natl Cancer Inst 1995;87:280.

13. Wang D, Dubois RN. Prostaglandins and cancer. Gut 2006;55(1):115–22.

14. Kantoff PW, Higano CS, Shore ND, et al. Sipuleucel-T immunotherapy for castration-resistant prostate cancer. N Engl J Med 2010;363:411.

15. Small EJ, Schellhammer PF, Higano CS, et al. Placebo-controlled phase III trial of immunologic therapy with sipuleucel-T (APC8015) in patients with metastatic, asymptomatic hormone refractory prostate cancer. J Clin Oncol 2006;24:3089.

16. Kantoff PW, Schuetz TJ, Blumenstein BA, et al. Overall survival analysis of a phase II randomized controlled trial of a Poxviral-based PSA-targeted immunotherapy in metastatic castration-resistant prostate cancer. J Clin Oncol 2010;28:1099.

17. Kaufman HL, Wang W, Manola J, et al. Phase II randomized study of vaccine treatment of advanced prostate cancer (E7897): a trial of the Eastern Cooperative Oncology Group. J Clin Oncol 2004;22:2122.

18. Gulley JL, Arlen PM, Madan RA, et al. Immunologic and prognostic factors associated with overall survival employing a poxviral-based PSA vaccine in metastatic castrate-resistant prostate cancer. Cancer Immunol Immunother 2010;59:663.

19. Arlen PM, Gulley JL, Parker C, et al. A randomized phase II study of concurrent docetaxel plus vaccine versus vaccine alone in metastatic androgen-independent prostate cancer. Clin Cancer Res 2006;12:1260.

20. Noguchi M, Kakuma T, Uemura H, et al. A randomized phase II trial of personalized peptide vaccine plus low dose estramustine phosphate (EMP) versus standard dose EMP in patients with castration resistant prostate cancer. Cancer Immunol Immunother 2010;59:1001.

21. Higano CS, Saad F, Curti BD, et al. A phase III trial of GVAX immunotherapy for prostate cancer versus docetaxel plus prednisone in asymptomatic, castration-resistant prostate cancer (CRPC). Genitourinary Cancers Symposium [abstract LBA150]. Orlando (FL): February 26–28, 2009.

22. Small E, Demkow, T, Gerritsen, WR, et al. A phase III trial of GVAX immunotherapy for prostate cancer in combination with docetaxel versus docetaxel plus prednisone in symptomatic, castration-resistant prostate cancer (CRPC). Proceedings Genitourinary Cancer Symposium [abstract 7]. Orlando (FL): 2009.

23. Higano CS, Schellhammer PF, Small EJ, et al. Integrated data from 2 randomized, double-blind, placebo-controlled, phase 3 trials of active cellular immunotherapy with sipuleucel-T in advanced prostate cancer. Cancer 2009;115:3670.

24. Small EJ, Higano CS, Kantoff PW, et al. Time to disease-related pain after sipuleucel-T in asymptomatic patients with metastatic castrate-resistant prostate cancer (mCRPC): results from three randomized phase III trials [abstract: 4661]. J Clin Oncol 2011;29(Suppl).

25. Nabhan C, Gomella LG, DeVries T, et al. An analysis to quantify the overall survival (OS) benefit of sipuleucel-T accounting for the crossover in the control arm of the IMPACT study [abstract: 144]. J Clin Oncol 2012;30(Suppl 5).

26. Sheikh NA, Wesley JD, Chadwick E, et al. Characterization of antigen-specific T-cell activation and cytokine expression induced by sipuleucel-T [abstract: 155]. J Clin Oncol 2011;29(Suppl 7).

27. Beer TM, Bernstein GT, Corman JM, et al. Randomized trial of autologous cellular immunotherapy with sipuleucel-T in androgen dependent prostate cancer. Clin Cancer Res 2011;17:4558.

28. Beer TM, Schellhammer PF, Corman JM, et al. Quality-of-life assessment in a randomized, double-blind study of sipuleucel-T in men with androgen-dependent prostate cancer [abstract: 4648]. J Clin Oncol 2011;29(Suppl).

29. Rini BI, Weinberg V, Fong L, et al. Combination immunotherapy with prostatic acid phosphatase pulsed antigen-presenting cells (Provenge) plus bevacizumab in patients with serologic progression of prostate cancer after definitive local therapy. Cancer 2006;107:67.

30. Fong L, Weinberg VK, Corman JM, et al. Immune responses in prostate tumor tissue following neo-adjuvant sipuleucel-T in patients with localized prostate cancer [abstract: 181]. J Clin Oncol 2012;30(Suppl 5).

31. Hanks BA, Jiang J, Singh RA, et al. Re-engineered CD40 receptor enables potent pharmacological activation of dendritic-cell cancer vaccines in vivo. Nat Med 2005;11:130.

32. Lapteva N, Seethammagari MR, Hanks BA, et al. Enhanced activation of human dendritic cells by inducible CD40 and Toll-like receptor-4 ligation. Cancer Res 2007;67:10528.

33. Iuliucci JD, Oliver SD, Morley S, et al. Intravenous safety and pharmacokinetics of a novel dimerizer drug, AP1903, in healthy volunteers. J Clin Pharmacol 2001;41:870.

34. Sonpavde G, McMannis J, Bai Y, et al. Results of a phase I/II clinical trial of BPX-101, a novel drug-activated dendritic cell (DC) vaccine for metastatic castration-resistant prostate cancer (mCRPC) [abstract: 132]. J Clin Oncol 2011;29(Suppl 7).

35. Arlen PM, Kaufman HL, DiPaola RS. Pox viral vaccine approaches. Semin Oncol 2005;32:549.

36. Drake CG. Prostate cancer as a model for tumour immunotherapy. Nat Rev Immunol 2010; 10:580.

37. Harrington LE, Most Rv R, Whitton JL, et al. Recombinant vaccinia virus-induced T-cell immunity: quantitation of the response to the virus vector and the foreign epitope. J Virol 2002;76:3329.

38. Fakih M, Johnson CS, Trump DL. Glucocorticoids and treatment of prostate cancer: a preclinical and clinical review. Urology 2002;60:553.

39. Antonia SJ, Mirza N, Fricke I, et al. Combination of p53 cancer vaccine with chemotherapy in patients with extensive stage small cell lung cancer. Clin Cancer Res 2006;12:878.

40. Audia S, Nicolas A, Cathelin D, et al. Increase of CD4+ CD25+ regulatory T cells in the peripheral blood of patients with metastatic carcinoma: a Phase I clinical trial using cyclophosphamide and immunotherapy to eliminate CD4+ CD25+ T lymphocytes. Clin Exp Immunol 2007;150:523.

41. Wada S, Yoshimura K, Hipkiss EL, et al. Cyclophosphamide augments antitumor immunity: studies in an autochthonous prostate cancer model. Cancer Res 2009;69:4309.

42. Arlen PM, Gulley JL, Todd N, et al. Antiandrogen, vaccine and combination therapy in patients with nonmetastatic hormone refractory prostate cancer. J Urol 2005;174:539.

43. Koh YT, Gray A, Higgins SA, et al. Androgen ablation augments prostate cancer vaccine immunogenicity only when applied after immunization. Prostate 2009;69:571.

44. Madan RA, Mohebtash M, Arlen PM, et al. Ipilimumab and a poxviral vaccine targeting prostate-specific antigen in metastatic castration-resistant prostate cancer: a phase 1 dose-escalation trial. Lancet Oncol 2012;13:501.

45. Dreicer R, Stadler WM, Ahmann FR, et al. MVA-MUC1-IL2 vaccine immunotherapy (TG4010) improves PSA doubling time in patients with prostate cancer with biochemical failure. Invest New Drugs 2009;27:379.

46. van Luijn MM, Chamuleau ME, Ressing ME, et al. Alternative Ii-independent antigen-processing pathway in leukemic blasts involves TAP-dependent peptide loading of HLA class II complexes. Cancer Immunol Immunother 2010;59:1825.

47. Hirano F, Kaneko K, Tamura H, et al. Blockade of B7-H1 and PD-1 by monoclonal antibodies potentiates cancer therapeutic immunity. Cancer Res 2005;65:1089.

48. Iwai Y, Terawaki S, Honjo T. PD-1 blockade inhibits hematogenous spread of poorly immunogenic tumor cells by enhanced recruitment of effector T cells. Int Immunol 2005;17:133.

49. Smith-Garvin JE, Koretzky GA, Jordan MS. T cell activation. Annu Rev Immunol 2009;27:591.

50. Hodi FS, O'Day SJ, McDermott DF, et al. Improved survival with ipilimumab in patients with metastatic melanoma. N Engl J Med 2010;363:711.

51. Langer LF, Clay TM, Morse MA. Update on anti-CTLA-4 antibodies in clinical trials. Expert Opin Biol Ther 2007;7:1245.

52. O'Mahony D, Morris JC, Quinn C, et al. A pilot study of CTLA-4 blockade after cancer vaccine failure in patients with advanced malignancy. Clin Cancer Res 2007;13:958.

53. Slovin SF, Beer TM, Higano CS, et al. Initial phase II experience of ipilimumab (IPI) alone and in combination with radiotherapy (XRT) in patients with metastatic castration-resistant prostate cancer (mCRPC) [abstract: 5138]. J Clin Oncol 2009; 27(Suppl):15s.

54. Chakraborty M, Abrams SI, Camphausen K, et al. Irradiation of tumor cells up-regulates Fas and enhances CTL lytic activity and CTL adoptive immunotherapy. J Immunol 2003;170:6338.

55. Demaria S, Kawashima N, Yang AM, et al. Immune-mediated inhibition of metastases after treatment with local radiation and CTLA-4 blockade in a mouse model of breast cancer. Clin Cancer Res 2005;11:728.

56. Garnett CT, Palena C, Chakraborty M, et al. Sublethal irradiation of human tumor cells modulates phenotype resulting in enhanced killing by cytotoxic T lymphocytes. Cancer Res 2004;64:7985.

57. Harris TJ, Hipkiss EL, Borzillary S, et al. Radiotherapy augments the immune response to prostate cancer in a time-dependent manner. Prostate 2008;68:1319.

58. Apetoh L, Ghiringhelli F, Tesniere A, et al. Toll-like receptor 4-dependent contribution of the immune system to anticancer chemotherapy and radiotherapy. Nat Med 2007;13:1050.

59. Chakraborty M, Abrams SI, Coleman CN, et al. External beam radiation of tumors alters phenotype of tumor cells to render them susceptible to vaccine-mediated T-cell killing. Cancer Res 2004; 64:4328.

60. van den Eertwegh AJ, Versluis J, van den Berg HP, et al. Combined immunotherapy with granulocyte-macrophage colony-stimulating factor-transduced allogeneic prostate cancer cells and ipilimumab in patients with metastatic castration-resistant prostate cancer: a phase 1 dose-escalation trial. Lancet Oncol 2012;13:509.

61. Zang X, Allison JP. The B7 family and cancer therapy: costimulation and coinhibition. Clin Cancer Res 2007;13:5271.

62. Nishimura H, Okazaki T, Tanaka Y, et al. Autoimmune dilated cardiomyopathy in PD-1 receptor-deficient mice. Science 2001;291:319.

63. Brahmer JR, Drake CG, Wollner I, et al. Phase I study of single-agent anti-programmed death-1 (MDX-1106) in refractory solid tumors: safety, clinical activity, pharmacodynamics, and immunologic correlates. J Clin Oncol 2010;28:3167.

64. Brahmer JR, Tykodi SS, Chow LQ, et al. Safety and activity of anti-PD-L1 antibody in patients with advanced cancer. N Engl J Med 2012;366:2455.

65. Topalian SL, Hodi FS, Brahmer JR, et al. Safety, activity, and immune correlates of anti-PD-1 antibody in cancer. N Engl J Med 2012;366:2443.

66. Morris MJ, Divgi CR, Pandit-Taskar N, et al. Pilot trial of unlabeled and indium-111-labeled anti-prostate-specific membrane antigen antibody J591 for castrate metastatic prostate cancer. Clin Cancer Res 2005;11:7454.

67. Milowsky MI, Nanus DM, Kostakoglu L, et al. Vascular targeted therapy with anti-prostate-specific membrane antigen monoclonal antibody J591 in advanced solid tumors. J Clin Oncol 2007;25:540.

68. Jeske SJ, Milowsky MI, Smith CR, et al. Phase II trial of the anti-prostate specific membrane antigen (PSMA) monoclonal antibody (mAb) J591 plus low-dose interleukin-2 (IL-2) in patients (pts) with recurrent prostate cancer (PC). J Clin Oncol 2007; 25(Suppl 18). ASCO Annual Meeting Proceedings Part I, [abstract: 15558].

69. Galsky MD, Eisenberger M, Moore-Cooper S, et al. Phase I trial of the prostate-specific membrane antigen-directed immunoconjugate MLN2704 in patients with progressive metastatic castration-resistant prostate cancer. J Clin Oncol 2008;26:2147.

70. Bander NH, Milowsky MI, Nanus DM, et al. Phase I trial of 177lutetium-labeled J591, a monoclonal antibody to prostate-specific membrane antigen, in patients with androgen-independent prostate cancer. J Clin Oncol 2005;23:4591.

71. Milowsky MI, Nanus DM, Kostakoglu L, et al. Phase I trial of yttrium-90-labeled anti-prostate-specific membrane antigen monoclonal antibody J591 for androgen-independent prostate cancer. J Clin Oncol 2004;22:2522.

72. Tagawa ST, Milowsky MI, Morris M, et al. Phase II trial of 177Lutetium radiolabeled anti-prostate-specific membrane antigen (PSMA) monoclonal antibody J591 (177Lu-J591) in patients (pts) with metastatic castrate-resistant prostate cancer (metCRPC) [abstract: 5140]. J Clin Oncol 2008; 26(Suppl 15):284s.

73. Tagawa ST, Vallabhajosula S, Osborne J, et al. Phase I trial of fractionated-dose 177lutetium radiolabeled anti-prostate-specific membrane antigen (PSMA) monoclonal antibody J591 (177Lu-J591) in patients (pts) with metastatic castration-resistant prostate cancer (metCRPC) [abstract: 4667]. J Clin Oncol 2010;28(Suppl 15).

74. McNeel DG, Dunphy EJ, Davies JG, et al. Safety and immunological efficacy of a DNA vaccine encoding prostatic acid phosphatase in patients with stage D0 prostate cancer. J Clin Oncol 2009; 27:4047.

75. Pavlenko M, Roos AK, Lundqvist A, et al. A phase I trial of DNA vaccination with a plasmid expressing prostate-specific antigen in patients with hormone-refractory prostate cancer. Br J Cancer 2004;91:688.

76. Becker JT, Olson BM, Johnson LE, et al. DNA vaccine encoding prostatic acid phosphatase (PAP) elicits long-term T-cell responses in patients with recurrent prostate cancer. J Immunother 2010;33:639.

77. Higano CS, Corman JM, Smith DC, et al. Phase 1/2 dose-escalation study of a GM-CSF-secreting, allogeneic, cellular immunotherapy for metastatic hormone-refractory prostate cancer. Cancer 2008; 113:975.

78. Small EJ, Sacks N, Nemunaitis J, et al. Granulocyte macrophage colony-stimulating factor–secreting allogeneic cellular immunotherapy for hormone-refractory prostate cancer. Clin Cancer Res 2007; 13:3883.

79. Cell Genesys Halts VITAL-2 GVAX Trial in Advanced Prostate Cancer. Available at: http://phx.corporate-ir.net/phoenix.zhtml?c=98399&p=irol-newsArticle&ID=1191052. Accessed January 3, 2010.

80. Eaton JD, Perry MJ, Nicholson S, et al. Allogeneic whole-cell vaccine: a phase I/II study in men with hormone-refractory prostate cancer. BJU Int 2002;89:19.

81. Noguchi M, Mine T, Komatsu N, et al. Assessment of immunological biomarkers in patients with advanced cancer treated by personalized peptide vaccination. Cancer Biol Ther 2011;10:1266.

82. Nakada T, Noguchi Y, Satoh S, et al. NY-ESO-1 mRNA expression and immunogenicity in advanced prostate cancer. Cancer Immun 2003;3:10.

83. Zeng G, Li Y, El-Gamil M, et al. Generation of NY-ESO-1-specific CD4+ and CD8+ T cells by a single peptide with dual MHC class I and class II specificities: a new strategy for vaccine design. Cancer Res 2002;62:3630.

84. Zeng G, Wang X, Robbins PF, et al. CD4(+) T cell recognition of MHC class II-restricted epitopes from NY-ESO-1 presented by a prevalent HLA DP4 allele: association with NY-ESO-1 antibody production. Proc Natl Acad Sci U S A 2001;98:3964.

85. Komatsu N, Matsueda S, Tashiro K, et al. Gene expression profiles in peripheral blood as a biomarker in cancer patients receiving peptide vaccination. Cancer 2012;118:3208.

86. Elzey BD, Siemens DR, Ratliff TL, et al. Immunization with type 5 adenovirus recombinant for a tumor antigen in combination with recombinant canarypox virus (ALVAC) cytokine gene delivery induces

destruction of established prostate tumors. Int J Cancer 2001;94:842.

87. Siemens DR, Elzey BD, Lubaroff DM, et al. Cutting edge: restoration of the ability to generate CTL in mice immune to adenovirus by delivery of virus in a collagen-based matrix. J Immunol 2001;166:731.

88. Lubaroff DM, Konety BR, Link B, et al. Phase I clinical trial of an adenovirus/prostate-specific antigen vaccine for prostate cancer: safety and immunologic results. Clin Cancer Res 2009;15:7375.

89. Aragon-Ching JB, Williams KM, Gulley JL. Impact of androgen-deprivation therapy on the immune system: implications for combination therapy of prostate cancer. Front Biosci 2007;12:4957.

90. Drake CG, Doody AD, Mihalyo MA, et al. Androgen ablation mitigates tolerance to a prostate/prostate cancer-restricted antigen. Cancer Cell 2005;7:239.

91. Mercader M, Bodner BK, Moser MT, et al. T cell infiltration of the prostate induced by androgen withdrawal in patients with prostate cancer. Proc Natl Acad Sci U S A 2001;98:14565.

92. Roden AC, Moser MT, Tri SD, et al. Augmentation of T cell levels and responses induced by androgen deprivation. J Immunol 2004;173:6098.

93. Sutherland JS, Goldberg GL, Hammett MV, et al. Activation of thymic regeneration in mice and humans following androgen blockade. J Immunol 2005;175:2741.

94. Geary SM, Lemke CD, Lubaroff DM, et al. Tumor immunotherapy using adenovirus vaccines in combination with intratumoral doses of CpG ODN. Cancer Immunol Immunother 2011;60:1309.

95. Pamer EG. Immune responses to Listeria monocytogenes. Nat Rev Immunol 2004;4:812.

96. Shahabi V, Reyes-Reyes M, Wallecha A, et al. Development of a Listeria monocytogenes based vaccine against prostate cancer. Cancer Immunol Immunother 2008;57:1301.

97. Maciag PC, Radulovic S, Rothman J. The first clinical use of a live-attenuated Listeria monocytogenes vaccine: a phase I safety study of Lm-LLO-E7 in patients with advanced carcinoma of the cervix. Vaccine 2009;27:3975.

98. Le DT, Brockstedt DG, Nir-Paz R, et al. A live-attenuated Listeria vaccine (ANZ-100) and a live-attenuated Listeria vaccine expressing mesothelin (CRS-207) for advanced cancers: phase i studies of safety and immune induction. Clin Cancer Res 2012;18:858.

99. Eisenhauer EA, Therasse P, Bogaerts J, et al. New response evaluation criteria in solid tumours: revised RECIST guideline (version 1.1). Eur J Cancer 2009;45:228.

100. Arlen PM, Bianco F, Dahut WL, et al. Prostate Specific Antigen Working Group guidelines on prostate specific antigen doubling time. J Urol 2008;179:2181.

101. de Bono JS, Scher HI, Montgomery RB, et al. Circulating tumor cells predict survival benefit from treatment in metastatic castration-resistant prostate cancer. Clin Cancer Res 2008;14:6302.

102. Hoos A, Eggermont AM, Janetzki S, et al. Improved endpoints for cancer immunotherapy trials. J Natl Cancer Inst 2010;102:1388.

103. Wolchok JD, Hoos A, O'Day S, et al. Guidelines for the evaluation of immune therapy activity in solid tumors: immune-related response criteria. Clin Cancer Res 2009;15:7412.

104. Arlen P, Tsang KY, Marshall JL, et al. The use of a rapid ELISPOT assay to analyze peptide-specific immune responses in carcinoma patients to peptide vs. recombinant poxvirus vaccines. Cancer Immunol Immunother 2000;49:517.

105. Kreher CR, Dittrich MT, Guerkov R, et al. CD4+ and CD8+ cells in cryopreserved human PBMC maintain full functionality in cytokine ELISPOT assays. J Immunol Methods 2003;278:79.

106. Whiteside TL. Immunologic monitoring of clinical trials in patients with cancer: technology versus common sense. Immunol Invest 2000;29:149.

107. Bilusic M, Gulley JL. Endpoints, patient selection, and biomarkers in the design of clinical trials for cancer vaccines. Cancer Immunol Immunother 2012;61:109.

108. Chang MH, You SL, Chen CJ, et al. Decreased incidence of hepatocellular carcinoma in hepatitis B vaccinees: a 20-year follow-up study. J Natl Cancer Inst 2009;101:1348.

109. Garland SM, Hernandez-Avila M, Wheeler CM, et al. Quadrivalent vaccine against human papillomavirus to prevent anogenital diseases. N Engl J Med 2007;356:1928.

110. Sonpavde G, Thompson TC, Jain RK, et al. GLIPR1 tumor suppressor gene expressed by adenoviral vector as neoadjuvant intraprostatic injection for localized intermediate or high-risk prostate cancer preceding radical prostatectomy. Clin Cancer Res 2011;17:7174.

Moving Toward Personalized Medicine in Castration-Resistant Prostate Cancer

Eliezer M. Van Allen, MD[a,b], Mark Pomerantz, MD[a,]*

KEYWORDS

- Castration-resistant prostate cancer • CRPC • Personalized medicine • Androgen receptor • ETS
- Next-generation sequencing

KEY POINTS

- Next-generation sequencing has allowed improved characterization of castration-resistant prostate cancer.
- Novel targeted therapies can focus on insights into the biology of androgen receptor and the androgen synthesis pathways.
- Novel therapies target genomic susceptibilities of distinct subgroups.
- Tailored immunotherapy is another personalized approach to therapy.
- New methods to implement these technologies in prospective clinical settings are underway.

INTRODUCTION

Across cancer types, recent genomic studies have revealed genetic polymorphisms and mutations that may serve as therapeutic targets.[1,2] Based on these findings and the increasing ability to identify biologically and clinically relevant genetic alterations, the era of personalized cancer treatment is achievable. This potential shift in clinical practice represents a transformation in oncology that may dramatically improve outcomes for patients who have cancer. Personalized approaches to cancer care have recently demonstrated clinically significant benefit, including targeting the activation of the gene BRAF in metastatic melanoma[3] and the EML4-ALK gene fusion in metastatic non–small-cell lung cancer.[4] By defining subpopulations of patients based on specific genetic, "druggable" alterations (ie, genetic alterations for which therapies exist), these examples demonstrate not only the feasibility but often the superiority of a personalized approach to cancer care when compared with nonpersonalized standard therapies.

Prostate cancer (CaP) is the most common solid tumor in men in the United States. CaP is considered a hormone-dependent tumor in which malignant cells express the androgen receptor (AR) and require its activation for survival. Castration-resistant prostate cancer (CRPC) refers to the clinical state in which resistance to androgen deprivation therapy (ADT) has emerged and disease progression results despite castrate levels of testosterone (typically defined as ≤50 ng/dL).[5] Castration resistance is associated with a poor prognosis and metastatic CRPC is generally considered lethal.[6] Traditional therapeutic approaches to CRPC have included primarily cytotoxic chemotherapy, specifically docetaxel plus prednisone, yielding a median overall survival of approximately 18 months in the metastatic setting.[7,8]

However, an improved understanding of the biologic mechanisms leading to ADT resistance and CRPC emergence has resulted in multiple novel therapeutic approaches targeting specific vulnerabilities of the tumor cell. These include

a Department of Medical Oncology, Dana-Farber Cancer Institute, 450 Brookline Avenue, Boston, MA 02115, USA; b The Broad Institute of Harvard and MIT, 7 Cambridge Center, Cambridge, MA 02142, USA
* Corresponding author.
E-mail address: Mark_Pomerantz@dfci.harvard.edu

Urol Clin N Am 39 (2012) 483–490
http://dx.doi.org/10.1016/j.ucl.2012.07.005
0094-0143/12/$ – see front matter © 2012 Published by Elsevier Inc.

innovative androgen-based therapies, building on the full genomic characterization of CRPC, and immunotherapy-based approaches, targeting CRPC-related antigens (**Table 1**). Taken together, these approaches form the basis for targeted therapies for CRPC and will be described sequentially in detail.

PERSONALIZED MEDICINE IN ONCOLOGY

To realize the potential of personalized medicine in CRPC, an appreciation of this approach in other cancers is worthwhile. One prominent recent example involves a new treatment paradigm for metastatic melanoma. Before there was a clear understanding of the potential drivers of this disease, standard first-line therapy included nonspecific cytotoxic chemotherapy or immunotherapy and no systemic therapy-demonstrated improved overall survival.

However, once activating mutations in the BRAF gene were discovered in approximately 50% of patients with advanced melanoma,[9] targeted therapies directed specifically at that alteration were developed and studied specifically in those patients who harbored the recurrent activating mutation in BRAF. These efforts culminated in the development of vemurafenib (Zelboraf), an agent directed at a specific activating mutation in BRAF that demonstrated improved overall survival in advanced melanoma.[10] Vemurafenib is now Food and Drug Administration (FDA) approved, along with a diagnostic test that identifies the activating BRAF alteration that warrants use of this agent. Patients with newly diagnosed metastatic melanoma are routinely tested for this mutation to choose the appropriate first-line therapy.

This approach can be summarized as follows: (1) define a clinical cohort of patients whose tumors harbor specific molecular alterations, (2) utilize agents that selectively target those alterations, and (3) match patients to drugs. This tailored therapy method serves as a model for similar efforts in CRPC, using the numerous pathways and alterations involved in this disease.

TARGETING THE ANDROGEN PATHWAY

In CRPC, despite depleted circulating androgen, AR activity is restored by numerous mechanisms. Clinically, this phenomenon is manifested by rising prostate-specific antigen (PSA) levels and, recently, the underlying biologic processes have been characterized. These mechanisms of increased AR activity include (1) AR amplification or overexpression, (2) activating AR mutations, (3) alternative sources of androgen production, (4) AR coactivator overexpression, and (5) indirect AR activation.[11] Globally, these mechanisms involve either an increase in AR ligand or AR activation. Multiple novel approaches are in development to specifically target these events.

Table 1
Targeted therapies for CRPC

Target	Agent	Stage of Therapy
Androgen production	Abiraterone	FDA approved
—	Tak-700	Early-phase clinical trials
—	Tok-001	Early-phase clinical trials
AR binding	MDV-3100	Phase III trials
—	ARN-509	Early-phase clinical trials
—	Tok-001	Early-phase clinical trials
ETS-positive	PARP1 inhibitors	Early-phase clinical trials
SPINK1 overexpressed	Cetuximab	Early-phase clinical trials
—	Erlotinib	Early-phase clinical trials
PI3K pathway[a]	PI3K inhibitors	Early-phase clinical trials
—	AKT inhibitors	Early-phase clinical trials
—	mTOR inhibitors	Early-phase clinical trials
MAPK pathway	RAF inhibitors	Early-phase clinical trials
—	MEK inhibitors	Early-phase clinical trials
Immunotherapy	Sipuleucel-T	FDA approved
—	Ipilimumab	Phase III trials

[a] Many trials also include combined AR inhibition.

AR Ligand Reduction

Traditional approaches to androgen depletion in the treatment of prostate cancer include GnRH agonists, which desensitize gonadotropin release and suppress testicular androgen production. In addition, the antifungal agent ketoconazole has long been used to suppress the contribution of androgen from the adrenal gland. Neither approach is particularly specific to AR ligand reduction, nor are they associated with common side effects such as decreased bone density or clinical adrenal insufficiency.

With the discovery that nontesticular sources of androgen maintain some androgen production and promote prostate cancer progression,[12] multiple targeted approaches have emerged to translate this resistance pathway into a susceptibility. The most developed therapy targeting residual androgen deprivation is abiraterone acetate (Zytiga), a highly selective irreversible inhibitor of CYP17A1 (17α–hydroxylase/C17,20-lyase), an enzyme involved in androgen synthesis. Ketoconazole more crudely inhibits this enzyme along with additional enzymes in adrenal biosynthesis pathways.

In a phase II study of CRPC patients who had already progressed despite docetaxel, administration of abiraterone acetate resulted in a PSA decline of greater than or equal to 30% in 32 of 47 patients and was quite well tolerated.[13] A subsequent phase III study involving this patient population demonstrated a significant improvement in overall survival in the abiraterone acetate arm, with a 14.8 month (vs 10.9 months) overall survival and a hazard ratio of 0.646.[14] Additional therapies targeting CYP17 that are currently in development and clinical study include Tak-700 (Millennium Pharmaceuticals, Cambridge, MA, USA and Takeda, Osaka, Japan)[15] and Tok-001 (Tokai Pharmaceuticals, Cambridge, MA, USA), which also acts as an AR antagonist.[16]

AR Deactivation

Direct inhibition of AR remains a frequently used therapeutic maneuver and a logical treatment strategy. However, first-generation AR antagonists, such as bicalutamide, or mixed agonists-antagonists, such as flutamide, have had limited clinical benefit. One potential mechanism of resistance to these therapies is that alternative splicing of AR leads to alteration or loss of the ligand-binding domain to which traditional AR-targeted therapies bind.[17] Another resistance mechanism invokes AR copy number amplification, which may affect AR coactivators and result in the medications functioning predominantly as agonists

instead of than antagonists. In this setting, antiandrogens can promote instead of than inhibit tumor growth.[18]

As a result, two new AR antagonists have been developed to potentially circumvent these resistance mechanisms. MDV3100 (Medivation, San Francisco, CA, USA) is a small-molecule antagonist of AR that binds to AR with higher affinity than traditional antiandrogens. In addition, it inhibits AR translocation to the nucleus and blocks AR–DNA binding.[19] A phase I-II study of 42 patients with CRPC and progressive disease demonstrated a 50% or greater reduction in PSA in 56% of patients.[20] Based on these findings, multiple phase III trials have been initiated in the before and after chemotherapy settings, with preliminary results expected in the next 1 to 2 years.

ARN-509 (Aragon, San Diego, CA, USA) is a competitive AR inhibitor that is antagonistic to AR overexpression and, unlike traditional AR antagonists, lacks agonist activity in preclinical CRPC models.[21] It functions by binding to AR, inhibiting cell growth and androgen-mediated transcription in CaP that overexpresses AR, thereby suppressing tumor growth. Phase II studies of this agent are ongoing. Finally, Tok-001 combines CYP17 inhibition with AR targeting and is in clinical trials.

Current AR Precision Therapy Limitations

Though a better understanding of AR biology has led to multiple therapies targeting susceptibilities in this pathway, there is not yet a method to identify in advance which CRPC patients may benefit most from targeting this pathway or which specific targets within the pathway deserve the most attention in an individual patient. Although there is no clinical test for quantifying AR copy number amplification to predict which patients may benefit the most from AR antagonists, predictive assays such as this may prove beneficial in the future. In addition, incorporation of serial biopsies of patient lesions after initial resistance to ADT therapy may help determine which resistance mechanism developed in that patient's tumor and what AR-targeted agent, if any, might be clinically useful. Recent genetic sequencing of CRPC tumor samples suggest that mutations in AR and other key genes in its pathway occur as the disease progresses and may offer clues about how to attack ADT-resistant disease.[22]

In sum, discoveries in AR biology have led to multiple therapies strategically designed to attack CRPC-related susceptibilities. As a class of agents, these newer androgen-related therapies are more specific than their predecessors in targeting AR and the androgen pathway. Although they demonstrate a great step in the direction of truly personalized CRPC therapy, they are still clinically used without specific knowledge of the individual patient's tumor profile. However, when combined with some additional findings (see later discussion), these agents will likely form the foundation of a personalized approach to CRPC management. Furthermore, as data are accumulated on inherited variation in androgen synthesis pathways, such as genetic polymorphisms in CYP17 and their impact on survival, it is conceivable that selection of these agents will be based on a patient's predicted ability to respond to such agents.[23] Studies addressing variations in the androgen pathway are ongoing.

TARGETING NOVEL PATHWAYS IN CRPC

Beyond focusing on novel characteristics of androgen production and AR activation for more tailored approaches to CRPC treatment, numerous insights into the genetics underlying CRPC development and progression have led to additional treatment strategies. Each biologic insight results in carving out subpopulations of CRPC patients with unique genetic signatures for whom tailored therapies beyond the androgen-oriented ones discussed previously may be considered.

Targeted Therapies Based on E–Twenty-Six Transcription Factors

Roughly 50% of CaP demonstrate the gene fusion of the oncogenic E–twenty-six (ETS) transcription factor ERG to TMPRSS2, which is an androgen-regulated gene.[24] In addition to ERG, other ETS transcription factors have been found in CaP, including ETV1, ETV4, and ETV5.[25] After an ETS fusion is formed via gene rearrangement, the ETS gene is overexpressed and contributes to acceleration of prostate carcinogenesis.[26,27] Currently, these fusions can be identified clinically via traditional pathology techniques on primary prostate resection samples using fluorescence in situ hybridization. However, as with many other alterations (see later discussion), they can also be identified on primary or metastatic lesions using next-generation sequencing technologies that can survey the genomic landscape of alterations and isolate all relevant lesions at the individual level (**Table 2**).

Unfortunately, transcription factors, including ETS, are notoriously difficult to target directly using conventional approaches.[28] However, efforts to target associated enzymes involved in ERG function suggest viable therapeutic

Table 2 Tumor profiling techniques and definitions	
Term	**Definition**
Next-generation sequencing	DNA sequencing methods that produce millions of short sequence DNA reads in a parallel process
Exome	The sequence of known exons of an individual
Transcriptome	The sequence of expressed genes of an individual
Genome	The entire DNA sequence of an individual
Germline polymorphism	Variation at a specific locus in a genome

targets specifically for patients with documented TMPRSS2:ERG fusion. For example, a recent study demonstrated that the TMPRSS2:ERG fusion interacts in a DNA-independent manner with poly(ADP-ribose)polymerase 1 (PARP1), and in preclinical models, pharmacologic inhibition of PARP1 inhibits ETS-positive prostate cancer in tumors grown in xenografts.[25] Given the numerous PARP1 inhibitors currently in development, clinical trials to evaluate the impact of this therapy in ETS-positive CRPC are underway. Although clinical validation of PARP1 inhibition in ETS-positive CRPC is necessary, such findings highlight the importance of identifying subgroups based on unique genomic profiles before initiation of specific therapies.

Additional Targeted Therapies for ETS Fusion-Negative CRPC

For the other 50% of CaP that are ETS fusion-negative, efforts to ascertain additional genomic susceptibilities have yielded multiple novel findings for which personalized therapies are in development.

SPINK1-overexpressed CRPC

SPINK1 encodes a secreted serine protease inhibitor and is thought to have a role in modulating the activity of cancer-related proteases. It was shown that overexpressed SPINK1 CaP defined an aggressive molecular subtype of ETS fusion-negative prostate cancers, encompassing roughly 10% of all cases.[29] Because SPINK1 encodes an extracellular secreted protein, it is more amenable to direct therapeutic targeting when compared with ETS-positive disease. As such, preclinical models demonstrated the therapeutic potential of an anti-SPINK1 monoclonal antibody on prostate cancer models with overexpressed SPINK1.[30] Although humanized SPINK1 monoclonal antibodies are not yet available for human testing, there is a clear therapeutic rationale for its development.

It has also been demonstrated that SPINK1 partially mediates its effects through interaction with epidermal growth factor receptor (EGFR). Administration of cetuximab (Erbitux), anti-EGFR monoclonal antibody, to mice xenografts modeling this disease subtype resulted in attenuation of tumor growth.[30] Even though previous phase I-II clinical trials of cetuximab in metastatic CRPC were disappointing,[31] certain subgroups did have a significant benefit and it has been postulated that these may have been overexpressed SPINK1 cohorts. It is conceivable that if anti-EGFR agents are tested specifically on the overexpressed SPINK1 subgroup, there may be significant benefits to this therapy. Studies have begun to test for this alteration prospectively to select these patients for EGFR-targeted therapies such as cetuximab.

MAPK Pathway–Activated CRPC

To identify other subgroups of CRPC that may benefit from individualized therapies, ETS fusion-negative prostate cancers were sequenced for additional novel and druggable gene fusions. Expression of two gene fusions in prostate cells, one involving BRAF and the other involving RAF1, resulted in neoplasia and were found in 1% to 2% of a large cohort of patient samples. Furthermore, these cells were sensitive to RAF and MEK inhibitors.[32] As a result, clinical trials involving these agents for this subgroup of CRPC have been initiated.

PI3K Pathway–Activated CRPC

Finally, the PI3K signaling pathway is known to be activated in CRPC. Approximately 70% of metastatic CRPC have genomic alterations in the PI3K signaling pathway, mostly via loss of PTEN.[33–35] Given the availability of multiple PI3K pathway inhibitors currently in clinical development, including PI3K inhibitors, AKT inhibitors, and mTOR1/2 inhibitors, multiple studies have begun to address the potential therapeutic benefit of these therapies in CRPC patients who harbor genetic alterations in this pathway.

Furthermore, a recent notable finding demonstrated that there is cross-regulation of AR pathways and PI3K pathways by reciprocal feedback, such that both pathways coordinately support survival.[36] As a result, studies are also underway exploring combined AR antagonism using AR-targeted therapies (see previous discussion) with PI3K pathway inhibitors for potential complementary and synergistic effect. By prospectively testing CRPC patients for these alterations, it will be feasible to funnel patients toward particular therapies that best attack the drivers of their tumors at the level of AR and at the level of the genome for potential synergistic effects.

Other Novel Pathways Under Investigation

Moving beyond these pathways, multiple next-generation sequencing studies have implicated additional potential targets. One group recently performed whole exome sequencing of 50 pre-treated metastatic CRPC patient samples.[22] In addition to targets in the pathways, multiple additional alterations were nominated for further study and possible therapeutic targeting. These include mutations in FOXA1, which repress androgen signaling and increase tumor growth, and mutations in MLL2, a gene that interacts with AR and is required for AR signaling. There are no treatments currently available to specifically target these alterations; however, they are priorities for future study.

Furthermore, a whole exome sequencing study of 112 primary prostate tumor and normal pairs identified subsets of patients with recurrent mutations in SPOP, among others, that may define additional new molecular subtypes of prostate cancer.[37] However, the functional significance of genes such as SPOP remains unclear and therapeutic strategies tailored to these alterations will require further study.

Limitations to Pathway-Oriented Therapy

Importantly, these large sequencing studies highlight the current challenges of personalizing therapy for CRPC. Despite deep genomic characterization of numerous CRPC tumors, no new prominent activating driver mutations (such as with BRAF mutations in melanoma) for which a targeted therapy already exists or is in development have been identified. As such, although each of the alterations discussed previously represents a subset of patients who may benefit from a tailored therapy based on tumor characteristics, these subsets are generally small and further studies are necessary to determine whether broader driver alterations exist beyond the level of the genome in CRPC.

IMMUNOTHERAPY

Beyond personalizing therapy based on AR characteristics or genomic subclassifications, efforts to advance prostate-specific immunotherapy have yielded benefits for CRPC. The most mature effort involves sipuleucel-T (Provenge). Sipuleucel-T is created by using mature, autologous antigen-presenting cells obtained from individual patients that are cocultured with a fusion protein containing prostatic acid phosphatase. The resulting product is then infused back into the specific patient, demonstrating truly individualized therapy from an immunologic perspective. A phase III trial of sipuleucel-T in metastatic CRPC patients without visceral metastases demonstrated an improvement in overall survival by 3.9 months,[38] and it was FDA-approved in 2011 for this patient population.

Additional novel approaches involving immunologic therapies to target the interaction between CRPC cells and the immune system include ipilimumab (Yervoy), which is an anti–cytotoxic T lymphocyte-associated antigen 4 antibody. Early studies in patients with metastatic CRPC have suggested a clinical benefit to this approach[39] and have prompted a phase III trial. Unfortunately, a third approach involving a cellular vaccine created from two modified prostate cell lines, GVAX, did not demonstrate clinical benefit in two large phase III trials despite promising preliminary findings.[40]

RESISTANCE TO TARGETED THERAPIES

Moving beyond personalized therapies targeting specific AR susceptibilities, genomic alterations, or immunologic properties, additional studies aim to identify resistance mechanisms to these approaches, which invariably occur across treatment strategies. In addition to studying preclinical models, comprehensive genomic profiling of patient samples before and after developing resistance to targeted therapies, such as abiraterone acetate or PARP1 inhibitors, is ongoing. These studies involve pretreatment CT-guided bone marrow biopsies of metastatic lesions, followed by administration of the study protocol therapies. On demonstration of disease progression, patients undergo a second biopsy. The pretreatment and posttreatment specimens, along with normal blood, are then genomically characterized. A goal with these studies is to identify sources of resistance that in turn can be specifically targeted.

INTEGRATION OF PERSONALIZED MEDICINE INTO THE CRPC CLINICAL ENVIRONMENT
General Approaches

Given that many of personalized therapies for CRPC require specific genomic characterizations to nominate the appropriate choice of agent, such as identifying the splice site variant of AR that might invoke second generation AR antagonists or SPINK1 overexpression to suggest usage of anti-EGFR monoclonal antibodies, innovations in implementing comprehensive genomic characterization for clinical usage are also undergoing study. One robust example, the Michigan Oncology Sequencing Center, uses whole exome and transcriptome sequencing of patients that yield genetic alteration and expression data at the individual patient level. Following data analysis pipelines, the results are interpreted by a sequencing tumor board that makes recommendations for treatment

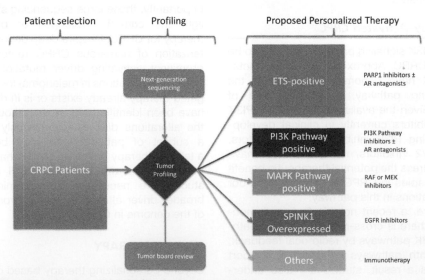

Fig. 1. Workflow for achieving individualized CRPC treatment.

decisions based on specific alterations identified in the genomic characterization.[41]

That approach, although not specific to CRPC patients, outlines a method for translating these advanced characterization techniques for individual patients (**Fig. 1**). It has prompted similar efforts for CRPC patients to prospectively study whether advanced knowledge of patient-specific tumor susceptibilities advances care. The expectation is that these experiments will define a workflow for allowing translation of promising findings into effective therapies for CRPC.

CRPC-Specific Potential Approach

One potential workflow is:

1. All CRPC patients begin with AR-oriented therapies while initial genomic characterization occurs.
2. At the time of resistance to the initial AR therapy, a review of the patient's tumor genomic data may nominate tailored therapies based on pathway alterations versus additional AR-oriented therapies.
3. Once AR and tailored therapies have been exhausted, immunotherapy or standard cytotoxic therapies may be initiated while repeat tumor genomic characterization occurs via biopsy of a resistant lesion.

The goal with this approach is to continually update the patient's potential treatment options using the individual's tumor data in the relevant clinical scenario. Although this strategy does not yet exist in standard clinical environments and may be subject to change, it remains a potential model for truly personalized therapy.

SUMMARY

Until recently, most CRPC patients were treated with nonspecific chemotherapy agents or hormonal treatments. However, in the last few years numerous advances in personalized approaches to CRPC treatment have emerged that may dramatically impact care. These include targeted androgen and AR therapies, novel treatments based on genomic subclassifications of CRPC patients, and unique immunotherapy approaches that use patient-derived tissue to generate individualized treatments. Furthermore, as patients develop resistance to these therapies, studies exploring the mechanisms of resistance will help inform additional therapeutic approaches.

Innovations in clinical-grade characterization techniques to nominate potential targets at the patient-by-patient level are in development, as are numerous clinical trials aimed at determining which of these targeted approaches yields clinical benefit. Overall, the rapid understanding of CRPC subgroups has led to a host of promising treatment strategies aimed at unique susceptibilities and this approach shows great promise in dramatically altering the way CRPC is treated moving forward.

REFERENCES

1. Macconaill LE, Garraway LA. Clinical implications of the cancer genome. J Clin Oncol 2010;28(35): 5219–28.
2. McDermott U, Downing JR, Stratton MR. Genomics and the continuum of cancer care. N Engl J Med 2011;364(4):340–50.
3. Flaherty KT, Puzanov I, Kim KB, et al. Inhibition of mutated, activated BRAF in metastatic melanoma. N Engl J Med 2010;363(9):809–19.
4. Kwak EL, Bang YJ, Camidge DR, et al. Anaplastic lymphoma kinase inhibition in non-small-cell lung cancer. N Engl J Med 2010;363(18):1693–703.
5. Ryan CJ, Tindall DJ. Androgen receptor rediscovered: the new biology and targeting the androgen receptor therapeutically. J Clin Oncol 2011;29(27): 3651–8.
6. Yap TA, Zivi A, Omlin A, et al. The changing therapeutic landscape of castration-resistant prostate cancer. Nat Rev Clin Oncol 2011;8(10):597–610.
7. Petrylak DP, Tangen CM, Hussain MH, et al. Docetaxel and estramustine compared with mitoxantrone and prednisone for advanced refractory prostate cancer. N Engl J Med 2004;351(15):1513–20.
8. Tannock IF, de Wit R, Berry WR, et al. Docetaxel plus prednisone or mitoxantrone plus prednisone for advanced prostate cancer. N Engl J Med 2004; 351(15):1502–12.
9. Davies H, Bignell GR, Cox C, et al. Mutations of the BRAF gene in human cancer. Nature 2002; 417(6892):949–54.
10. Chapman PB, Hauschild A, Robert C, et al. Improved survival with vemurafenib in melanoma with BRAF V600E mutation. N Engl J Med 2011; 364(26):2507–16.
11. Knudsen KE, Scher HI. Starving the addiction: new opportunities for durable suppression of AR signaling in prostate cancer. Clin Cancer Res 2009;15(15):4792–8.
12. Stanbrough M, Bubley GJ, Ross K, et al. Increased expression of genes converting adrenal androgens to testosterone in androgen-independent prostate cancer. Cancer Res 2006;66(5):2815–25.
13. Reid AH, Attard G, Danila DC, et al. Significant and sustained antitumor activity in post-docetaxel, castration-resistant prostate cancer with the CYP17

inhibitor abiraterone acetate. J Clin Oncol 2010; 28(9):1489–95.

14. de Bono JS, Logothetis CJ, Molina A, et al. Abiraterone and increased survival in metastatic prostate cancer. N Engl J Med 2011;364(21):1995–2005.

15. Kaku T, Hitaka T, Ojida A, et al. Discovery of orteronel (TAK-700), a naphthylmethylimidazole derivative, as a highly selective 17,20-lyase inhibitor with potential utility in the treatment of prostate cancer. Bioorg Med Chem 2011;19(21):6383–99.

16. Bruno RD, Vasaitis TS, Gediya LK, et al. Synthesis and biological evaluations of putative metabolically stable analogs of VN/124-1 (TOK-001): head to head anti-tumor efficacy evaluation of VN/124-1 (TOK-001) and abiraterone in LAPC-4 human prostate cancer xenograft model. Steroids 2011;76(12):1268–79.

17. Guo Z, Yang X, Sun F, et al. A novel androgen receptor splice variant is up-regulated during prostate cancer progression and promotes androgen depletion-resistant growth. Cancer Res 2009;69(6):2305–13.

18. Chen CD, Welsbie DS, Tran C, et al. Molecular determinants of resistance to antiandrogen therapy. Nat Med 2004;10(1):33–9.

19. Tran C, Ouk S, Clegg NJ, et al. Development of a second-generation antiandrogen for treatment of advanced prostate cancer. Science 2009; 324(5928):787–90.

20. Scher HI, Beer TM, Higano CS, et al. Antitumour activity of MDV3100 in castration-resistant prostate cancer: a phase 1-2 study. Lancet 2010;375(9724):1437–46.

21. Clegg NJ, Wongvipat J, Joseph JD, et al. ARN-509: a novel antiandrogen for prostate cancer treatment. Cancer Res 2012;72(6):1494–503.

22. Grasso CS, Wu YM, Robinson DR, et al. The mutational landscape of lethal castration-resistant prostate cancer. Nature 2012;487(7406):239–43.

23. Todenhofer T, Schwentner C, Stenzl A. Personalized treatment of prostate cancer based on inherited variations of steroid pathway-related genes. Eur Urol 2012;62(1):97–9 [Epub 2012 Jan 3].

24. Kumar-Sinha C, Tomlins SA, Chinnaiyan AM. Recurrent gene fusions in prostate cancer. Nat Rev Cancer 2008;8(7):497–511.

25. Brenner JC, Ateeq B, Li Y, et al. Mechanistic rationale for inhibition of poly(ADP-ribose) polymerase in ETS gene fusion-positive prostate cancer. Cancer Cell 2011;19(5):664–78.

26. Carver BS, Tran J, Gopalan A, et al. Aberrant ERG expression cooperates with loss of PTEN to promote cancer progression in the prostate. Nat Genet 2009; 41(5):619–24.

27. King JC, Xu J, Wongvipat J, et al. Cooperativity of TMPRSS2-ERG with PI3-kinase pathway activation in prostate oncogenesis. Nat Genet 2009;41(5):524–6.

28. Darnell JE Jr. Transcription factors as targets for cancer therapy. Nat Rev Cancer 2002;2(10):740–9.

29. Tomlins SA, Rhodes DR, Yu J, et al. The role of SPINK1 in ETS rearrangement-negative prostate cancers. Cancer Cell 2008;13(6):519–28.

30. Ateeq B, Tomlins SA, Laxman B, et al. Therapeutic targeting of SPINK1-positive prostate cancer. Sci Transl Med 2011;3(72):72ra17.

31. Slovin SF, Kelly WK, Wilton A, et al. Anti-epidermal growth factor receptor monoclonal antibody cetuximab plus Doxorubicin in the treatment of metastatic castration-resistant prostate cancer. Clin Genitourin Cancer 2009;7(3):E77–82.

32. Palanisamy N, Ateeq B, Kalyana-Sundaram S, et al. Rearrangements of the RAF kinase pathway in prostate cancer, gastric cancer and melanoma. Nat Med 2010;16(7):793–8.

33. Taylor BS, Schultz N, Hieronymus H, et al. Integrative genomic profiling of human prostate cancer. Cancer Cell 2010;18(1):11–22.

34. Reid AH, Attard G, Ambroisine L, et al. Molecular characterisation of ERG, ETV1 and PTEN gene loci identifies patients at low and high risk of death from prostate cancer. Br J Cancer 2010;102(4):678–84.

35. El Sheikh SS, Romanska HM, Abel P, et al. Predictive value of PTEN and AR coexpression of sustained responsiveness to hormonal therapy in prostate cancer—a pilot study. Neoplasia 2008;10(9):949–53.

36. Carver BS, Chapinski C, Wongvipat J, et al. Reciprocal feedback regulation of PI3K and androgen receptor signaling in PTEN-deficient prostate cancer. Cancer Cell 2011;19(5):575–86.

37. Barbieri CE, Baca SC, Lawrence MS, et al. Exome sequencing identifies recurrent SPOP, FOXA1 and MED12 mutations in prostate cancer. Nat Genet 2012;44(6):685–9.

38. Kantoff PW, Higano CS, Shore ND, et al. Sipuleucel-T immunotherapy for castration-resistant prostate cancer. N Engl J Med 2010;363(5):411–22.

39. Fong L, Kwek SS, O'Brien S, et al. Potentiating endogenous antitumor immunity to prostate cancer through combination immunotherapy with CTLA4 blockade and GM-CSF. Cancer Res 2009;69(2):609–15.

40. Lee DJ, Cha EK, Dubin JM, et al. Novel therapeutics for the management of castration-resistant prostate cancer (CRPC). BJU Int 2012;109(7):968–85.

41. Roychowdhury S, Iyer MK, Robinson DR, et al. Personalized oncology through integrative high-throughput sequencing: a pilot study. Sci Transl Med 2011;3(111):111ra21.

Palliative Care in Castrate-Resistant Prostate Cancer

Michael W. Rabow, MD[a],*, Michael Xiang Lee, MD, MPH[b]

KEYWORDS

- Palliative care • Castrate-resistant prostate cancer • Symptom management

KEY POINTS

- Men with castrate-resistant prostate cancer commonly experience distress across physical, emotional, social, and existential realms.
- Interdisciplinary palliative care teams of clinicians (including physicians, nurses, social workers, chaplains, pharmacists, psychologists, physical therapists, and nutritionists) focused on symptom management and patients' goals of care can collaborate with prostate cancer surgeons, oncologists, and radiation oncologists to provide the best care for men at all stages of cancer treatment, including at the end of life.
- Palliative care should be offered concurrently with disease-directed treatments.
- Basic palliative care interventions include communication, education, and simple emotional support.
- Interdisciplinary palliative care teams can provide necessary assistance with management of complex pain, fatigue depression, anxiety, existential crisis, and caregiver distress.

INTRODUCTION

Prostate cancer is the second leading cause of cancer death in men after lung cancer.[1] For patients with metastatic castration-resistant prostate cancer, the median survival in recent phase 3 clinical trials ranges from 12.2 to 21.7 months.[2–8] Although localized prostate cancer typically is asymptomatic, significant symptoms and suffering are associated with advanced prostate cancer and its treatments. This article reviews the benefits of palliative care comanagement in helping patients with castrate-resistant prostate cancer and their family caregivers manage symptoms and distress. Working to relieve distressing symptoms and improve quality of life (QOL) for patients and family throughout the course of their disease are the goals of palliative care, which should be pursued along with ongoing disease management efforts.

CONCURRENT PALLIATIVE AND ONCOLOGIC CARE

The World Health Organization (WHO) defines palliative care in cancer as an approach that improves QOL of patients and their families facing the problems associated with life-threatening illness, through prevention and relief of suffering by means of early identification and impeccable assessment and treatment of pain and other problems, physical, psychological, and spiritual.[9] Palliative care improves QOL and reduces unnecessary costs of health care with its focus on management of symptoms, psychological support, and assistance in goal-setting and the decision-making process for patients facing serious illness.[10–12]

Traditionally, palliative care has been used only late in the course of disease and often delivered only in the hospital setting. Years ago, clinicians

Disclosures: None (both authors).

[a] Symptom Management Service, Helen Diller Family Comprehensive Cancer Center, University of California San Francisco, Suite 313, 1545 Divisadero Street, San Francisco, CA 94143-0320, USA; [b] Division of Hematology/Oncology, Department of Medicine, University of California San Francisco, Moffitt 1286, Box 1270, 505 Parnassus Avenue, San Francisco, CA 94143-1270, USA

* Corresponding author.

E-mail address: mrabow@medicine.ucsf.edu

Urol Clin N Am 39 (2012) 491–503

http://dx.doi.org/10.1016/j.ucl.2012.07.006

viewed palliative care as an alternative to aggressive treatment of cancer and, in fact, hospice regulations require forgoing disease-directed treatments. However, palliative care includes much more than hospice care and comfort-only care for patients at the end of life. Palliative care provides an extra layer of support to improve quality of life for patients with any prognosis that can be offered concurrently with disease-directed treatments. Controlled trials of early palliative care provided concurrently with cancer-directed treatment show its efficacy in improving quality of life for patients undergoing active cancer treatment, and even in prolonging survival.[13,14] In a randomized trial, Temel and colleagues[14] showed that early palliative care in addition to usual chemotherapy for patients with metastatic non–small cell lung cancer led to significant improvement in quality of life and mood, decreased aggressive care at the end of life, and prolonged survival compared with usual cancer treatment. Patients need not have to choose between curative attempts and palliative care. The American Society of Clinical Oncology (ASCO), the National Cancer Policy Board, and the National Comprehensive Cancer Network (NCCN) all recommend concurrent palliative care as standard of care for all patients undergoing treatment for advanced cancer.[15–17]

SYMPTOMS IN ADVANCED PROSTATE CANCER
Epidemiology of Prostate Cancer Symptoms

Men with advanced prostate cancer experience physical and mental health morbidity and impaired quality of life as a result of both their illness and its treatment. Disease- and treatment-related symptoms include those in all domains of the bio-psycho-socio-spiritual model of comprehensive care.

Disease morbidity

In advanced metastatic prostate cancer that is castrate-resistant, pain is the predominant physical symptom. Prostate cancer most commonly metastasizes to bone (particularly the pelvis and spine), potentially causing debilitating pain and pathologic fractures. Bone metastases occur in 70% of men with advanced disease and 90% of men who die of prostate cancer. Approximately half of patients with bone metastases experience a skeletal complication. Patients with advanced disease are also at risk for lymphedema, urinary tract obstruction, and spinal cord compression. Among men with castrate-resistant disease, 10% develop cord compression.

Fatigue is among the most common and distressing complaints of men with advanced prostate cancer.[18–20] Prominent psychosocial symptoms include depression and anxiety.[21–24] Although data are limited, studies have found depression in up to half of men with prostate cancer, with anxiety shown to be even more prevalent.[25,26] Among men with prostate cancer, suicide has been associated with depression, recent diagnosis, pain, and being foreign-born.[27] Advanced prostate cancer creates numerous challenges to men's coping ability, including an altered view of self, lack of empowerment, altered view of the future, and disrupted partner intimacy. Very little is known with certainty about existential and spiritual distress among this population.[28]

Treatment morbidity

Ongoing evaluation, treatment decisions, and treatment itself for castrate-resistant prostate cancer also create burdensome symptoms. Many men who received prior treatment for localized disease already may have common symptoms associated with a particular treatment. Radical prostatectomy can lead to pain, erectile dysfunction (ED), and urinary incontinence. Nerve-sparing procedures lessen the risk of ED, but less so in older men. After bilateral nerve-sparing surgery by an experienced surgeon, approximately one-half of men will return to pretreatment erectile functioning. External-beam radiotherapy is associated with ED (approximately 50% of men), urinary incontinence, bowel dysfunction (including rectal urgency and mucus discharge), fatigue, and rectal pain. Brachytherapy is associated with ED (around 25% of men), urinary incontinence and burning, and pain. Depression, anxiety, and impaired QOL are common across treatments. Worsened QOL is clearly associated with sexual and urinary dysfunction and pain.

Androgen deprivation therapy can cause ED, loss of libido, hot flashes, depression, osteoporosis, fatigue, weight gain, and loss of mental acuity.[29] Bisphosphonates for skeletal lesions carry the risk of renal toxicity and osteonecrosis.

Chemotherapy side effects from taxane-based agents can include fatigue, anemia, pancytopenia, pneumonitis, and edema around spinal metastatic lesions that can create cord compression.

Quality of Life and Spiritual Distress

Ultimately, disease- and treatment-related symptoms and distress impact the quality of a patient's life.[30,31] Health-related quality of life (HRQOL) may be defined as the impact of illness and health care on a patient's function, daily activities, and emotional well-being. ASCO considers patient

QOL second only to survival in importance. QOL influences treatment satisfaction. Notably, QOL may be predictive of patient disease outcomes, including survival.[32] HRQOL declines during the final year of life for men with advanced prostate cancer.

HRQOL research has mostly focused on physical outcomes, and less so on psychological ones. Little research describes the spiritual distress that the diagnosis or treatment of prostate cancer causes in men and their family caregivers, but most clinicians recognize the potential for and frequency of profound existential issues engendered by the diagnosis of prostate cancer, the complications of its treatment, and the poor prognosis of castrate-resistant prostate cancer.

Limitations of the Evidence Base for and Barriers to Palliative Care

Consensus exists among professional organizations and clinical and academic leaders that patients with cancer face a significant symptom burden that should be a prime focus of management. Given all the morbidities across multiple domains involving both disease and treatment, most patients with advanced prostate cancer require symptom management services and benefit from palliative care.[18,33] Pain, depression, and quality of life must be assessed and interventions offered to treat, manage, or improve them throughout the course of illness and at the end of life.

The current system has major limitations to providing this care, and inadequately proven models proposed to remedy the situation.[34,35] These limitations include the lack of data about what types of care are best, the limited ability of cancer clinicians to implement symptom management care, and the lack of data about the feasibility and efficacy of care delivery models for improving symptom management. The evidence base for treatment of many physical, emotional, and existential prostate cancer morbidities is limited. The ability of prostate cancer clinicians to provide optimal symptom management is hampered by time constraints, lack of training in providing expert symptom management, and patient expectations and willingness to discuss symptom issues with their cancer physician. Even with the recognition that cancer symptom management is likely best performed in an oncologic/palliative care comanagement model, numerous elements of this model have yet to be evaluated rigorously, including feasibility, efficacy of interventions, staffing, health care use, and costs.

SYMPTOM MANAGEMENT AND PALLIATIVE CARE STRATEGIES IN CASTRATE-RESISTANT PROSTATE CANCER

Principles of symptom management are analogous to those for other treatment goals. First, symptom assessment requires identifying the bothersome symptoms with a good history and physical examination. Second, identifying the underlying cause of the symptom to treat it is a primary goal. Third, symptom-directed treatment is a priority even while correctable underlying causes are still being sought. Fourth, anticipating symptoms and preparing for them and their treatment is necessary. Fifth, symptoms that are continuous should be treated with round-the-clock medication dosing, rather than as-needed dosing. In general, it is easier to keep a patient's symptoms controlled than to get control of a symptom. Sixth, symptom treatments can create their own symptoms. The classic example is constipation from opioid analgesics used for pain. Seventh, many symptoms are best treated through a coordination of modalities, including pharmacologic and nonpharmacologic interventions. Eighth, preparation and education are key to help patients cope with the burden of symptoms. Information needs are paramount for most patients.

Principles and Tools of Palliative Care for Prostate Cancer

The first step in symptom management is to accurately identify the presence and severity of symptoms. In general, a 2-step approach to symptom identification and assessment is reasonable—brief, initial screening followed by more extensive, targeted evaluation. Brief screening questions to assess symptoms can be asked during routine oncologic visits.[36,37] Some practices include these screening questions as part of routine previsit or waiting-room surveys. Normalizing the possibility of symptoms can help alleviate patient embarrassment about pain, sexual dysfunction, or relationship distress. Simple screening questions for common symptoms in prostate cancer and treatment are given in **Table 1**.

Bothersome symptoms (as defined by patients themselves or by pre-determined survey thresholds) can be further assessed in detail. In general, symptoms can be assessed in terms of their severity, the level of bother they create, and the impact of the symptom on patient functioning. A simple 0 to 10 severity scale (such as the Edmonton Symptom Assessment Scale) or a "distress thermometer" are readily understood by most patients, useful for tracking patients'

Table 1
Symptom screening questions

Symptom	Screening Questions
Pain	Are you having any pain?
Fatigue	How is your energy level?
Urinary incontinence	Do you have trouble with leaking urine?
Bowel dysfunction	Do you have trouble with your bowels?
Erectile dysfunction	Many men have difficulty with getting or maintaining erections; how have things been for you?
Loss of libido	Are you satisfied with your sex life? How is your interest in sex?
Anxiety	Many men worry about various things when they get prostate cancer; are you feeling anxious or stressed?
Depression	How is your mood? Are you feeling sad or depressed? Have you lost interest in things that used to give you pleasure?
Relationship strain	How are things at home?
Spiritual distress	Are you at peace spiritually?
Poor quality of life	How is your quality of life overall?

Table 2
Validated symptom screening instruments

Symptom	Scale
Pain	0–10 scale Distress Thermometer Brief Pain Inventory
Fatigue	Functional Assessment of Chronic Illness Therapy–Fatigue
Urinary function	UCLA Prostate Cancer Index International Prostate Symptom Score
Erectile dysfunction	UCLA Prostate Cancer Index
Bowel function	UCLA Prostate Cancer Index
Anxiety	Hospital Anxiety and Depression Scale Distress thermometer Generalized Anxiety Disorder-7 (GAD-7)
Depression	Hospital Anxiety and Depression Scale Distress Thermometer Patient Health Questionnaire-9 (PHQ-9)
Spiritual distress	Spiritual Well-Being Scale Functional Assessment of Chronic Illness Therapy–Spirituality (FACIT-Sp-12)
Poor quality of life	UCLA Prostate Cancer Index European Organisation for Research and Treatment of Cancer Quality of Life Questionnaire Core 30 Medical Outcomes Study 36-Item Short-Form Health Survey (SF-36)

symptoms over time, and recommended by specialty organizations. Several validated symptom surveys have proven feasible in clinical settings. Examples of validated symptom assessment tools are given in **Table 2**.

Although screening for psychosocial distress for men with cancer is widely recommended (including by the Institute of Medicine[38] and NCCN[17]), treating clinicians often do not follow these recommendations, citing lack of time and limited referral resources more commonly than patients' unwillingness to discuss distress.[36]

Treatment of Physical Symptoms

This section provides specific treatment strategies for common physical symptoms experienced by men with castrate-resistant prostate cancer,[39] including pain, fatigue, hot flashes, osteoporosis and skeletal events, and nausea and vomiting. ED and incontinence are also considered, because they are common complications associated with

the treatment of localized prostate cancer that likely persist through the end of life for men with castration-resistant disease.

Pain

Pain is typically from bony metastases. Severe radicular pain with sensory/motor deficits or neurogenic bladder suggests cord compression and must be evaluated emergently for more definitive treatment. Several general pain management principles can direct the team's interventions:

1. A good history and physical examination is important to identify treatable causes of the pain and the type of pain present. In particular, nociceptive pain ("dull," "pounding," "aching" pain from tissue injury) must be distinguished

from neuropathic pain ("shooting," "stabbing," "burning," or "electrical" pain from nerve injury or dysfunction).

2. Patients' pain is a subjective experience that cannot be verified by clinicians. Patients ultimately must determine what level of pain management is acceptable to them.

3. Given the side effects of pain medications, patients typically must balance sedation and pain control. Improved function and control of pain adequate to participate in important life activities is the goal for most patients.

4. Typically, the experience of pain includes the physiologic experience (which may have gender and racial determinants) and the cultural, existential, and psychological implications of pain, pain tolerance, and pain treatment. This concept of physiologic distress plus emotional and existential suffering is known as "total pain."

5. It is easier to keep a patient out of pain than to get a patient out of pain. For round-the-clock pain, round-the-clock pain treatment is necessary, preferably with a long acting analgesic.

6. Pain management requires frequent assessment and reassessment, focusing on patients' evaluation of the severity of their pain, side effects, QOL, and function.

Many nonpharmacologic pain treatments are safe and can be recommended to almost all patients, including ice, heat, massage, physical therapy, transcutaneous electrical nerve stimulation, visualization, and acupuncture. Intensive nonpharmacologic treatments, such as radiation and surgery, are particularly important for bony metastases causing pain, cord compression, and imminent fractures requiring stabilization.

Pharmacologic pain treatments include 4 broad categories: nonopioid, opioid, neuropathic, and other analgesic medications. Chemotherapy that reduces tumor bulk may also be considered a symptomatic treatment.

Nonopioid medications such as nonsteroidal anti-inflammatory drugs (NSAIDs) and acetaminophen are often used for mild pain. Each has a significant side-effect profile that may limit their use. However, NSAIDs may be uniquely beneficial for bony pain. NSAIDs, including cyclooxygenase (COX)-2 inhibitors, carry the risk of gastrointestinal bleeding and renal and cardiac toxicity. Proton-pump inhibitors may help patients avoid gastric upset and bleeding. Acetaminophen carries the risk of hepatic toxicity with dosages greater than 3 g/d (2 g/d for the elderly). When NSAIDs or acetaminophen are combined with opioids (in formulations such as acetaminophen with codeine or

hydrocodone with acetaminophen), dosing will be limited by these nonopioid toxicities.

Opioid agonists are the mainstay of treatment for moderate to severe pain. There is no maximum dose of opioids. Opioid are available in short-acting and long-acting formulations. Short-acting medications (eg, immediate-release morphine sulfate, oxycodone, hydromorphone) typically are dosed every 4 hours. However, once a medication has reached its maximum concentration (usually after approximately 45–60 minutes for oral administration), short-acting medications can be re-dosed if a patient is still experiencing significant pain. Long-acting medications include methadone and controlled release formulations of morphine sulfate, oxycodone, and oxymorphone. Fentanyl is available intravenously, as a short-acting oral transmucosal or buccal formulation, or as a very long-acting transdermal formulation that is dosed every 3 days. Typically, a long-acting pain medication should be combined with a short-acting medication for "breakthrough" pain. Breakthrough dosing can be approximated as 10% of the total daily dose of morphine equivalent. When stable, the total 24-hour need for breakthrough pain medication can be calculated and used to adjust the long-acting medication dose. A useful listing of opioid medications, dosing, routes of administration, and widely promoted practice guidelines is available at http://www.nccn.org/.[40]

A key principle is the concept of equianalgesic dosing—the dosing of any one opioid may be translated into the dosing of another opioid using the equivalencies in **Table 3**. Because of incomplete cross-tolerance, starting with 50% to 75% of the calculated equianalgesic dose is prudent.

Special attention should be paid to methadone. Methadone has several distinct advantages. It is inexpensive, available in both pill and liquid formulations, has a long half-life, has limited risk for diversion, and, most importantly, binds both mu and N-methyl-D-aspartate receptors. As a consequence, methadone provides both nociceptive and neuropathic analgesia. Although it has a long half-life, for analgesic purposes it is typically dosed 3 to 4 times a day. Methadone's disadvantages are a potential risk of QT prolongation and its complexity in equianalgesic dosing. Because its opioid equivalency varies with the amount of opioid a patient has been exposed to previously, consultation with a palliative care or pain specialist is prudent before transitioning a patient between chronic opioids and methadone.

One of the most important clinical considerations in using opioids is to prevent and treat its major side effect: constipation. Nearly all patients with regular use of opioids require management

Table 3
Equianalgesic dosing of opioids

Opioid Analgesic	Equianalgesic Dose (mg)	
	Oral	Parenteral
Morphine	30 (short- or long-acting)	10
Hydromorphone	7.5	1.5
Oxycodone	20 (short- or long-acting)	—
Methadone	20 (acute), variable (chronic)	10 (acute), variable (chronic)
Hydrocodone (available only with acetaminophen as Vicodin, Lortab, or Norco)	30	—
Codeine (30 mg of codeine is combined with acetaminophen in Tyco #3)	180–200	130
Fentanyl	—	0.1
Fentanyl transdermal	a	—

[a] For transdermal fentanyl, the dose in micrograms per hour is approximately equivalent to one-half to one-quarter of the total daily morphine dose in milligrams.

of constipation. A reasonable regimen is a stimulant laxative (such as senna [8.6–51.6 mg twice daily] or bisacodyl [5–30 mg daily]) titrated to having an easy bowel movement approximately every day. The stool softener docusate sodium has traditionally been used along with stimulant laxatives but likely adds little clinical efficacy.[41] If necessary, polyethylene glycol 3350, lactulose, or milk of magnesia can be added as needed. Subcutaneous methylnaltrexone can be used for severe opioid constipation unrelieved by oral agents. Additionally, all patients should be encouraged to drink plenty of fluids, eat fruits and vegetables, and be physically active to allow optimum bowel function. Significant fiber supplementation may increase gastrointestinal discomfort in opioid-induced constipation.

Although constipation is the most common side effect of opioids, numerous others are possible, including sedation, pruritis, nausea/vomiting, and respiratory depression. Although respiratory depression is often feared by patients and clinicians alike, it is preceded by significant sedation, alerting patients and caregivers to its possibility. Pain can almost always be relieved at opioid doses much lower than those that might affect respiratory function. For all of these opioid side effects, time, reducing the dose, or changing the opioid to an alternate one (opioid "rotation") are generally sufficient to ameliorate the symptom. Although physical dependence (ie, withdrawal symptoms with sudden discontinuation of the opioid) and tolerance (ie, requiring increased dosages of medication to achieve the same effect) are expected because of the pharmacology of opioids, addiction (ie, misuse

of the medication for purposes other than analgesia and despite evidence of harm) is rare. Patients who display anger and demanding behavior when their usual medication is refused or delayed are likely to be displaying "pseudo-addiction" (ie, irritability that indicates physiologic withdrawal) rather than addiction.

Neuropathic analgesics are a class of medications with a particular ability to treat neuropathic pain. As coanalgesics, they may help minimize the dose of opioid medications, and research shows that the combination of neuropathic and opioid analgesics is more effective than a single agent and at lower doses. The most widely used neuropathic medications are shown in **Table 4**.

Other analgesic medications include steroids, radioisotopes, regional analgesia, and bisphosphonates. Glucocorticoids (prednisone, 20–40 mg/d or dexamethasone, 2–4 mg once to 4 times daily) are helpful for pain caused by swelling, including cerebral edema, and pain with an inflammatory component, such as metastatic bony pain. The analgesia from glucocorticoids is generally short-lived, making them appropriate particularly as a bridge to more definitive treatments and at the end of life. Caution should be used when considering glucocorticoids for patients already on NSAIDs because of gastrointestinal toxicity. Strontium 89 can be infused intravenously to treat pain from disseminated tumors. Anesthesia-based pain consultants can be helpful at providing regional analgesia for back pain with epidural injections or pump-administered infusions of opioids, muscle-relaxants, and anesthetics. Bisphosphonates, in particular potent intravenous formulations such as

Table 4
Neuropathic analgesics

Class	Medications	Typical Dose Range
Opioids	See **Table 3**, especially methadone	0.3 mg/kg morphine orally q3–4 h, no maximum dose in chronic use
Antidepressants	Amitriptyline	10–150 mg qhs
	Nortriptyline	10–150 mg qhs
	Desipramine	10–200 mg qhs
	Duloxetine	60 mg qd
Anticonvulsants	Gabapentin	300–1200 mg tid
	Pregabalin	50–100 mg tid
Others	Lidocaine transdermal	One to three 5% patches applied daily for 12 h
	Tramadol hydrochloride	50–100 mg bid–qid

zoledronic acid, can improve pain, decrease osteoporosis, and decrease the risk of painful skeletal-related events such as fracture.

Fatigue

A careful history and limited laboratory testing are key to identifying potentially treatable underlying causes of fatigue,[42] such as anemia, depression, pain, delirium (including from medications, dehydration, renal or hepatic failure, brain metastases, or hypoxia), medication toxicity (including opioid sedation, opioid neurotoxicity, benzodiazepines, tricyclic antidepressants, selective serotonin-reuptake inhibitors [SSRIs], and muscle relaxants), malnutrition, and deconditioning. Dose reduction or dose rotation of opioids, stimulants such as caffeine or methylphenidate, and multispecialty treatment of pain may help reduce the fatigue associated with opioid sedation or neurotoxicity. Some evidence shows that treatment of depression may improve fatigue disproportionate to improvement in mood. Appetite stimulants may help with appetite, although their benefit in improving energy does not seem related to changes in nutritional parameters.

Treating an underlying cause of fatigue can be curative, although most cases are not so simply dealt with. Among men with castrate-resistant prostate cancer, fatigue may be experienced as a side effect of androgen deprivation therapy, chemotherapy, medication side effects, a complication of radiotherapy or surgery, or a symptom of the anorexia-cachexia syndrome of metastatic cancer. Nonpharmacologic approaches to its management include energy conservation (saving energy for prioritized activities during the day), exercise, and adequate nutrition. Consultation with a physical and occupational therapist may be helpful, as might mobility assistive devises (including canes and wheelchairs).

Pharmacologic intervention may be desired by some men. Caffeine may be tried. Additionally, low-dose psychostimulants may be effective,[43] including methylphenidate, dextroamphetamine, and modafinil. Methylphenidate can be used as needed by patients, although most use it twice a day with the second dose before 3 PM to avoid interruption of sleep. Although methylphenidate is widely used and supported by evidence, some studies do not support its use. However, no evidence shows that methylphenidate has any negative impact on the progression of prostate cancer, and therefore an empiric trial may be warranted. A listing of symptomatic treatment options for fatigue is provided in **Table 5**.

Hot flashes

Patients with castrate-resistant prostate cancer often continue to receive gonadotropin-releasing hormone agonist therapy and second-line antiandrogen agents. Androgen deprivation therapy can create hot flashes that many find distressing. Nonpharmacologic management includes use of a fan, light clothing, and relaxation techniques. Proven pharmacologic treatments include the antidepressants venlafaxine,[44] escitalopram, and

Table 5
Symptomatic treatments for fatigue

Medication	Starting Dose
Methylphenidate	2.5 mg bid
Dextroamphetamine	2.5 mg bid
Modafinil	200 mg/d
Corticosteroids	Dexamethasone, 8 mg/d
Megestrol acetate	480–800 mg/d

sertraline, and hormonal therapy with megestrol (20 mg twice daily), cyproterone, diethylstilbestrol, and estradiol patches. Hormonal treatments carry the potential risk of stimulating prostate cancer growth and megestrol has been associated with rising prostate-specific antigen. Recent placebo-controlled evidence shows that gabapentin at 900 mg/d is helpful. Most men with hot flashes do not prefer to use medication to treat them. Although many foods and supplements have been tried for menopausal hot flashes in women (including soy and black cohash), rigorous study does not support their use. Limited evidence shows that acupuncture may be an effective treatment.

Osteoporosis and skeletal events
Weight-bearing exercise, quitting cigarette smoking, vitamin D, calcium, pamidronate, and bisphosphonates are useful in the context of androgen deprivation therapy. Weekly oral bisphosphonates are effective at preventing bone loss. Potent intravenous bisphosphonates can increase bone density and are effective at decreasing skeletal events.[4] The use of zoledronic acid must be weighed against the possible side effects of osteonecrosis of the jaw and renal insufficiency. Estrogens, which also treat hot flashes, may also help with osteoporosis. The development of markers of bone metabolism to help identify patients for whom potent bisphosphonates are most useful is eagerly awaited.

Nausea and vomiting
Nausea and vomiting can stem from advanced prostate cancer or its treatments. The 5-HT3 antagonist ondansetron is the most widely used antiemetic agent and one of the most effective, especially for chemotherapy-induced nausea and vomiting. Ondansetron can be given orally (including an orally disintegrating formulation) or intravenously. The recommended dose is 24 mg given as 8 mg three times daily as needed. Common side effects include headache, constipation, and QTc prolongation. Other potent antiemetic agents used for treatment and prevention of chemotherapy-induced nausea and vomiting include palonosetron, granisetron, aprepitant, and fosaprepitant. Additionally, prochlorperazine (which may be as effective an antiemetic as ondansetron), metoclopramide, haloperidol, dexamethasone, cannabinoids, and nonpharmacologic therapy such as acupuncture[45] can add to the armamentarium of treatment for nausea and vomiting. Benzodiazepines such as lorazepam are particularly effective for anticipatory nausea with chemotherapy.

ED
ED in men with advanced prostate cancer is common. For most patients, the cause is multifactorial. Treatment of early-stage prostate cancer with prostatectomy or radiotherapy leads to ED in a significant number of patients. Androgen deprivation therapy alters levels of testosterone, creating a risk for ED. Chemotherapy with its accompanied toxicities further adds to the prevalence and severity of this condition. Men with advanced prostate cancer often experience anxiety, depression, and loss of self-esteem that can further contribute to ED and affect overall satisfaction with sexual activity.

Treatment of ED requires a multimodality approach that addresses both psychological and physical causes, many of which are addressed later.[46] Specific treatment for ED include phosphodiesterase-5 (PDE-5) inhibitors, penile injections, transurethral prostaglandins, vacuum constriction devices, and counseling. Treatment must be individualized depending on patient preferences, patient motivation, and other medical comorbidities.

Urinary dysfunction
Urinary incontinence is a common complication after treatment of localized prostate cancer, and continues for men with advanced cancer. Prostatectomy is most commonly associated with stress incontinence; radiotherapy with urge incontinence. The number of incontinence pads used per day is a simple assessment of the severity of incontinence. As most men have improvement over time, simple education about the natural history of incontinence after treatment may help relieve anxiety and distress about the symptom. In addition, the concept of incontinence may have significant negative meaning for many, forcing men to recognize the seriousness of their disease, the inevitability of their aging, or their overall lack of control in the face of cancer. Many may find this symptom particularly embarrassing in their personal, social, and work lives. Education, normalization, and support may be useful, and can be provided by the physician and nurse and/or in individual counseling or peer support groups.

To accelerate improved urinary function, pelvic floor (Kegel) exercises are recommended. Stopping urine midstream is a simple instruction to offer, but referral for biofeedback or to a pelvic physical therapist for training also may be helpful. Other strategies recommended for incontinence include timed voiding, drinking less, avoiding excess fluids at night, and avoiding caffeine. Transrectal neuromuscular electrical stimulation is effective but requires active patient participation. Urethral collagen injection is a temporary approach to incontinence that may be helpful for a few months. An artificial urethral sphincter is effective in most men. Surgical creation of a bulbourethral sling can be used for more definitive treatment.

For urinary irritation, as is common after radiotherapy, α-blockers are typically used to improve urine flow. Bladder antispasmodic medication such as oxybutynin is helpful for urge incontinence.

Treatment of Emotional Symptoms

Emotional distress is common and can be effectively treated. In the setting of the severe stress associated with receiving the news of treatment failure or metastatic or castrate-resistant disease, men may be overwhelmed by feelings of sadness, anger, worry, and fear. In this setting, "adjustment reaction" (which can have either depressive or anxiety symptoms or both) may be the appropriate diagnosis, rather than "major depression" or "anxiety." Men are often relieved to hear that their emotions and adjustment reaction are a "normal reaction to abnormal stress," rather than hearing that they have depression, which might be considered an "abnormal reaction to normal life stresses." Premorbid mental illness increases the risk of mood disorders in men with prostate cancer. Reassuring men and their loved ones of the commonality of emotional distress, normalizing treatment for it, and reassuring men that they are not going "crazy" and are likely to improve can all be helpful. Reassurance, relaxation techniques, psychotherapy, psychoeducation, cognitive behavioral therapy, anxiolytics (eg, benzodiazepines), antidepressants, and patient support and education programs are effective.[47]

Depression

Depression and adjustment disorder with depressed mood are common in prostate cancer. Depression may be a sequela of some of the complications of early cancer treatment (such as ED), a side effect of androgen deprivation therapy, or a reaction to the poor prognosis of castrate-resistant disease. However, depression in the setting of end-stage prostate cancer is not inevitable; when present, it should be treated. Pain increases the risk of depression. Because men with widely metastatic disease may have many of the "vegetative" signs of depression (eg, anorexia, low energy), diagnosing depression in this setting must focus on the psychological signs (including hopelessness and self-reproach). Clinicians treating depressed patients should remain alert to the increased risk of suicide associated with increased age, social isolation, substance abuse, poor physical functioning, life-threatening illness, pain, and history of prior attempts.

Treatment of depression in men with prostate cancer is similar to that in other settings. Antidepressant medications, psychotherapy, and support groups are the mainstays of therapy. Although most men do not want to take antidepressant medication, most will do so if advised by their physician. First-line antidepressant medications are the SSRIs. Escitalopram and citalopram have the lowest incidence of sexual side effects. Mirtazapine may have the added benefit of antiemetic properties for men who also experience nausea and vomiting. Venlafaxine may be ideal for men with depression and hot flashes. Duloxetine may be ideal for those with depression and neuropathic pain. Methylphenidate may be appropriate as initial treatment, especially for men with short life expectancies, because its onset of effect is a matter of days. For others it is often started concurrently with an SSRI and used as symptomatic relief during the 3 to 4 weeks before the onset of therapeutic effect of the SSRI. Emerging evidence indicates that the anesthetic ketamine also may be helpful for depression at the end of life.[48]

Anxiety

In the setting of a worrisome diagnosis, fear of progression, and great uncertainty, anxiety is common. Anxiety may accompany treatment with steroids. Although benzodiazepines may be particularly useful to quell the intensity of acute or intermittent anxiety and panic, treating chronic anxiety should be accomplished with cognitive-behavioral therapy and/or medication. SSRI antidepressants are first-line agents for anxiety.

Sexuality and identity distress

Palliative care includes helping men cope with challenges to their self-concept around sexuality, role, and identity. With loss of libido, ED, fatigue, gynecomastia, and muscle weakness, men may feel they are "not the man they used to be." They may speak of loss of "vitality" or "life force." Self-concept and confidence for some men may be tightly linked to erectile function. To be attentive to these issues, oncologic clinicians can try some simple normalization and empathic responses and then coordinate with psychologists, nurses, and clinical social workers to help patients redefine themselves and find sources of strength and self-efficacy. Cognitive-behavioral therapy may be useful, as may support groups. In peer support groups, men may find acceptance and role modeling for defining values beyond erectile function. Simple education and couples therapy may help men understand that they and their partners can enjoy satisfying sexual activity and intimacy without penetration.

Addressing Interpersonal, Social, and Spiritual Distress

Relationships with loved ones are impacted deeply by illness. In addition to losses in physical functioning, a change in role or relationship can be distressing. Men may be uncomfortable with the need to quit work or rely on others for personal care needs, financial support, transportation, or emotional support. Financial instability, job insecurity, and difficulty with insurability create stress and the possible need for consultation with social workers, financial counselors, and lawyers. Facing uncertainty, loss of control, challenge to self-image and identity, debility, and fear of dying associated with prostate cancer commonly raise deep existential questions for men. Generally, though, *answers* to interpersonal, social, and spiritual questions may not be necessary or appropriate. Openness and *responsiveness* (bearing witness) to these issues and referrals to the palliative care team may be sufficient involvement for oncologists or surgeons seeking to provide comprehensive care.

END-OF-LIFE CARE FOR PATIENTS AND FAMILY CAREGIVERS

Most patients with castrate-resistant prostate cancer will die of their disease. Therefore, it is imperative that patients have an accurate understanding of their prognosis, engage in communication about end-of-life care with their providers and family, and participate in advance care planning.[49–51] It is well documented that physicians consistently overestimate the duration of patient survival.[52] Although physicians' ability to predict life expectancy is often inaccurate, it is clinically useful to consider the possibilities. Communication of prognosis by treating physicians is critical in preparing patients to make informed decisions about disease-specific treatment and preparing for the end of life. Strong evidence suggests that patients and families prefer honest, detailed prognostic information. Excellent communication is necessary to support patients in making the best decisions about when to discontinue ineffective treatments and focus on comfort care exclusively.[53]

Advance care planning allows patients to consider, determine, and communicate the type of care they want at the end of life and to appoint a surrogate decision-maker to act on their behalf if they lose decision-making capacity. Advance care planning documents are most useful if they indicate a patient's values and goals beyond simple care preferences for specific clinical scenarios. However, advance care planning has not fully realized its goal of improving patients' end-of-life care, because treating physicians and patients often do not discuss advance care preferences, or physicians may ignore them. In one study, hospitalized patients with cancer often had advanced care preferences that they shared with family or documented but not with the treating oncologists.[54] A recent systemic review reported good evidence that multicomponent interventions increase advance care planning.[55] Engaging values, involving skilled facilitators, and including patients, caregivers, and providers could increase practice and effectiveness of communication about end-of-life goals and advance care planning.

A palliative care team approach often is needed to manage the complex needs of dying patients and their family members. Hospice care (ie, palliative care only for patients at the end of life) improves quality of care through providing effective palliation of symptoms; psychological, social, and spiritual support to patients and family; and bereavement counseling for family and friends.[56] Hospice care helps patients remain comfortable, allows them to die at home (where most wish to die), increases patient and family satisfaction, may help prolong life, and is cost-effective.[57–59] Family members of patients with home hospice services reported higher satisfaction, fewer concerns with care, and fewer unmet needs. Notably, care in hospice ameliorates the increased risk of mortality for bereaved family caregivers.[60] Simple recognition of the burdens on family caregivers and helping them to orchestrate appropriate assistance at home, such as home nursing care, home health aides, and hospice, are among the most important physician interventions for supporting family caregivers.[61]

SUMMARY

Palliative care (including symptom management) for men with castrate-resistant prostate cancer is key to address disease and treatment morbidity, and should be offered to men concurrently with disease-directed treatment. Men commonly experience distress across the physical, emotional, existential, and social realms. Increasingly, with advances in treatment efficacy, men can live with symptoms for long periods. Interdisciplinary palliative care teams focused on symptom management and giving careful attention to patients' goals of care can collaborate with prostate cancer surgeons, oncologists, and radiation oncologists to provide the best care for men at all stages of cancer treatment. Basic interventions include scrupulous communication, education, emotional support, and the simple but powerful act of bearing witness. Palliative care teams, working in concert with cancer clinicians, can provide necessary assistance with management of complex pain, fatigue, depression, anxiety, caregiver distress, and existential crisis. At the end of life, palliative care may become the patient's sole goal of care.

REFERENCES

1. Jemal A, Siegel R, Ward E, et al. Cancer statistics, 2009. CA Cancer J Clin 2009;59:225–49.

2. Higano C, Saad F, Somer B, et al. A phase III trial of GVAX immunotherapy for prostate cancer versus docetaxel plus prednisone in asymptomatic, castration-resistant prostate cancer (CRPC). Presented at the 2009 Genitourinary Cancers Symposium; February 26–28, 2009; Orlando, Florida.

3. Small E, Demkow T, Gerritsen WR, et al. A phase III trial of GVAX immunotherapy for prostate cancer in combination with docetaxel versus docetaxel plus prednisone in symptomatic, castration-resistant prostate cancer (CRPC). Presented at the 2009 Genitourinary Cancers Symposium; February 26–28, 2009; Orlando, Florida.

4. Saad F, Gleason DM, Murray R, et al. A randomized, placebo-controlled trial of zoledronic acid in patients with hormone-refractory metastatic prostate carcinoma. J Natl Cancer Inst 2002;94:1458–68.

5. Carducci MA, Saad F, Abrahamsson PA, et al. A phase 3 randomized controlled trial of the efficacy and safety of atrasentan in men with metastatic hormone-refractory prostate cancer. Cancer 2007; 110:1959–66.

6. Sternberg CN, Petrylak DP, Sartor O, et al. Multinational, double-blind, phase III study of prednisone and either satraplatin or placebo in patients with castrate-refractory prostate cancer progressing after prior chemotherapy: the SPARC trial. J Clin Oncol 2009;27:5431–8.

7. Petrylak DP, Tangen CM, Hussain MH, et al. Docetaxel and estramustine compared with mitoxantrone and prednisone for advanced refractory prostate cancer. N Engl J Med 2004;351:1513–20.

8. Tannock IF, de Wit R, Berry WR, et al. Docetaxel plus prednisone or mitoxantrone plus prednisone for advanced prostate cancer. N Engl J Med 2004; 351:1502–12.

9. WHO definitions of palliative care. World Health Organization Web site. Available at: http://www.who.int/cancer/palliative/definition/en. Accessed August 14, 2012.

10. Bakitas M, Lyons KD, Hegel MT, et al. Effects of a palliative care intervention on clinical outcomes in patients with advanced cancer: the Project ENABLE II randomized controlled trial. JAMA 2009; 302:741–9.

11. Elsayem A, Swint K, Fisch MJ, et al. Palliative care inpatient service in a comprehensive cancer center: clinical and financial outcomes. J Clin Oncol 2004; 22(10):2008–14.

12. Homsi J, Walsh D, Nelson KA, et al. The impact of a palliative medicine consultation service in medical oncology. Support Care Cancer 2002; 10(4):337–42.

13. Elsayem A, Smith ML, Parmley L, et al. Impact of a palliative care service on in-hospital mortality in a comprehensive cancer center. J Palliat Med 2006;9(4):894–902.

14. Temel JS, Greer JA, Muzikansky A, et al. Early palliative care for patients with metastatic non-small-cell lung cancer. N Engl J Med 2010;363:733–42.

15. Smith TJ, Temin S, Alesi ER, et al. American Society of Clinical Oncology provisional clinical opinion: the integration of palliative care into standard oncology care. J Clin Oncol 2012;30(8):880–7.

16. National Cancer Policy Board and Institute of Medicine. In: Foley KM, Gelband H, editors. Improving palliative care for cancer. Washington, DC: National Academy Press; 2001.

17. Levy MH, Back A, Benedetti C, et al. NCCN clinical practice guidelines in oncology: palliative care. J Natl Compr Canc Netw 2009;7(4):436–73.

18. Yennurajalingam S, Atkinson B, Masterson J, et al. The impact of an outpatient palliative care consultation on symptom burden in advanced prostate cancer patients. J Palliat Med 2012; 15(1):20–4.

19. Stone PC, Minton O. Cancer-related fatigue. Eur J Cancer 2008;44(8):1097–104.

20. Portnoy RK, Itrl L. Cancer-related fatigue. Oncologist 1999;4:1–10.

21. Balderson N, Towell T. The prevalence and predictors of psychological distress in men with prostate cancer who are seeking support. Br J Health Psychol 2003;8(Pt 2):125–34.

22. Cliff AM, MacDonagh RP. Psychosocial morbidity in prostate cancer: II. A comparison of patients and partners. BJU Int 2000;86(7):834–9.

23. Hervouet S, Savard J, Simard S, et al. Psychological functioning associated with prostate cancer: cross-sectional comparison of patients treated with radiotherapy, brachytherapy, or surgery. J Pain Symptom Manage 2005;30(5):474–84.

24. Lintz K, Moynihan C, Steginga S, et al. Prostate cancer patients' support and psychological care needs: survey from a non-surgical oncology clinic. Psychooncology 2003;12(8):769–83.

25. Weber BA, Sherwill-Navarro P. Psychosocial consequences of prostate cancer: 30 years of research. Geriatr Nurs 2005;26(3):166–75.

26. Bennett G, Badger TA. Depression in men with prostate cancer. Oncol Nurs Forum 2005;32:545–56.

27. Llorente MD, Burke M, Gregory GR, et al. Prostate cancer: a significant risk factor for late-life suicide. Am J Geriatr Psychiatry 2005;13:195–201.

28. Krupski TL, Kwan L, Fink A, et al. Spirituality influences health related quality of life in men with prostate cancer. Psychooncology 2006;15(2):121–31.

29. Chen AC, Petrylak DP. Complications of androgen-deprivation therapy in men with prostate cancer. Curr Urol Rep 2005;6(3):210–6.

30. Litwin MS, Lubeck DP, Stoddard ML, et al. Quality of life before death for men with prostate cancer: results from the CaPSURE database. J Urol 2001; 165(3):871–5.

31. Penson DF, Feng Z, Kuniyuki A, et al. General quality of life 2 years following treatment for prostate cancer: what influences outcomes? Results from the prostate cancer outcomes study. J Clin Oncol 2003;21(6):1147–54.

32. Collette L, van Andel G, Bottomley A, et al. Is baseline quality of life useful for predicting survival with hormone-refractory prostate cancer? A pooled analysis of three studies of the European Organisation for Research and Treatment of Cancer Genitourinary Group. J Clin Oncol 2004;22(19):3877–85.

33. Steginga SK, Occhipinti S, Dunn J, et al. The supportive care needs of men with prostate cancer. Psychooncology 2001;10(1):66–75.

34. Fisch MJ, Lee JW, Weiss M, et al. Prospective, observational study of pain and analgesic prescribing in medical oncology outpatients with breast, colorectal, lung, or prostate cancer. J Clin Oncol 2012;30(16):1980–8.

35. Green JS. An investigation into the use of palliative care services by patients with prostate cancer. Am J Hosp Palliat Care 2002;19(4):259–62.

36. Pirl WF, Muriel A, Hwang V. Screening for psychosocial distress: a national survey of oncologists. J Support Oncol 2007;5(10):499–504.

37. Roth AJ, Kornblith AB, Batel-Copel L, et al. Rapid screening for psychologic distress in men with prostate carcinoma: a pilot study. Cancer 1998;82(10): 1904–8.

38. Institute of Medicine. Cancer care for the whole patient: meeting psychosocial health needs. Washington, DC: The National Academies Press; 2007.

39. Ok J, Meyers FJ, Evans CP. Medical and surgical palliative care of patients with urological malignancies. J Urol 2005;174:1177–82.

40. Swarm R, Abernethy AP, Anghelescu DL, et al. NCCN Adult Cancer Pain. J Natl Compr Canc Netw 2010;8(9):1046–86.

41. Hawley PH, Byeon JJ. A comparison of sennosides-based bowel protocols with and without docusate in hospitalized patients with cancer. J Palliat Med 2008;11(4):575–81.

42. Maliski SL, Kwan L, Orecklin JR, et al. Predictors of fatigue after treatment for prostate cancer. Urology 2005;65(1):101–8.

43. Kerr CW, Drake J, Milch RA, et al. Effects of methylphenidate on fatigue and depression: a randomized, double-blind, placebo-controlled trial. J Pain Symptom Manage 2012;43(1):68–77.

44. Quella SK, Loprinzi CL, Sloan J. Pilot evaluation of venlafaxine for the treatment of hot flashes in men undergoing androgen ablation therapy for prostate cancer. J Urol 1999;162(1):98–102.

45. Ezzo J, Vickers A, Richardson MA, et al. Acupuncture-point stimulation for chemotherapy-induced nausea and vomiting. J Clin Oncol 2005;23(28):7188.

46. Schover LR, Fouladi RT, Warneke CL, et al. The use of treatments for erectile dysfunction among survivors of prostate carcinoma. Cancer 2002;95(11): 2397–407.

47. Giesler RB, Given B, Given CW, et al. Improving the quality of life of patients with prostate carcinoma: a randomized trial testing the efficacy of a nurse-driven intervention. Cancer 2005;104(4):752–62.

48. Connolly KR, Thase ME. Emerging drugs for major depressive disorder. Expert Opin Emerg Drugs 2012;17(1):105–26.

49. Reynolds PM, Sanson-Fisher RW, Poole AD, et al. Cancer and communication: information-giving in an oncology clinic. BMJ 1981;282:1449–51.

50. Derdiarian AK. Informational needs of recently diagnosed cancer patients. Nurs Res 1986;35:276–81.

51. Hagerty RG, Butow PN, Ellis PA, et al. Cancer patient preferences for communication of prognosis in the metastatic setting. J Clin Oncol 2004;22(9): 1721–30.

52. Glare P, Virik K, Jones M, et al. A systematic review of physicians' survival predictions in terminally ill cancer patients. BMJ 2003;327:195.

53. Earle CC, Neville BA, Landrum MB, et al. Trends in the aggressiveness of cancer care near the end of life. J Clin Oncol 2004;22(2):315–21.

54. Lamont EB, Siegler M. Paradoxes in cancer patients' advance care planning. J Palliat Med 2000;3(1):27–35.

55. Lorenz KA, Lynn J, Dy SM, et al. Evidence for improving palliative are at the end of life: a systematic review. Ann Intern Med 2008;148(2):147–59.

56. Valdimarsdóttir U, Helgason AR, Fürst CJ, et al. Need for and access to bereavement support after loss of a husband to urologic cancers: a nationwide follow-up of Swedish widows. Scand J Urol Nephrol 2005;39(4):271–6.

57. Connor SR, Pyenson B, Fitch K, et al. Comparing hospice and nonhospice patient survival among patients who die within a three-year window. J Pain Symptom Manage 2007;33(3):238–46.

58. Wallston KA, Burger C, Smith RA, et al. Comparing the quality of death for hospice and non-hospice cancer patients. Med Care 1988;26(2):177–82.

59. Mor V, Kidder D. Cost savings in hospice: final results of the National Hospice Study. Health Serv Res 1985;20(4):407–22.

60. Christakis NA, Iwashyna TJ. The health impact of health care on families: a matched cohort study of hospice use by decedents and mortality outcomes in surviving, widowed spouses. Soc Sci Med 2003; 57(3):465–75.

61. Rabow MW, Hauser JM, Adams J. Supporting family caregivers at the end of life: "they don't know what they don't know". JAMA 2004;291(4): 483–91.

Quality of Life with Advanced Metastatic Prostate Cancer

Matthew J. Resnick, MD[a,b,*], David F. Penson, MD, MPH[a,b]

KEYWORDS

- Prostate cancer • Metastatic • Castrate-resistant • Quality of life • Functional status • Palliation

KEY POINTS

- Health-related quality of life (HRQOL) is a patient reported outcome measure that represents the patient's overall perception of his disease and its treatment, and captures evaluations of the patient's physical, psychological, and social functioning.
- Prostate cancer disease burden is associated with more significant declines in HRQOL.
- Androgen deprivation therapy results in HRQOL declines in various domains.
- Chemotherapy for metastatic castrate-resistant prostate cancer often results in improvements in pain and functional status.
- While skeletal-related events result do appear to negatively impact HRQOL, the effect of osteoclast-targeted therapy on HRQOL remains largely unknown.
- Emerging therapies may result in significant HRQOL improvements in this population at risk for poor patient-reported outcomes.

INTRODUCTION

Prostate cancer remains the most commonly diagnosed noncutaneous malignancy in the United States, with an estimated 241,700 new cases in 2012, resulting in an estimated 28,840 deaths in the same year.[1] Localized prostate cancer is frequently characterized by a lengthy natural history and relatively indolent clinical course. This is in stark contrast to advanced disease, which commonly results in a considerable symptom burden to patients. Indeed, both disease burden and treatment may result in significant changes in patients' health-related quality of life (HRQOL), a patient-reported outcome measure (PRO) that represents the patient's overall perception of his disease and its treatment and captures evaluations of the patient's physical, psychological, and social functioning.[2] This article will discuss commonly used instruments in the evaluation of

HRQOL among cancer patients, the HRQOL implications of advanced metastatic prostate cancer, and incremental changes in HRQOL associated with treatment.

HRQOL INSTRUMENTS

HRQOL is assessed using surveys, known as instruments, that query the patient regarding different areas, or domains, of his quality of life. Questions on the instruments are often referred to as items and are often grouped into scales, which generate summary scores for a particular domain. Individual instruments measure either general or disease-specific HRQOL. General HRQOL domains tend to be applicable to all patients, regardless of their underlying illnesses. General HRQOL focuses on general health perceptions, sense of overall well being, and function in the physical, emotional, and social domains.

[a] Department of Urologic Surgery, Center for Surgical Quality and Outcomes Research, Vanderbilt University, Nashville, TN, USA; [b] VA Tennessee Valley Geriatric Research Education and Clinical Center (GRECC), 1310 24th Avenue South, Nashville, TN 37212-2637, USA
* Corresponding author. Department of Urologic Surgery, Vanderbilt University, A-1302 Medical Center North, Nashville, TN 37232.
E-mail address: matthew.resnick@vanderbilt.edu

Urol Clin N Am 39 (2012) 505–515
http://dx.doi.org/10.1016/j.ucl.2012.07.007
0094-0143/12/$ – see front matter © 2012 Elsevier Inc. All rights reserved.

On the contrary, disease-specific HRQOL instruments such as the University of California Los Angeles (UCLA) Prostate Cancer Index (UCLA-PCI) evaluate domains germane to a particular disease. Examples would include measurement of erectile function and urinary control in prostate cancer patients.[3,4]

There are a number of general and disease-specific instruments commonly used in the evaluation of HRQOL in men with advanced prostate cancer. Perhaps the most commonly used general HRQOL instrument is the RAND 36-Item Short Form Health Survey (SF-36), which assesses 8 health concepts: physical functioning, bodily pain, role limitations due to physical health problems, role limitations due to personal or emotional problems, general mental health, social functioning, energy/fatigue, and general health perceptions.[5,6] The SF-36 may be scored as 2 separate physical (PCS) and mental (MCS) composite scores to allow the physician or investigator to identify differences between physical and mental dysfunction.[6] More recently the SF-12, an abbreviated version of the SF-36, has been introduced, which can be self-administered in 2 minutes or less. The SF-12 has been found to reproduce the vast majority of the variance found in the SF-36 PCS and MCS measures, and it is a useful alternative in studies in which the SF-36 is too cumbersome.[7] Other commonly used general HRQOL instruments include the Quality of Well-Being scale (QWB),[8-10] the Sickness Impact Profile (SIP),[1,11-13] and Nottingham Health Profile (NHP).[14]

In addition to the commonly used general HRQOL instruments, there are various cancer-specific instruments that measure changes in HRQOL related to malignancy. One such tool is the European Organization for the Research and Treatment of Cancer Quality of Life Questionnaire (EORTC QLQ-C30). The EORTC QLQ-C30 is a 30-item scale that incorporates 5 functional scales (physical, role, cognitive, emotional, social), 3 symptom scales (pain, fatigue, nausea/vomiting), and a global health and quality-of-life scale. Additionally, there are a number of single-item questions related to common symptoms among cancer patients.[15] While the EORTC instrument was initially tested in patients with unresectable lung cancer, it has undergone validation in patients with various tumor types, including prostate.[16] There is a prostate cancer module, the EORTC QLQ–PR25, that specifically addresses urinary, sexual, and bowel symptoms and function as well as adverse effects of androgen deprivation therapy (ADT). The PR25 instrument has been evaluated in prostate cancer populations with both localized and metastatic disease.[17]

The Functional Assessment of Cancer Therapy (FACT) is another commonly used cancer-specific HRQOL instrument. The FACT is a 2-part instrument that evaluates general HRQOL measures related to cancer and cancer therapy (FACT-G) and tumor-specific measures related to the disease of interest. The 28-item FACT-G includes a total score and subscale scores for physical, functional, social, and emotional well being, as well as satisfaction with the treatment relationship.[18] There is a specific module for prostate cancer (FACT-P) that includes items related to sexual function, urinary function, and bowel function.[19] Additionally, the Cancer Rehabilitation Evaluation System Short Form (CARES-SF) is an instrument dedicated to the evaluation of general HRQOL in cancer patients. The CARES-SF contains 59 items and has 5 multi-item subscales including physical, psychosocial, medical interaction, marital interaction, and sexual function.[20,21]

One unique instrument that is often used in assessments of HRQOL in cancer patients is the EQ5D/EuroQol instrument. The EQ5D/EuroQol instrument combines self-assessment with valuation of a standard set of health states. The EQ5D/EuroQol instrument is unique in that it evaluates patients' specific utilities, and has the potential to provide some insight into the value assigned to specific domains among patients with specific disease states. The EQ5D/EuroQol instrument measures well being in 5 dimensions: mobility, self-care, usual activities, pain/discomfort, and anxiety/depression, and responses are weighted to generate a summary index.[22,23]

Evaluation of HRQOL in patients with advanced metastatic prostate cancer is generally performed using 1 of the instruments developed for the measurement of general HRQOL in cancer patients. Nonetheless, there exist multiple prostate cancer-specific HRQOL instruments that merit discussion. Certainly, the UCLA-PCI and the Expanded Prostate Cancer Index-50 (EPIC-50) are 2 such instruments that have been well studied. The UCLA-PCI is a 20-item instrument that is generally coadministered with the RAND SF-36 to men with early stage prostate cancer. The instrument contains 6 subscales, including urinary function, urinary bother, sexual function, sexual bother, bowel function, and bowel bother.[24] The UCLA-PCI was broadened to develop the EPIC-50. The expanded instrument includes such as the assessment of hormonal symptoms, irritative urinary symptoms, and multi-item scores quantifying bother between the sexual, urinary, hormonal, and bowel domains.[25] There is an abbreviated version of the EPIC-50, the EPIC-26, which has demonstrated internal consistency and reliability in patients with localized prostate cancer. The application of prostate cancer-specific instruments to advanced metastatic disease is certainly valuable for assessment of prostate cancer-specific domains; however, these instruments fail to provide the same degree of global assessment as the general cancer instruments such as the FACT-G/P, EORTC-C30, and the CARES-SF. It is for this reason that these instruments are not commonly encountered in the metastatic prostate cancer literature.

Metastatic prostate cancer frequently results in significant pain, and pain measurement is common in HRQOL evaluation, particularly among advanced prostate cancer patients. There are several pain scales that are commonly used to evaluate chronic pain. The McGill Pain Questionnaire evaluates sensory, affective, evaluative, and temporal aspects of the patient's pain condition. Based upon the answers to various questions, sensory, affective, and total pain indices are calculated.[26,27] The Present Pain Intensity (PPI) scale is part of the McGill Pain Questionnaire and uses verbal pain descriptors and scores pain from 0 to 5, with higher scores representing worse pain.[26] The Brief Pain Inventory (BPI) was developed from the Wisconsin Brief Pain Questionnaire. The BPI evaluates pain severity, the degree of interference with function, and relief from current pain regimen.[27,28] The BPI uses a numeric rating scale, with higher scores representing more severe pain.

HRQOL IMPLICATIONS OF METASTATIC PROSTATE CANCER

Both disease burden and treatment may contribute to changes in HRQOL. It is clear from numerous series that patients with metastatic prostate cancer suffer from significant decrements in numerous HRQOL domains. Curran and colleagues[16] evaluated HRQOL using the EORTC-C30 instrument in men enrolled in 3 different EORTC phase 3 studies: locoregional disease (EORTC 30,891), poor prognosis metastatic disease (EORTC 30,893), or painful progressive hormone-resistant disease (30,903). Patients in the hormone-resistant study and the poor prognosis metastatic trials reported significantly worse pain scores, role functioning scores, physical functioning scores, and global health status than patients in the locoregional trial. These data suggest that disease burden is inversely related to HRQOL in patients with prostate cancer. These data are supported by data from Albertsen and colleagues,[29] who studied HRQOL in 113 men with metastatic prostate cancer, 60 of whom were in remission and 53 of whom had progressive

disease. Not surprisingly, patients in remission had more favorable overall quality of life as measured with the EORTC QLQ-C30. Patients in remission demonstrated a significantly higher level of physical function and had fatigue, pain, weight loss, and appetite loss. The investigators then stratified the cohort by disease burden into 3 categories: those with minimal disease in remission, those with extensive disease in remission, and those with extensive disease in progression. Patients with minimal disease in remission reported similar scores on the SF-36 to the general US population. When compared with patients with extensive disease in progression, those with extensive disease in remission had more favorable physical functioning, fatigue, pain, and appetite loss. Sullivan and colleagues[30] administered multiple HRQOL questionnaires to an observational cohort with metastatic castrate-resistant prostate cancer (CRPC) over time. The study revealed significant declines in the FACT-P PCS, EQ5D/EuroQol, and in 10 of 14 domains of the EORTC QLQ-C30 from baseline to 3, 6, and 9 months (**Fig. 1**). Patients reported increasing pain, fatigue, and appetite loss as a function of time. Taken together, these data suggest inverse dose-dependent changes in HRQOL with increasing disease burden.

Changes in HRQOL among men with metastatic prostate cancer continue through the end of life. Certainly, death from prostate cancer is often characterized by significant pain and functional limitations. Sandblom and colleagues[31] found that men dying from prostate cancer reported significantly more severe pain than those dying of other causes. Additionally, patients in the last year of life reported declines in multiple general HRQOL measures including the EQ5D/EuroQol; however, measures of general HRQOL were similar between those dying from prostate cancer and those dying of other causes. Melmed and colleagues[32] evaluated changes in general HRQOL at the end of life in men with metastatic prostate cancer. Nearly all domains revealed declines in HRQOL toward the end of life. Interestingly, however, the investigators found differential decrements in various HRQOL domains by marital status and socioeconomic status. Specifically, those who were married or in a relationship experienced significant declines in emotional well being at the end of life, whereas single men experienced more rapid declines in physical function. Furthermore, men of lower socioeconomic status were more likely to experience rapid deterioration in the physical domains but slower deterioration in the emotional domains. Conversely, men of higher socioeconomic status were more likely to

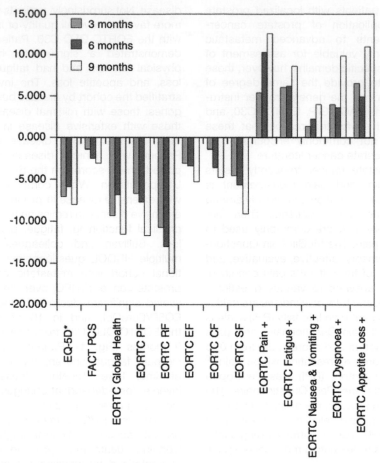

Fig. 1. Mean change in HRQOL scores from baseline to 3, 6, and 9 months for the EQ-5D, FACT-P PCS and EORTC QLQ-C30 domains. Higher scores in domains denoted with (+) represent less favorable HRQOL. (*Reproduced from* Sullivan PW, Mulani PM, Fishman M, et al. Quality of life findings from a multicenter, multinational, observational study of patients with metastatic hormone-refractory prostate cancer. Qual Life Res 2007;16:574; with permission.)

experience rapid declines in the emotional well being, social function, and general health perception domains. Improving the understanding of those factors associated with HRQOL changes may allow practitioners to provide intervention to at-risk populations and improve the overall quality of care administered to prostate cancer patients throughout their disease course.

HRQOL CHANGES WITH ADT

While this article focuses on men with advanced metastatic CRPC, a complete assessment of HRQOL in this cohort requires some attention to changes imposed with the administration of ADT. The introduction of ADT, either in the form of medical or surgical castration, has considerable downstream HRQOL implications in men with

prostate cancer. Certainly, initiating ADT in asymptomatic men results in unfavorable changes in a number of HRQOL domains. Alibhai and colleagues[33] evaluated both physical function and HRQOL using the SF-36 in men with prostate cancer on ADT, men with prostate cancer not on ADT, and a healthy control group. The study revealed numerous declines in objective measures of physical function as well as in the physical function, role-physical, bodily pain, and vitality domains. These findings have been supported by Sadetsky and colleagues[34] who, using CaPSURE, found worse physical well being in patients receiving ADT. Furthermore, patients receiving primary ADT suffered more severe HRQOL declines than those receiving combination ADT and local therapy. Indeed, numerous series in diverse populations have revealed declines in both general HRQOL and prostate cancer-specific HRQOL with the introduction of ADT.[35–40]

There appears to be little difference in HRQOL outcomes between patients who undergo medical versus surgical castration. Litwin and colleagues[41] evaluated HRQOL outcomes in 63 men with metastatic prostate cancer who underwent either surgical castration or combined medical castration using both the SF-36 and the UCLA-PCI. The study found no differences in either general or prostate cancer-specific HRQOL between treatment groups. Interestingly, Potosky and colleagues[42] evaluated outcomes among men in the Prostate Cancer Outcomes Study who underwent either medical or surgical castration and found that those men on luteinizing hormone-releasing hormone (LHRH) therapy experienced breast swelling, physical discomfort, and worry because of cancer more frequently than did those men who underwent orchiectomy. Nonetheless, there were no differences in general HRQOL, as measured by the SF-36, between treatment groups. Similarly, Nygard and colleagues[13] found no difference in HRQOL between those undergoing medical or surgical castration.

It follows that, if ADT use is associated with worse HRQOL, then increasing time off of ADT may have beneficial effects on HRQOL. Other possible advantages of intermittent ADT include reducing the morbidity of ADT associated with long-term therapy, monitoring the course of prostate cancer with prostate-specific antigen (PSA) testing, and the possibility of delaying hormone resistance.[44] Additionally, considering the multitude of HRQOL impairments associated with ADT, it is possible that intermittent therapy ameliorates many of these adverse effects. In their phase 3 study of continuous versus intermittent ADT, Calais da Salva and colleagues[44] measured the EORTC QLQ-C30 and found few differences in general HRQOL between patients receiving continuous and intermittent ADT. Interestingly, patients in both the intermittent and continuous arms experienced declines in sexual function; however, decline was more severe in the continuous group. Furthermore, upon withdrawal of ADT in the intermittent cohort, sexual function returned to near baseline. Multiple phase 2 studies have documented recovery in the sexual function domain while off therapy,[45–47] leading many to advocate for intermittent therapy, particularly among men who assign high utility to sexual function. Certainly, the decision to pursue intermittent ADT depends on numerous factors including patient preference, extent of disease, and burden of comorbidity.

CHANGES IN HRQOL WITH CHEMOTHERAPY FOR METASTATIC CRPC
Mitoxantrone

While the administration of ADT in men with metastatic castrate-sensitive prostate cancer is often associated with improvement in pain and functional status, many such men ultimately will suffer from disease progression secondary to hormone resistance. Given the negative effect of disease progression on HRQOL, a great deal of interest has been given to HRQOL-related endpoints in chemotherapy trials. One such chemotherapeutic agent approved for palliation in patients with symptomatic hormone refractory prostate cancer is mitoxantrone. Tannock and colleagues[48] randomized 161 patients to receive either mitoxantrone with prednisone or prednisone alone. Using improvement in pain as a primary endpoint, the study found that 29% of those treated with mitoxantrone achieved a satisfactory palliative response, defined as a 2-point decrease in pain level on a 6-point scale for minimum of 6 weeks, compared with 12% of those treated with prednisone alone. The duration of palliation was longer in those patients treated with mitoxantrone with prednisone compared with prednisone alone, at 43 weeks and 18 weeks, respectively. Furthermore, the pain subscale of the EORTC QLQ-30 was significantly higher in those treated with mitoxantrone.

A follow-up study using the same cohort more specifically detailed changes in HRQOL with treatment using the EORTC QLQ-C30 and the QOLM-P14, a 14-item instrument designed to evaluate HRQOL in men with metastatic CRPC. Patients treated with mitoxantrone and prednisone experienced improvement in multiple HRQOL domains including pain, fatigue, physical, emotional, and global quality of life. Additionally, through the study time period, patients in the mitoxantrone with prednisone cohort experienced continued improvement in such domains. While patients treated with prednisone alone did experience some improvement from baseline to 6 weeks in a number of HRQOL domains, these patients did not experience any further improvement after 6 weeks. Finally, the addition of mitoxantrone to prednisone in those patients who failed prednisone resulted in significant improvements in pain, pain impact, pain relief, insomnia, and global quality of life.[49]

The cancer and leukemia group B (CALGB) 9182 trial randomized 242 men with metastatic CRPC to mitoxantrone with hydrocortisone or hydrocortisone alone. While global HRQOL, sexual and urologic function, problems of daily activity, and pain summary score were similar between treatment groups, there were subtle differences between those treated with mitoxantrone and hydrocortisone and hydrocortisone alone. Specifically, the Functional Living Index Cancer (FLIC) emotional state and family disruption subscales, as well as pain frequency and severity, were significantly improved in those treated with mitoxantrone and hydrocortisone. While the CALGB study also failed to document any overall survival differences between treatment groups, a small difference in time to progression favored mitoxantrone and hydrocortisone.[50] Despite negligible differences in survival associated with treatment, mitoxantrone achieved US Food and Drug Administration (FDA) approval for symptom relief in men with metastatic CRPC.

Docetaxel

While mitoxantrone was found to improve various HRQOL domains in patients with CRPC, there remained a clear void in the therapeutic algorithm for this group of patients given the lack of survival improvement associated with treatment. Docetaxel was the first chemotherapeutic agent to have a documented survival advantage in patients with M1 CRPC, and it was approved by the FDA in 2004. The studies that documented this survival benefit also included HRQOL and various PROs as secondary endpoints. TAX 327 randomized 1006 men with metastatic CRPC to docetaxel with prednisone or mitoxantrone with prednisone. In addition to measuring survival as the primary endpoint (and documenting the effectiveness of docetaxel in prolonging survival), the study measured pain response and FACT-P to evaluate changes in HRQOL with treatment. Patients were defined as having improvement in HRQOL if they had at least a 16-point improvement in their FACT-P score on 2 measurements at least 2 weeks apart. The likelihood of pain reduction was significantly higher in the cohort of patients treated with docetaxel every 3 weeks than in those receiving mitoxantrone, with 33% and 22% experiencing pain reduction, respectively. There was no difference in the risk of pain reduction between patients treated with weekly docetaxel and mitoxantrone. Furthermore, the duration of pain reduction did not differ between groups. Patients receiving docetaxel were significantly more likely to experience HRQOL improvement, with 22% of patients receiving docetaxel every 3 weeks and 23% of patients receiving weekly docetaxel reported improvement in HRQOL compared with 13% of those receiving mitoxantrone.[51]

In addition to the TAX 327 study, Southwest oncology group (SWOG) 9916 randomized 770 men with metastatic CRPC to receive either docetaxel with estramustine or mitoxantrone with prednisone. As in TAX 327, the primary endpoint of SWOG 9916 was overall survival, which again was found to favor treatment with docetaxel and estramustine. Unlike the TAX 327 trial, however, there was no difference between treatment groups with regard to pain relief.[52] SWOG 9916 measured HRQOL and pain using the EORTC QLQ-C30, the QLQ-PR25, and the McGill Pain Questionnaire Short Form. There were no detected differences in pain response between treatment groups. Furthermore, no differences in general quality of life were identified between groups; however, the number of participants with at least a 10-point improvement in general quality of life at 1 year was significantly greater in the docetaxel with estramustine cohort. The implications of this finding remain unclear given the large amount of missing data at the same time point. There were no differences in prostate cancer-specific symptoms, as measured by the QLQ-PR25, between groups; however, the rates of nausea and vomiting were significantly higher in the docetaxel with estramustine group after cycles 4 and 8.[53]

Other Agents

Various other agents have been studied in patients with CRPC at various stages in treatment. Abratt and colleagues[54] studied vinorelbine in in combination with ADT versus ADT alone in 414 men with CRPC. The study demonstrated an improvement in progression-free survival in the absence of an overall survival benefit. Both cohorts experienced modest improvements in general HRQOL as measured by the EORTC QLQ-C30. Specifically, the pain, fatigue, and nausea/vomiting items improved in both groups as a function of time. There were no observed differences between treatment groups. Certainly, those patients with progressive disease following docetaxel-based chemotherapy are at risk for progressive declines in HRQOL. The TROPIC study randomized men with progressive disease after docetaxel treatment to either cabazitaxel or mitoxantrone. While men receiving cabazitaxel did derive a small survival benefit, there was no difference in the likelihood of pain response or median time to pain response.[55] Nonetheless, the administration of abiraterone acetate to patients with CRPC refractory to docetaxel therapy does appear to result in improvement in functional status. Danila and colleagues[56] reported phase 2 data from 58 men who had progressive disease despite docetaxel therapy. The administration of abiraterone was associated with an improvement in European organisation for research and treatment of cancer (ECOG) performance status in 28% of patients. Additionally, while some have suggested that there may be HRQOL improvements with the administration of sipuleucel-T, there are no definitive data to support this claim. While second-line agents such as cabazitaxel do appear to have modest benefits with regard to disease control, they do not appear to impact HRQOL parameters in this population with progressive disease. Certainly, more investigation is essential to optimize functional and HRQOL benefits in patients with progressive disease despite first-line therapies.

HRQOL IMPACT OF SKELETAL-RELATED EVENTS AND BONE-TARGETED THERAPIES

Patients with metastatic CRPC are at risk for skeletal-related events (SREs), including pathologic fracture, need for bone radiation, spinal cord compression, or change in antineoplastic agent to treat bone pain. Not surprisingly, patients suffering from SREs have significant declines in various HRQOL domains secondary to both pain as well as reduction in specific patients' abilities to perform activities of daily living. Weinfurt and colleagues[57] evaluated HRQOL changes associated with SREs using FACT-G, EuroQol/EQ5D, and BPI. The study revealed statistically and clinically significant declines in physical well being after radiation to bone and pathologic fracture,

functional well being after radiation, and emotional well being after radiation and pathologic fracture. Interestingly, there was an improvement in pain after radiation to bone, but there were no other significant changes in pain after any other SRE (Fig. 2).

Osteoclast-Targeted Agents

Considering the declines in HRQOL associated with SREs, any effort to reduce bone complications should, in theory, improve HRQOL in this at-risk population. Perhaps the best-studied bone-targeted agent in patients with metastatic CRPC is zoledronic acid, which has been found to reduce both the incidence of SREs and the time to first SRE in randomized phase 3 trials.[58,59] Despite the reduction in risk of SRE over the study period, general HRQOL, as measured by the FACT-G and EURO-QOL instruments, did not differ between treatment groups.[58] Long-term follow-up revealed improvement in pain scores at every study time point in the high-dose zoledronic acid arm as well as at the 21- and 24-month time points in standard-dose zoledronic acid arm when compared with placebo. Despite these improvements, no difference between treatment groups was detected with regard to change from baseline analgesic score.[59] Galvez and colleagues[60] evaluated pain, functional status, and general HRQOL in 218 men with metastatic prostate cancer treated with zoledronic acid. The study

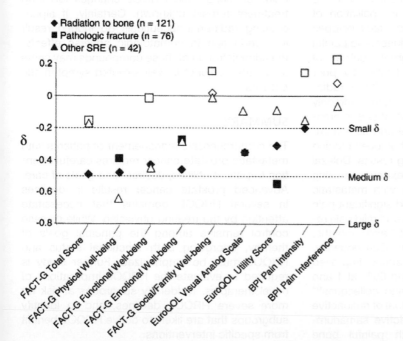

Fig. 2. Impact of SREs on FACT-G, EuroQOL, and BPI. Standardized effect sizes were calculated using the mean change in HRQOL domain divided by standard deviation. Effect sizes significantly different from baseline ($P<.05$) are indicated by closed symbols. (Reproduced from Weinfurt KP, Li Y, Castel LD, et al. The significance of skeletal-related events for the health-related quality of life of patients with metastatic prostate cancer. Ann Oncol 2005;16:582; with permission.)

found improvement in at-rest and on-movement pain scores from baseline in patients with both castrate-sensitive and castrate-resistant disease. Despite significant changes in pain scores over the study period, neither ECOG performance status nor Karnofsky Index improved significantly. Nonetheless, the study did identify significant improvement in the physical component score of the SF-36 over the study period, indicating some downstream functional improvement.

More recently denosumab, a RANK-ligand targeted monoclonal antibody, was approved by the FDA for the prevention of SREs in patients with bone metastases from solid tumors. In a randomized phase 3 trial of denosumab versus zoledronic acid in men with CRPC, there was a significant improvement time to first SRE with denosumab treatment.[61] Despite the phase 3 data supporting the use of denosumab in patients with metastatic CRPC, there are few data that specifically address changes in pain or HRQOL with therapy. While there are ample data to support the use of bone-targeted agents for SRE risk-reduction, this risk reduction does not clearly translate into improvements in functional status or HROQL. Further investigation is imperative to identify subgroups of patients who stand to benefit from these high-cost therapies.

Radiopharmaceutical Therapy

Systemic radiotherapy with bone-seeking radio-isotopes is an alternative treatment modality to external palliative radiotherapy for palliation of bone pain in osseous metastasis. Radioisotopes may be particularly useful with widespread painful bone lesions or in situations where the delivery of external beam radiotherapy is limited by prior treatment and cumulative dose.[62] The 2 radio-pharmaceuticals that have been most commonly administered for diffuse bone metastases in prostate cancer include strontium-89 and samarium-153. More recently, radium-223 has been studied in prostate cancer with promising results. Dolezal and colleagues[63] reported their experience using samarium-153 to treat 32 men with metastatic CRPC. The investigators reported significant pain relief in 44% and 38% of patients and mild pain relief in 25% and 28% of patients at 1 and 3 months, respectively, after administration. Consequently, mean Karnofsky performance status improved from 57% at baseline to 67% and 68% at 1 and 3 months, respectively. Sartor and colleagues[64] reported the results of a phase 3 trial of radioactive samarium-153 versus nonradioactive samarium-153 in men with CRPC with painful bone

metastases. The study found significant improvements in pain scores and analgesic requirement in those treated with the radioactive compound. Multiple other reports have documented pain relief in patients with both metastatic prostate and breast cancer.[65–67] None of these studies, however, have specifically addressed changes in HRQOL with treatment.

Myelosuppression is the most common adverse effect of samarium-153 and strontium-89, owing to their properties as beta-emitting radio-isotopes with several millimeters of energy deposition. Alpha-emitting radioisotopes deliver higher-energy radiation with a range of approximately 100 μM and thus have the theoretical advantage of reduced myelosuppression. One such alpha-emitting radioisotope is radium-223. Phase 2 trials of radium-223 in patients with metastatic CRPC have yielded promising results. Nilsson and colleagues[68] recently reported a significant dose–response relationship between dose and reduction in pain index. Of responders, nearly 52% in the highest dose subgroup experienced complete or marked reduction in pain index. The phase 3 alpharadin in symptomatic prostate cancer (ALSYMPCA) trial, which had randomized men with metastatic CRPC to radium-223 and standard care, closed early after meeting the study's primary endpoint of overall survival. Indeed, patients randomized to receive radium-223 enjoyed a median survival of 14.0 months compared with 11.2 months for standard care.[69] These data are not published, and the pain, functional, and HRQOL changes following treatment remain unknown. Certainly, if alpha-emitting radiopharmaceuticals do indeed result in a reduction in hematologic adverse effects, the administration of these compounds may serve as a useful adjunct in well-selected symptomatic patients.

SUMMARY

The comprehensive management of patients with metastatic prostate cancer requires careful attention to patient utilities, desires, and goals of care. Advanced prostate cancer results in declines in several HRQOL domains that necessitate attention by the treating physician. While disease control remains among the principal goals of therapy, improving both functional status and HRQOL must be emphasized. Further study is required to evaluate the HRQOL implications of novel therapies, to identify subgroups at risk for more severe HRQOL declines, and to identify subgroups that are likely to derive HRQOL benefit from specific interventions.

REFERENCES

1. Siegel R, Naishadham D, Jemal A. Cancer statistics, 2012. CA Cancer J Clin 2012;62:10–29.

2. Arpinelli F, Bamfi F. The FDA guidance for industry on PROs: the point of view of a pharmaceutical company. Health Qual Life Outcomes 2006;4:85.

3. Patrick DL, Deyo RA. Generic and disease-specific measures in assessing health status and quality of life. Med Care 1989;27:S217–32.

4. Wein AJ, Kavoussi LR, Novick AC, et al. Campbell-Walsh urology. Philadelphia: W B Saunders Co; 2011.

5. Ware JE, Sherbourne CD. The MOS 36-Item Short-Form Health Survey (SF-36). I. Conceptual framework and item selection. Med Care 1992;30:473–83.

6. Hays RD, Sherbourne CD, Mazel RM. The RAND 36-Item Health Survey 1.0. Health Econ 1993;2:217–27.

7. Ware J, Kosinski M, Keller SD. A 12-Item Short-Form Health Survey: construction of scales and preliminary tests of reliability and validity. Med Care 1996; 34:220–33.

8. Kaplan RM, Bush JW, Berry CC. Health status: types of validity and the index of well-being. Health Serv Res 1976;11:478–507.

9. Kaplan RM, Anderson JP. A general health policy model: update and applications. Health Serv Res 1988;23:203–35.

10. Kaplan RM, Ganiats TG, Sieber WJ, et al. The quality of well-being scale: critical similarities and differences with SF-36. Int J Qual Health Care 1998;10:509–20.

11. Bergner M, Bobbitt RA, Pollard WE, et al. The sickness impact profile: validation of a health status measure. Med Care 1976;14:57–67.

12. Pollard WE, Bobbitt RA, Bergner M, et al. The sickness impact profile: reliability of a health status measure. Med Care 1976;14:146–55.

13. Bergner M, Bobbitt RA, Carter WB, et al. The sickness impact profile: development and final revision of a health status measure. Med Care 1981;19:787–805.

14. Hunt SM, McEwen J, McKenna SP. Measuring health status: a new tool for clinicians and epidemiologists. J R Coll Gen Pract 1985;35:185–8.

15. Aaronson NK, Ahmedzai S, Bergman B, et al. The European Organization for Research and Treatment of Cancer QLQ-C30: a quality-of-life instrument for use in international clinical trials in oncology. J Natl Cancer Inst 1993;85:365–76.

16. Curran D, Fossa S, Aaronson N, et al. Baseline quality of life of patients with advanced prostate cancer. European Organization for Research and Treatment of Cancer (EORTC), Genito-Urinary Tract Cancer Cooperative Group (GUT-CCG). Eur J Cancer 1997;33:1809–14.

17. Van Andel G, Bottomley A, Fosså SD, et al. An international field study of the EORTC QLQ-PR25: a questionnaire for assessing the health-related quality of life of patients with prostate cancer. Eur J Cancer 2008;44:2418–24.

18. Cella DF, Tulsky DS, Gray G, et al. The functional assessment of cancer therapy scale: development and validation of the general measure. J Clin Oncol 1993;11:570–9.

19. Esper P, Mo F, Chodak G, et al. Measuring quality of life in men with prostate cancer using the functional assessment of cancer therapy–prostate instrument. Urology 1997;50:920–8.

20. Schag CA, Heinrich RL. Development of a comprehensive quality of life measurement tool: CARES. Oncology (Williston Park) 1990;4:135–8 [discussion: 147].

21. Schag CA, Ganz PA, Wing DS, et al. Quality of life in adult survivors of lung, colon and prostate cancer. Qual Life Res 1994;3:127–41.

22. EuroQol—a new facility for the measurement of health-related quality of life. The EuroQol Group. Health Policy 1990;16:199–208.

23. Brooks R. EuroQol: the current state of play. Health Policy 1996;37:53–72.

24. Litwin MS, Hays RD, Fink A, et al. The UCLA Prostate Cancer Index: development, reliability, and validity of a health-related quality of life measure. Med Care 1998;36:1002–12.

25. Wei JT, Dunn RL, Litwin MS, et al. Development and validation of the expanded prostate cancer index composite (EPIC) for comprehensive assessment of health-related quality of life in men with prostate cancer. Urology 2000;56:899–905.

26. Melzack R. The McGill Pain Questionnaire: major properties and scoring methods. Pain 1975;1:277–99.

27. Breivik H, Borchgrevink PC, Allen SM, et al. Assessment of pain. Br J Anaesth 2008;101:17–24.

28. Daut RL, Cleeland CS, Flanery RC. Development of the Wisconsin Brief Pain Questionnaire to assess pain in cancer and other diseases. Pain 1983;17:197–210.

29. Albertsen PC, Aaronson NK, Muller MJ, et al. Health-related quality of life among patients with metastatic prostate cancer. Urology 1997;49:207–16 [discussion: 216–7].

30. Sullivan PW, Mulani PM, Fishman M, et al. Quality of life findings from a multicenter, multinational, observational study of patients with metastatic hormone-refractory prostate cancer. Qual Life Res 2007;16:571–5.

31. Sandblom G, Carlsson P, Sennfält K, et al. A population-based study of pain and quality of life during the year before death in men with prostate cancer. Br J Cancer 2004;90:1163–8.

32. Melmed GY, Kwan L, Reid K, et al. Quality of life at the end of life: trends in patients with metastatic prostate cancer. Urology 2002;59:103–9.

33. Alibhai SM, Breunis H, Timilshina N, et al. Impact of androgen-deprivation therapy on physical function and quality of life in men with nonmetastatic prostate cancer. J Clin Oncol 2010;28:5038–45.

34. Sadetsky N, Greene K, Cooperberg MR, et al. Impact of androgen deprivation on physical well-being in patients with prostate cancer: analysis from the CaPSURE (Cancer of the Prostate Strategic Urologic Research Endeavor) registry. Cancer 2011; 117:4406–13.

35. Lubeck DP, Grossfeld GD, Carroll PR. The effect of androgen deprivation therapy on health-related quality of life in men with prostate cancer. Urology 2001;58:94–100.

36. Basaria S, Lieb J, Tang AM, et al. Long-term effects of androgen deprivation therapy in prostate cancer patients. Clin Endocrinol (Oxf) 2002;56: 779–86.

37. Dacal K, Sereika SM, Greenspan SL. Quality of life in prostate cancer patients taking androgen deprivation therapy. J Am Geriatr Soc 2006;54:85–90.

38. Herr HW, O'Sullivan M. Quality of life of asymptomatic men with nonmetastatic prostate cancer on androgen deprivation therapy. J Urol 2000;163: 1743–6.

39. van Andel G, Kurth KH. The impact of androgen deprivation therapy on health related quality of life in asymptomatic men with lymph node positive prostate cancer. Eur Urol 2003;44:209–14.

40. Green HJ, Pakenham KI, Headley BC, et al. Coping and health-related quality of life in men with prostate cancer randomly assigned to hormonal medication or close monitoring. Psychooncology 2002;11: 401–14.

41. Litwin MS, Shpall AI, Dorey F, et al. Quality-of-life outcomes in long-term survivors of advanced prostate cancer. Am J Clin Oncol 1998;21:327–32.

42. Potosky AL, Knopf K, Clegg LX, et al. Quality-of-life outcomes after primary androgen deprivation therapy: results from the Prostate Cancer Outcomes Study. J Clin Oncol 2001;19:3750–7.

43. Nygård R, Norum J, Due J. Goserelin (Zoladex) or orchiectomy in metastatic prostate cancer? A quality of life and cost-effectiveness analysis. Anticancer Res 2001;21:781–8.

44. Calais da Silva FE, Bono AV, Whelan P, et al. Intermittent androgen deprivation for locally advanced and metastatic prostate cancer: results from a randomised phase 3 study of the South European Uroncological Group. Eur Urol 2009;55:1269–77.

45. Malone S, Perry G, Segal R, et al. Long-term side effects of intermittent androgen suppression therapy in prostate cancer: results of a phase II study. BJU Int 2005;96:514–20.

46. Spry NA, Kristjanson L, Hooton B, et al. Adverse effects to quality of life arising from treatment can recover with intermittent androgen suppression in men with prostate cancer. Eur J Cancer 2006;42: 1083–92.

47. Bruchovsky N, Klotz L, Crook J, et al. Quality of life, morbidity, and mortality results of a prospective phase II study of intermittent androgen suppression for men with evidence of prostate-specific antigen relapse after radiation therapy for locally advanced prostate cancer. Clin Genitourin Cancer 2008; 6:46–52.

48. Tannock IF, Osoba D, Stockler MR, et al. Chemotherapy with mitoxantrone plus prednisone or prednisone alone for symptomatic hormone-resistant prostate cancer: a Canadian randomized trial with palliative end points. J Clin Oncol 1996;14:1756–64.

49. Osoba D, Tannock IF, Ernst DS, et al. Health-related quality of life in men with metastatic prostate cancer treated with prednisone alone or mitoxantrone and prednisone. J Clin Oncol 1999;17:1654–63.

50. Kantoff PW, Halabi S, Conaway M, et al. Hydrocortisone with or without mitoxantrone in men with hormone-refractory prostate cancer: results of the cancer and leukemia group B 9182 study. J Clin Oncol 1999;17:2506–13.

51. Tannock IF, de Wit R, Berry WR, et al, TAX 327 Investigators. Docetaxel plus prednisone or mitoxantrone plus prednisone for advanced prostate cancer. N Engl J Med 2004;351:1502–12.

52. Petrylak DP, Tangen CM, Hussain MH, et al. Docetaxel and estramustine compared with mitoxantrone and prednisone for advanced refractory prostate cancer. N Engl J Med 2004;351:1513–20.

53. Southwest Oncology Group, Berry DL, Moinpour CM, et al. Quality of life and pain in advanced stage prostate cancer: results of a Southwest Oncology Group randomized trial comparing docetaxel and estramustine to mitoxantrone and prednisone. J Clin Oncol 2006;24:2828–35.

54. Abratt RP, Brune D, Dimopoulos MA, et al. Randomised phase III study of intravenous vinorelbine plus hormone therapy versus hormone therapy alone in hormone-refractory prostate cancer. Ann Oncol 2004;15:1613–21.

55. de Bono JS, Oudard S, Ozguroglu M, et al, TROPIC Investigators. Prednisone plus cabazitaxel or mitoxantrone for metastatic castration-resistant prostate cancer progressing after docetaxel treatment: a randomised open-label trial. Lancet 2010;376: 1147–54.

56. Danila DC, Morris MJ, de Bono JS, et al. Phase II multicenter study of abiraterone acetate plus prednisone therapy in patients with docetaxel-treated castration-resistant prostate cancer. J Clin Oncol 2010;28:1496–501.

57. Weinfurt KP, Li Y, Castel LD, et al. The significance of skeletal-related events for the health-related quality of life of patients with metastatic prostate cancer. Ann Oncol 2005;16:579–84.

58. Saad F, Gleason DM, Murray R, et al, Zoledronic Acid Prostate Cancer Study Group. A randomized, placebo-controlled trial of zoledronic acid in patients with hormone-refractory metastatic prostate carcinoma. J Natl Cancer Inst 2002;94:1458–68.

59. Saad F, Gleason DM, Murray R, et al, Zoledronic Acid Prostate Cancer Study Group. Long-term efficacy of zoledronic acid for the prevention of skeletal complications in patients with metastatic hormone-refractory prostate cancer. J Natl Cancer Inst 2004;96:879–82.

60. Gálvez R, Ribera V, González-Escalada JR, et al. Analgesic efficacy of zoledronic acid and its effect on functional status of prostate cancer patients with metastasis. Patient Prefer Adherence 2008;2:215–24.

61. Fizazi K, Carducci M, Smith M, et al. Denosumab versus zoledronic acid for treatment of bone metastases in men with castration-resistant prostate cancer: a randomised, double-blind study. Lancet 2011;377:813–22.

62. Christensen MH, Petersen LJ. Radionuclide treatment of painful bone metastases in patients with breast cancer: a systematic review. Cancer Treat Rev 2012;38(2):164–71.

63. Dolezal J, Vizda J, Odrazka K. Prospective evaluation of samarium-153-EDTMP radionuclide treatment for bone metastases in patients with hormone-refractory prostate cancer. Urol Int 2007;78:50–7.

64. Sartor O, Reid RH, Hoskin PJ, et al, Quadramet 424Sm10/11 Study Group. Samarium-153-Lexidronam complex for treatment of painful bone metastases in hormone-refractory prostate cancer. Urology 2004;63:940–5.

65. Lewington VJ, McEwan AJ, Ackery DM, et al. A prospective, randomised double-blind crossover study to examine the efficacy of strontium-89 in pain palliation in patients with advanced prostate cancer metastatic to bone. Eur J Cancer 1991;27:954–8.

66. Laing AH, Ackery DM, Bayly RJ, et al. Strontium-89 chloride for pain palliation in prostatic skeletal malignancy. Br J Radiol 1991;64:816–22.

67. Dafermou A, Colamussi P, Giganti M, et al. A multicentre observational study of radionuclide therapy in patients with painful bone metastases of prostate cancer. Eur J Nucl Med 2001;28:788–98.

68. Nilsson S, Strang P, Aksnes AK, et al. A randomized, dose-response, multicenter phase II study of radium-223 chloride for the palliation of painful bone metastases in patients with castration-resistant prostate cancer. Eur J Cancer 2012;48:678–86.

69. Bayer's investigational compound radium-223 chloride met its primary end point of significantly improving overall survival in a phase III trial in patients with castration-resistant prostate cancer that has spread to the bone. Available at: http://www.pharma.bayer.com/html/pdf/news_room115.pdf.

Targeted Therapies in Metastatic Castration-Resistant Prostate Cancer
Beyond the Androgen Receptor

Yohann Loriot, MD[a], Amina Zoubeidi, PhD[a],
Martin E. Gleave, MD[a,b],*

KEYWORDS

- Prostate cancer • Cabazitaxel • Cabozantinib • Dasatinib • Clusterin • Hsp27 • OGX-011

KEY POINTS

- Many pathways are involved in cell survival or bone metastases, in addition to the AR pathway in CRPC.
- Tubulin-targeting agents are still under clinical investigation.
- Preclinical studies support DNA repair targeting in CRPC.
- Cell survival pathways are critical for resistance to endocrine therapies and chemotherapy in prostate cancer.
- MET and Src pathways are involved in many cellular processes leading to metastasis formation in prostate cancer, supporting their inhibition.

INTRODUCTION

Prostate Cancer (PCa) is the most common cancer in North America and the second leading cause of cancer-related death in men. Despite improved outcomes through early detection and treatment of localized PCa, many men still die of metastatic disease. Although androgen ablation remains the most effective management option for patients with advanced disease, most progress to castration-resistant prostate cancer (CRPC) within 2 years of treatment initiation.[1–4] CRPC progression is a complex process by which cells acquire the ability to survive and proliferate in the absence of testicular androgens. Many mechanisms have been postulated to account for androgen receptor (AR) activation in CRPC tumors, including (1) activation of AR by nonsteroids such as growth factors and cytokines via deregulated multiple signaling pathways; (2) genetic mutation(s) or amplification(s) of AR that render the receptor hyperactive, which sensitizes cells toward low levels of androgen; (3) altered expression of activity of AR coactivators or chaperone proteins; (4) expression of AR splice variants that lack the ligand-binding domain (LBD) and are constitutively active in a ligand-independent manner; and (5) intratumoral steroidogenesis. These proposed mechanisms are not mutually exclusive and they likely work in concert to drive CRPC. Despite the failure of maximal androgen blockade trials using first-generation nonsteroidal AR inhibitors like flutamide or bicalutamide, CRPC tumors are not uniformly hormone refractory and remain sensitive to therapies directed against the AR axis.[5] Hence, several new classes of AR-targeting agents are now in clinical development, including inhibitors of steroidogenesis (abiraterone)[6] and more potent AR antagonists (MDV3100).[7] Although enthusiasm for this

a Vancouver Prostate Centre, University of British Columbia, 899 12th Avenue West, Vancouver, British Columbia V5Z 1M9, Canada; b Department of Urological Sciences, University of British Columbia, Level 6, 2775 Laurel Street, Vancouver, British Columbia V5Z 1M9, Canada
* Corresponding author. Department of Urological Sciences, University of British Columbia, Level 6, 2775 Laurel Street, Vancouver, British Columbia V5Z 1M9, Canada.
E-mail address: m.gleave@ubc.ca

Urol Clin N Am 39 (2012) 517–531
http://dx.doi.org/10.1016/j.ucl.2012.07.008
0094-0143/12/$ – see front matter © 2012 Elsevier Inc. All rights reserved.

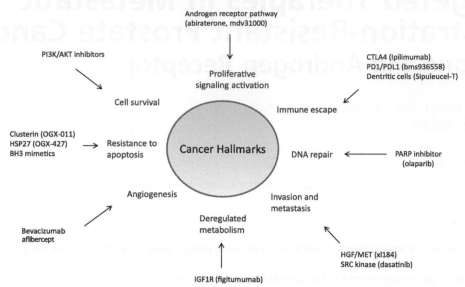

Fig. 1. Current targets in CRPC. CTLA4, cytotoxic T-lymphocyte antigen 4; IGF1R, insulin growth factor 1-receptor; PD1, programmed cell death protein 1; PDL1, programmed cell death protein ligand 1.

approach remains high, prostate tumor heterogeneity and adaptive responses that support development of resistance via alternative mechanisms create a critical need for other strategies to kill prostate cancer cells.

Improved understanding of prostate cancer biology is facilitating the identification of many pathways, aside from the AR, that drive CRPC progression by promoting invasion and metastasis, or by activating cell survival signaling. This article highlights the implications for practice, and focuses on those mediating cell survival, cell invasion, and cell proliferation (**Fig. 1**).[8]

TARGETING CELL PROLIFERATION
New Taxanes: Cabazitaxel

Preclinical data
Microtubules consist of tubulin heterodimers and radiate from the centrosome in the cytoplasm of interphase cells. They are involved in many cellular functions including cell motility, cell division, and intracellular transport. During the mitosis, microtubule networks ensure the correct attachment and segregation of chromosomes during cell division, making them attractive targets for anticancer drugs.[9] Docetaxel is a taxane that binds to β-tubulin of microtubules during the G_2-M phase of the cell cycle, leading to cell apoptosis in cycling cells. Recent studies have also shown additional effects of docetaxel on AR by preventing its translocation into the nucleus and thus inhibiting AR-induced signaling.[10,11] Docetaxel-based chemotherapy is standard first-line chemotherapy in patients with metastatic CRPC (mCRPC). Two randomized phase III trials have shown an improved overall survival in chemonaive patients with CRPC treated with docetaxel alone or in combination with estramustine compared with mitoxantrone. However, almost 50% of patients do not respond to docetaxel.[12,13]

Molecular mechanisms of resistance to docetaxel are multifactorial and involve decreased cellular drug accumulation caused by overexpression of membrane-bound efflux proteins (P-glycoprotein), expression of tubulin isotypes (overexpression of β-III tubulin) and defects in apoptosis.[14] Some gene expression signatures have been associated with docetaxel resistance of prostate cancer cells, but no single driver pathway that responds to drugs has emerged to target and circumvent such resistance.[15,16] New taxoid compounds have been developed as a low-affinity substrate for the P-glycoprotein efflux pump mechanism. Cabazitaxel (XRP6258, Jevtana) is a novel tubulin-binding taxane drug with antitumor activity in docetaxel-resistant cancers. Cabazitaxel promotes the assembly of tubulin and stabilizes microtubules against cold-induced depolymerization in vitro as potently as docetaxel.[17] Cabazitaxel showed potent antitumor activity comparable with docetaxel in docetaxel-sensitive cell lines and exhibited more potent cytotoxic activity than docetaxel in cancer cell lines with acquired resistance to docetaxel caused by P-glycoprotein overexpression. Cabazitaxel resulted in antitumor activity on a broad array of tumor xenografts.[17]

Clinical data

Phase 1 and 2 clinical studies reported that neutropenia is the primary dose-limiting toxicity, a recommended phase 2 dose between 20 and 25 mg/m^2, and antitumor activity in solid tumors including docetaxel-refractory mCRPC, supporting further clinical investigations.[17,18] Given the precedent efficacy of docetaxel in CRPC, along with the safety profile and observed responses in the phase I trial, an international phase III trial was conducted without phase II in patients with CRPC. The TROPIC trial was an international randomized phase 3 trial assessing cabazitaxel in men with mCRPC whose disease had progressed during or after treatment with a docetaxel-based regimen.[19] Patients were randomly assigned to receive either cabazitaxel (25 mg mg/m^2 intravenously every 3 weeks) or mitoxantrone (12 mg/m^2 every 3 weeks). The primary end point was the overall survival (OS). This study showed that cabazitaxel improved median OS by 2.4 months (15.1 months vs 12.7 months) compared with the mitoxantrone group, with a hazard ratio (HR) reduction of 0.70 (95% confidence interval [CI] 0.59–0.83, $P<.0001$). Median progression-free survival (PFS) was also better in the cabazitaxel group (2.8 months, 95% CI 2.4–3.0) in the cabazitaxel group and 1.4 months (1.4–1.7 months) in the mitoxantrone group (HR 0.74, 0.64–0.86, $P<.0001$). The most common clinically significant grade 3 or higher adverse events were neutropenia (cabazitaxel 82% of patients vs mitoxantrone 58%) and diarrhea (6% vs <1%). A phase III trial is currently comparing cabazitaxel with docetaxel in chemonaive patients with mCRPC.

Epothilones

Preclinical data

Epothilones are, like taxanes, tubulin-binding agents but have different binding sites on the tubulin polymers.[20] They induce apoptosis in cancer cells by disrupting the dynamic characteristics of microtubules. The epothilones include natural epothilone B (EPO906; patupilone) and several semisynthetic epothilone compounds such as BMS-247550 (ixabepilone) and sagopilone (ZK-EPO). Epothilones have cytotoxic effects against human cancer cells with high expression of P-glycoprotein[20] and are also active in cancer cells resistant to taxanes because of tubulin mutations.[21] Studies have shown that the precise binding sites and mode of action of epothilones differ from taxanes[21]; for example, ixabepilone can bind multiple β-tubulin isoforms, suppressing the dynamic instability of class III β-tubulin and class II β-tubulin microtubules, whereas taxanes weakly link class III β-tubulin. Epothilones also have low susceptibility to classic taxane resistance mechanisms, such as P-glycoprotein or multidrug resistance protein efflux, tubulin mutations, and alterations in tubulin isotypes.[22]

Epothilone B (patupilone) has tumor activity in human prostate cancer DU-145 and PC-3 xenografts. Patupilone has antitumor activity against both paclitaxel-sensitive and paclitaxel-refractory cancers in vitro including in human cancer cell lines with P-glycoprotein overexpression and human cancer cell lines with tubulin mutations.[23,24] Like epothilone B, ixabepilone has potent antitumor activity in mouse xenograft models bearing paclitaxel-sensitive or paclitaxel-refractory tumors. However, published preclinical data in prostate cancer xenografts are currently limited. Many studies have reported that ixabepilone has a low susceptibility to mechanisms of resistance to taxanes such as tubulin mutations and overexpression of the efflux pumps.[25]

Sagopilone is a fully synthetic formulation of epothilone B. In vivo, sagopilone has shown activity in many cancers including prostate cancer, and cancer models with an multidrug-resistant phenotype and paclitaxel-resistant cells.[26]

Clinical data

Phase I clinical trials indicate that epothilone and ixabepilone are well tolerated in patients who have cancer both as a single agent or in combination. However, neuropathy has led to frequent dose reductions in patients treated with ixabepilone in phase I clinical trials. The phase II clinical trials assessing ixabepilone suggest antitumor activity in men with mCRPC as single agent or in combination with estramustine. These agents have shown better activity in men with chemotherapy-naive mCRPC than in men previously treated with docetaxel.[27–29] A phase II randomized study compared ixabepilone 35 mg/m^2 every 3 weeks with intravenous mitoxantrone 14 mg/m^2 every 3 weeks plus prednisone 5 mg twice daily in 82 patients with taxane-refractory CRPC. The efficacy end points were not different between the 2 arms.[30] However, another phase II study showed that the combination of ixabepilone and mitoxantrone is both feasible and active in CRPC.[31]

A phase II trial of patupilone (8 mg/m^2) was safe, had antitumor activity, and was associated with symptomatic improvement in patients previously treated with docetaxel. A prostate-specific antigen (PSA) decline of greater than or equal to 50% occurred in 47% of patients, whereas a partial measurable disease response occurred in 24% of assessable patients. A patient-reported pain response was also observed in 59% of assessable patients.[32] In a recent phase II study, the activity of sagopilone 16 mg/m^2 given intravenously over 3 hours every 21 days was investigated in chemotherapy-naive patients with mCRPC in combination with oral prednisone.[33] Of the 24 patients evaluable for response, 5 (21%) achieved a PSA response (reduction ≥50%) and 14 (58%) had a 30% PSA reduction within 3 months of enrollment. Among the 12 patients with measurable disease, there was 1 confirmed complete response (CR) and 1 confirmed partial response (PR), and 4 further patients achieved unconfirmed PRs.

Third-generation taxanes such as TPI 287 and agents targeting the mitotic process (ispinesib targets kinesin spindle protein, and danusertib targets the serine-threonine aurora kinase) are currently investigated in phase II clinical trials in men with mCRPC previously treated with docetaxel.

DNA Repair Inhibition

Preclinical data

DNA repair is essential because DNA is susceptible to spontaneous damage. Cellular DNA is susceptible to carcinogens, and the target of a broad range of anticancer agents. Several cancer susceptibility genes therefore encode for DNA repair and DNA damage response factors. DNA repair is coupled with DNA damage responses that are commonly referred to as checkpoint responses. Those checkpoints enable cell cycle arrest, which provides time for repair and avoids further damage until the DNA damaging agent is cleared from the cell. Because DNA-damaging agents target DNA similarly in normal and cancer tissues, the effects of those clinically approved chemotherapeutic agents is likely to result from tumor-specific defects in DNA repair and DNA damage repair pathways.

Recent studies in breast and ovarian cancers suggest that targeting DNA repair may represent an efficient strategy for improving outcome of patients with metastatic cancers. Poly(ADP-ribose) polymerase 1 (PARP1) is a constitutively expressed nuclear enzyme important in base excision repair of single-stranded DNA breaks.[34] In its absence, excessive single-strand breaks accumulate, leading to collapsed DNA replication forks and conversion of single-strand breaks to double-strand breaks (DSBs). BRCA1 and BRCA2 proteins repair double-strand DNA breaks by homologous recombination, and BRCA-defective cells are unable to repair these DSBs, resulting in tumor cell death.[35] Inhibition of PARP1 in BRCA-deficient cells uses the concept of synthetic lethality, whereby a mutation in either of 2 genes individually has no effect on cell survival but combining the mutations leads to cell death. Inhibitors of PARP1 may offer an additional therapeutic option for BRCA carriers in breast and ovarian cancers[36] Furthermore, expression of proteins involved in DNA repair pathways such as BRCA1/2, ERCC1, and MSH2 have been associated with response to platinum-based chemotherapy in lung cancer, bladder cancer, and triple-negative breast cancers.[37-39]

The incidence of DNA repair defects and their clinical relevance in PCa remain to be clarified. BRCA1 and BRCA2 mutation carriers have an increased risk of developing prostate cancer.[40] Germline BRCA mutations seem to predict aggressive disease, with carriers showing earlier progression through the prostate cancer clinical states model and increased prostate cancer–specific mortality than noncarriers.[41] Although the incidence of BRCA2 mutation in prostate cancer is low, BRCA-associated prostate cancer may represent a genetically defined subset of the disease that may be more sensitive to platinum-based chemotherapy as observed in patients with BRCA-associated breast and ovarian cancers. Treatment of BRCA-associated prostate cancer with PARP inhibition would represent an efficient strategy of treatment tailored to BRCA2 status. Clinical trials assessing platinum-based agents such as carboplatin, cisplatin, or, more recently, satraplatin failed to show any benefit in patients with prostate cancer.[42-45] In a recent retrospective study, response to taxane-based therapy defined by PSA nadir within 12 weeks of therapy was not associated with BRCA1/2 mutation status.[46]

Oncogenic gene fusions recently found in PCa may also impair DNA repair ability of cancer cells. Oncogenic ETS gene rearrangements involving sequences of TMPRSS2 (an androgen-regulated gene) with ETS-family transcription factor genes (ERG, ETV1, ETV4, or ETV4) have been reported in around 40% of prostate cancers.[47] Once an ETS gene fusion is formed through genomic rearrangement, the subsequent overexpression of an ETS gene fusion protein can contribute to cancer progression through various mechanisms. Overexpression of ERG leads to accelerated carcinogenesis in mouse prostates with deletion of the tumor suppressor PTEN.[48] However, its clinical relevance remains to be elucidated because no strong association with clinical outcome has been shown. A recent study showed that androgen signaling promotes corecruitment of AR and topoisomerase II β (TOP2B) to sites of TMPRSS2-ERG genomic breakpoints, triggering recombinogenic TOP2B-mediated DSBs.[49] Furthermore, androgen stimulation resulted in de novo production of *TMPRSS2-ERG* fusion transcripts in a process that required TOP2B and components of the DSB repair machinery. Another study showed that ERG interacts with the enzymes PARP1 and dependent protein kinase, catalytic subunit (DNAPKcs) involved in DNA repair pathways. Several PARP inhibitors such as olaparib or veliparib have been developed alone or in combination with conventional chemotherapy, especially in BRCA-mutated ovarian and breast cancers. In prostate cancer, pharmacologic inhibition of PARP1 preferentially sensitized ETS-overexpressing VCAP xenografts compared with ETS-negative xenografts (PC3, DU145, 22RV1), although the dose of olaparib (>10 μM) used in this study was probably beyond the recommended dose in the patients.[50]

Clinical data

In the phase I clinical trial assessing olaparib in patients with BRCA1 or BRCA2 mutations, a patient with CRPC who was a *BRCA2* mutation carrier had more than a 50% reduction in the PSA level and resolution of bone metastases, participating in the study for more than 58 weeks at the time of the cutoff date.[51] A phase II assessing the combination of veliparib and the DNA damage agent, temozolomide, was conducted and is now closed to accrual (NCT01085422). Preliminary data showed that 2 patients out of 25 had a confirmed PSA response; 1 patient had a 37% decrease in PSA and the other patient had a 96% decrease in PSA and a 40% reduction in tumor size. Median PFS was 2.1 months (95% CI 1.8, 3.9).[52]

TARGETING SURVIVAL PATHWAYS

Defects in the ability to appropriately regulate apoptotic processes are one of the fundamental properties underlying cancer.[8] Bcl-2 was the first identified member of a family of apoptotic regulators sharing at least 1 Bcl-2 homology domain. Bcl-2 family members include antiapoptotic proteins (eg, Bcl-2, Bcl-X_L, and Mcl-1), multidomain proapoptotic proteins (eg, Bax and Bak), and BH3-only proapoptotic proteins (eg, Bim, Bid, Noxa, and Puma).[9] Interactions between, and relative ratios of, proapoptotic and antiapoptotic Bcl-2 family members are key determinants of cellular sensitivity to multiple cell death triggers, including many standard chemotherapeutic agents and ionizing radiation (IR).[53] Bcl-2, Bcl-X_L, and Mcl-1 gene amplification have been shown to be associated with castration resistance.[54] Targeting such antiapoptotic proteins resulted in improvement of chemotherapy efficacy in PCa cell lines.

BCL-2

Preclinical data

Bcl-2 antisense oligodeoxynucleotides (ASO) (G3139, oblimersen sodium, Genasense) have been shown to be effective in reducing Bcl-2 expression in several cell lines including prostate cancer cells.[55] Bcl-2 ASO enhances chemotherapy and radiation-induced cytotoxicity in prostate cancer cell lines.[56] Recently, BH3 mimetics such as ABT-737 and AT-101 (R-(−)-gossypol) have been designed to inhibit heterodimerization of Bcl-2 or Bcl-X_L to proapoptotic BH3 family members (Bax, Bak), resulting in caspase-dependent apoptosis activation.[57]

The BH3 mimetic ABT-737 binds with high affinity to the hydrophobic cleft and BH3 receptor region of Bcl-2, Bcl-X_L, and Bcl-w, but not to the less homologous Bcl-2–related protein Mcl-1. This ABT-737/Bcl-2 interaction antagonizes the interaction of Bcl-2 with the BH3 domain of proapoptotic proteins, neutralizing Bcl-2. Although ABT-737 shows single-agent activity promoting apoptosis in human small cell lung cancer and lymphoma cell lines in vitro and in tumor xenografts, apoptosis is not triggered in most human cancer cell lines.[57] Expression of Mcl-1, which is not targeted by ABT-737, may explain the resistance in prostate and other cancer cell lines to apoptosis. However, combining ABT-737 with agents that target Mcl-1 sensitized prostate cancer cell lines with an apoptotic block to cell death in vitro.[58]

Clinical data

The phase I clinical trial combining oblimersen and docetaxel did not show any severe toxicities at recommended dose and showed evidence of Bcl-2 protein inhibition in tumor tissue, and encouraging antitumor activity in patients with CRPC.[59] However, a randomized, phase II study failed to confirm preliminary data, mostly because of its short tissue half-life and interruptions with its continuous infusion, leading to insufficient target inhibition.[60]

A phase I/II trial combining docetaxel day 1 every 21 days with AT-101 40 mg twice daily on days 1 to 3 in chemonaive men with mCRPC showed encouraging efficacy, with two-thirds of patients achieving a biochemical response defined as decline greater than or equal to 50% and some of them (45%) having a measurable PR.[61] However, these preliminary results were not confirmed in a phase 2 trial that recently reported that AT-101 failed to improve OS when combined with docetaxel-based chemotherapy (NCT00286793).[62] The more selective compound ABT-737 and its oral-derived enantiomer

ABT-263 are currently being assessed in many phase I and phase II clinical trials based on preclinical data. A phase I trial is investigating the combination of docetaxel and ABT-263 in solid tumors including PCa (NCT00888108). However, the frequent pitfalls of such studies are the unselected population of patients and an empiric treatment sequence when the Bcl-2/Bcl-X$_L$ inhibitors are given in combination.

Clusterin

Preclinical data

Stress-induced prosurvival gene and cytoprotective chaperone networks are mechanisms involved in resistance to androgen deprivation therapy and chemotherapy in prostate and other cancers.[63,64] Secretory clusterin (sCLU) is a multifunctional, stress-induced, adenosine triphosphate (ATP)–independent molecular chaperone involved in many biologic processes ranging from mammary and prostate gland involution to amyloidosis and neurodegenerative disease, as well as cancer progression and treatment resistance.[65] sCLU functions to protect cells from many varied therapeutic stressors that induce apoptosis, including androgen or estrogen withdrawal, radiation, cytotoxic chemotherapy, and biologic agents.[66] sCLUs interact with stressed cell surface proteins to inhibit proapoptotic signal transduction (**Fig. 2**).[67] sCLU inhibits endoplasmic reticulum (ER) stress, retrotranslocating from the ER to the cytosol to inhibit aggregation of intracellular proteins and prevent apoptosis.[68] sCLU inhibits mitochondrial apoptosis by increasing Akt phosphorylation levels and NF-κB nuclear transactivation.

In localized human PCa, sCLU levels are low in low-grade, untreated, hormone-naive tissues, but increase with higher Gleason score[69] and within weeks after androgen deprivation.[70] sCLU expression correlates with loss of the tumor suppressor gene Nkx3.1 during the initial stages of prostate tumorigenesis in Nkx3.1 knockout mice.[71] In more advanced prostate cancer, sCLU levels increase following castration and in CRPC models. sCLU is associated with resistance to a broad variety of therapies including chemotherapy, radiation, and endocrine therapies including the second generation of antiandrogen.[70] Overall, sCLU functions as an antiapoptotic gene upregulated by treatment stress that confers therapeutic resistance when overexpressed.

OGX-011 (custirsen) is a second-generation 2′-methoxyethyl (MOE) gapmer phosphorothioate ASO with a long tissue half-life of ~7 days that targets the translation initiation site of human exon II CLU. OGX-011 potently suppresses sCLU levels in vitro and in vivo, improving efficacy of chemotherapy, radiation therapy, and hormonal therapy by enhancing stress-induced apoptosis and inhibiting epithelial–mesenchymal transition (EMT) in preclinical xenograft models of prostate, lung, renal cell, breast, and other cancers.[72,73]

Clinical data The first-in-human phase I study with OGX-011 used a novel neoadjuvant design to identify effective biologic dosing of OGX-011 to inhibit sCLU expression in human cancer.[74] In this dose-escalation study, cohorts of 3 to 6 patients with localized PCa were treated with neoadjuvant androgen deprivation plus OGX-011

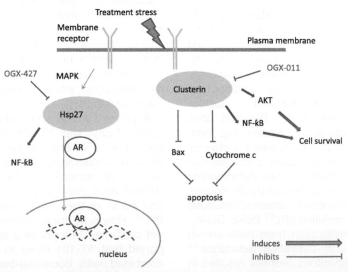

Fig. 2. Stress response pathway in prostate cancer. MAPK, mitogen-activated protein kinases; NFKB, nuclear factor kappa B.

in doses of up to 640 mg for 5 weeks before prostatectomy. The presurgery design was used to correlate changes in expression of sCLU to drug dose received and drug levels within the prostate tissue. In this study, treatment was well tolerated and, at doses of 320 mg and higher, high concentrations of full-length OGX-011 were achieved that were associated with preclinical activity. OGX-011 produced dose-dependent, greater than 90% knockdown of sCLU in normal and tumor tissue and increased apoptotic indices from 7.1% to 21.2%. Another phase I clinical trial combining OGX-011 with docetaxel showed that OGX-011 could be given at its full biologically effective single-agent dose of 640 mg with usual docetaxel schedules.[75] Toxic effects were primarily myelosuppression, fatigue, hair loss, gastrointestinal effects (expected docetaxel effects), as well as dose-related chills and fever (expected OGX-011 effects). OGX-011 had no effect on docetaxel pharmacokinetics. At the end of cycle 1, serum clusterin showed mean decreases of 34% and 38% (range, 15%–99%).

Randomized phase II studies were conducted in patients with CRPC because of limitations in interpreting antitumor responses of novel biologics when combined with chemotherapy.[76] Eighty-one patients with chemonaive, mCRPC were randomized to receive either docetaxel–OGX-011 or docetaxel alone.[77] There was evidence of pharmacodynamic effect with 18% decrease in mean serum sCLU in patients treated with docetaxel–OGX-011 versus 8% increase in controls ($P = .0005$). Median PFS was 7.3 months for docetaxel–OGX-011 and 6.1 months for the docetaxel-alone arm. Median OS on the docetaxel–OGX-011 arm was 23.8 months, ~7 months longer than those receiving docetaxel alone (16.9 months; HR = 0.49, $P = .012$), supporting ongoing phase III trial investigating OGX-011 in association with docetaxel in chemonaive patients (SYNERGY trial, NCT01188187).

Another phase II trial of docetaxel-recurrent CRPC randomized 42 patients to receive either docetaxel or mitoxantrone both combined with custirsen, suggested that custirsen could reverse docetaxel resistance or improve mitoxantrone efficacy in a chemoresistant population.[78] PSA declines of greater than or equal to 30% were seen in 55% of docetaxel-custirsen patients and 32% of mitoxantrone-custirsen patients. Pain responses were also seen in more than 50% of patients and, after a median follow-up of 13.3 months, 60% of patients were alive in both arms, supporting a phase III trial for second-line indication comparing cabazitaxel plus or minus OGX-011 in post–docetaxel-treated CRPC (AFFINITY trial, NCT01578655).

Hsp 27

Preclinical data

Hsp27 is an ATP-independent chaperone that is phosphoactivated by cell stress to maintain protein homeostasis and regulate activity of several transcriptional and signaling pathways, including AR,[79] insulinlike growth factor (IGF)-1,[80] and interleukin (IL)-6.[81] Higher levels of Hsp27 are commonly detected in many cancers, including prostate,[82] and is associated with metastasis, poor prognosis, and resistance to chemotherapy or radiation. Overexpression of Hsp27 in LNCaP cells suppressed castration-induced apoptosis and conferred androgen resistance.[83] OGX-427 is a second-generation ASO that inhibits expression of Hsp27. In vitro and in vivo pharmacologic studies have shown that OGX-427 has single-agent activity in reducing Hsp27 mRNA and protein, inhibiting cell proliferation, and inducing apoptosis in several human cancer cell lines.[83,84] OGX-427 also chemosensitizes several cytotoxic drugs, including docetaxel, to further delay tumor progression in vivo.[84] In vivo, OGX-427 induces downregulation of Hsp27 and AR protein levels, inducing rapid decreases in probasin-luciferase reporter–driven bioluminescence that correlated with early decreases in serum PSA and decreased LNCaP xenograft levels of AR and its chaperones, Hsp90 and Hsp27.[79]

Clinical data

In a phase I trial, OGX-427 was administered as a single agent in doses from 200 to 1000 mg with weekly infusions occurring after a loading dose period of 3 infusions within the first 10 days of initiating treatment.[85] OGX-427 treatment is well tolerated, with most adverse events and laboratory toxicities reported being grade 1 or grade 2, although a symptom complex of rigors, pruritus, and erythema during or shortly after infusion of drug has required steroid prophylaxis and/or treatment in some patients at higher doses. No maximum tolerated dose has been identified based on toxicity. OGX-427 is currently being assessed in a randomized phase II trial in patients with CRPC previously treated with docetaxel-based chemotherapy. Preliminary data on 22 chemonaive patients reported a PSA decline greater than or equal to 30% in 55% of patients and an acceptable safety profile.[86] In addition to pharmacokinetic and safety data, correlative studies using serial samples of circulating tumor cells (CTC) enumerated as an indicator of antitumor activity, as well as Hsp27 expression using immunofluorescence, were assessed. Decline of 50% or greater in both total and Hsp27+ CTCs were observed in more than half the patients in this phase I trial. Randomized phase II trials are ongoing in CRPC and bladder cancer.

TARGETING CELL INVASION
Targeting Met Kinase

Metastasis is one of the hallmarks of cancer. Growth and motility factor hepatocyte growth factor(HGF)/scatter factor (SF) and its receptor, the tyrosine kinase MET and Src, have been reported to play important roles in metastasis, thus providing a strong rationale for targeting these molecules in cancer. Hence, understanding the structure and function of HGF/SF, MET, and Src as well as associated signaling components has led to the successful development of blocking antibodies and a large number of small-molecule Met and Src kinase inhibitors with anticancer effects in several types of solid human tumors.

Preclinical data
Met is a receptor tyrosine kinase that is expressed in epithelial and endothelial cells. In normal cells, c-Met is activated by its ligand HGF/SF, which is produced by stromal cells such as fibroblasts, inducing a paracrine activation loop (**Fig. 3**).[87] Phosphorylated c-Met triggers the activation of downstream signaling pathways including the Ras-mitogen–activated protein kinase (MAPK) pathway, the phosphoinositide 3-kinases (PI3K)-Akt pathway. Both HGF and c-Met have been shown to regulate the metastatic process in many cancers.

MET and/or HGF overexpression are associated with prostate cancer metastasis, and, in preclinical studies, androgen ablation upregulated MET signaling, promoting tumor growth, invasion, and metastasis.[88,89]

Expression of c-Met is negatively regulated by androgens in AR-positive prostate cancer cells. The AR negatively regulates the c-Met promoter by repressing Sp1-induced c-Met promoter activity. AR interferes with Sp1 binding to the promoter region of c-Met. Knockdown of c-Met using specific c-Met siRNA inhibited the induction of c-Met expression by androgen depletion and repressed prostate cancer cell growth. These data were confirmed by in vivo data showing that castration induced the expression of c-Met expression in LNCaP cell xenografts.[89] Overexpression or gene alterations of c-Met are infrequent in nonadvanced prostate cancer but activation of c-Met pathway in PCa results from ligand-dependent mechanisms through a paracrine mode.[90] A growing body of evidence suggests that the Met pathway plays a critical role in advanced prostate cancers. Increased serum level of HGF is an independent prognostic indicator in patients with advanced-stage prostate cancer.[90–92] In addition, Met protein expression is observed more often in metastatic lesions than in primary tumors, with 100% of prostate bone metastases being Met positive.[90] These data support the inhibition of the activation of both HGF/c-Met and AR signaling pathways in the treatment of advanced PCa.

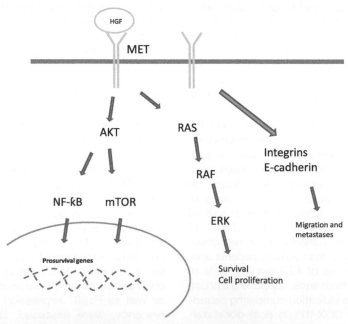

Fig. 3. MET pathway in prostate cancer. ERK, extracellular-signal-regulated kinases.

Preclinical data from Met inhibitors in prostate cancer

The role of the HGF/c-Met axis in promoting metastatic growth of PCa cells in the bone led to the testing of Met signaling pathway inhibitors in patients with mCRPC using small tyrosine kinase inhibitors and monoclonal antibodies.

BMS-777607, a selective and potent small-molecule Met kinase inhibitor, had little effect on tumor cell growth but inhibited cell scattering activated by exogenous HGF, and suppressed HGF-stimulated cell migration and invasion in Met-expressing PCa cell lines.[93] BMS-777607 blocked HGF-stimulated c-Met autophosphorylation and downstream activation of Akt and MAPK pathway. Cabozantinib (XL184) is an oral small-molecule inhibitor of multiple kinase signaling pathways, including MET, RET, VEGFR2/KDR, and KIT.[94] Cabozantinib is a potent inhibitor of Met and VEGFR2 with inhibitory concentration of 50% (IC_{50}) values of ~1 nmol/L and 0.03 nmol/L respectively. Met-activating kinase domain mutations Y1248H, D1246N, or K1262R are inhibited by cabozantinib as well as several kinases that have also been implicated in tumor oncogenesis, including KIT, RET, AXL, TIE2, and FLT3.

Treatment with cabozantinib inhibited Met and VEGFR2 phosphorylation in vitro and in tumor models in vivo, and led to significant reduction in cell invasion in vitro. In mouse models, cabozantinib decreased tumor and endothelial cell proliferation coupled with increased apoptosis and dose-dependent inhibition of tumor growth in breast, lung, and glioma tumor models.[94]

The c-Met inhibitors PHA-665752 and PF-2341066 decrease proliferation of AR-negative prostate cancer PC3 and DU145 cells as well as AR-positive PCa LNCaP and C4-2 cells.[95] PF-2341066 also suppressed growth of AR-positive, androgen-insensitive prostate cancer cells in xenograft mouse models.[95] Additional data showed that c-met inhibitor represses prostate cancer cell growth during progression of AR-positive prostate tumors in castrated mice. A significant 85% reduction in proliferation was observed when comparing PF-2341066–treated castrated mice versus control castrated mice using an LNCaP orthotopic model. This finding suggests that targeting of c-Met signaling in combination with androgen deprivation therapy may delay development of castration-resistant tumors.[95]

Clinical data

Phase I trial showed that cabozantinib has a manageable safety profile with angiogenic class-effect toxicities.[96] Preliminary data from a phase II randomized discontinuation trial assessing the efficacy and safety of cabozantinib in patients with measurable CRPC with or without bone metastases that had progressed after systemic chemotherapy were presented at the 2011 meeting of the American Society of Clinical Oncology.[97] Of 171 assessable patients, 43% had received prior docetaxel and 87% had bone metastases. At 12 weeks, 4% of patients had a confirmed tumor response and 79% had stable disease (SD). Of patients with measurable soft tissue lesions and at least 1 postbaseline assessment, 74% showed some evidence of tumor regression and randomization was suspended. Cabozantinib significantly improved median PFS compared with placebo (21 vs 6 weeks, respectively; HR 0.13; $P = .0007$). Median postrandomization PFS was 29 weeks in docetaxel-naive patients (n = 90) and 24 weeks in docetaxel-pretreated patients (n = 64). Of 108 patients assessable by bone scan, 75% had complete or partial resolution and 21% had stable scans. Of 83 patients with painful bone metastases, 67% had improved bone pain. Most patients had reductions in bone markers. However, there is currently a lack of functional data (changes in markers indicating bone metabolic or antitumor effects) that could explain the improved bone scans seen with cabozantinib. The most common toxicities with cabozantinib were fatigue (63%), decreased appetite (49%), diarrhea (46%), nausea (44%), and constipation (31%). Further phase III trials will be conducted both in chemonaive and chemotherapy-treated patients with CRPC.

Targeting Src Kinase

Src signaling

Src is a membrane-associated nonreceptor tyrosine kinase belonging to the Src family kinase group (SFK) including Lyn, Fyn, and Lck (**Fig. 4**).[98] SFK regulated signaling from transmembrane receptor-associated tyrosine kinases such as EGFR, PDGF, HER2, or IGF-1R leading to activation of intracellular

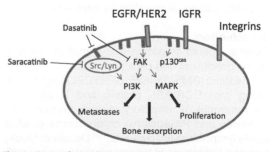

Fig. 4. Src pathway in prostate cancer. EGFR, epidermal growth factor receptor; FAK, focal adhesion kinase; HER2, human epidermal growth factor receptor 2.

target proteins. SFK phosphorylated key cellular components resulting in the activation of oncogenic signal transduction pathways in various human cancers. Focal adhesion kinase and Crk-associated substrate (p130^{CAS}) are 2 important substrates of SFKs and regulate cell adhesion, migration, and invasion (see **Fig. 4**). Src signaling is also involved in tumor cell proliferation and survival, in part via cell surface receptors such as EGFR, HER2, and IGF-1R, and Src inhibition leads to decreased proliferation and invasion of prostate and other cancer cell lines.

Of particular relevance to bone-specific metastatic cancers like prostate, Src kinase signaling pathways have been shown to promote osseous prostate cancer metastases by promoting bone activity. High Src activity has been found in mature osteoclast and Src activity inhibition prevents osteoclast formation. Furthermore, disruption of Src activity activates osteoblast proliferation and differentiation.[98]

A higher Src activity is also associated with CRPC and transition to castrate-resistant growth. Some studies show that Src is involved in AR transactivation after hormone deprivation.[99] Src inhibition has been found to block castrate-resistant growth in prostate cancer both in vitro and in vivo.[100] Increased phospho-Src (pSrc) was also recently associated with MDV3100 resistance in a prospective cohort assessing biomarkers of response to MDV3100 in bone metastases. Among men achieving a decrease in PSA of greater than 50% on MDV3100, mean pSrc expression was 10% (range 0%–30%), and more than 70% (range 0%–90%) for patients failing to having a decrease in PSA greater than 50% (P = .002).[101]

Src activity is also correlated with invasion and metastatic potential in prostate cancer.[102,103] Src inhibition suppresses prostate cancer cell migration in preclinical studies both in vitro and in vivo. Taken together, these data suggest that the Src signaling pathway is involved in many cellular processes leading to metastasis formation in prostate cancer, supporting its inhibition.

Src inhibitors

Several agents targeting Src signaling are now under preclinical and clinical evaluation.

Dasatinib (BMS-354825, SPRYCEL) targets SFK along with BCR-ABL protein and is approved for treatment of refractory chronic myelogenous leukemia and Philadelphia chromosome–positive acute lymphoblastic leukemia.[104] Dasatinib blocks Lyn and Src kinase in human prostate cancer cells at low (nanomolar) concentrations.[105] Moreover, focal adhesion kinase and p130^{CAS} signaling

downstream of SFKs are also inhibited. Dasatinib consequently suppresses cell adhesion, migration, and invasion of prostate cancer cells in vitro and in vivo, reducing growth and formation of lymph node metastases in androgen-sensitive and androgen-resistant tumors.[106] In a C42B orthotopic mouse model of prostate bone tumors, dasatinib decreased PSA, increased bone mineral density, decreased serum calcium, and potentiated the activity of docetaxel chemotherapy.[107] In bone resorption assays, dasatinib reduced osteoclast proliferation and calcium release. Some preclinical findings support cotargeting dasatinib with other pathways in prostate cancer; for example, IGF-1R pathway blockade might enhance antitumor activity from Src inhibition through PI3K inhibition.[108]

Saracatinib (AZD0530) is an inhibitor of Src and SFKs.[109] Saracatinib blocked osteoclast activation both in vitro and in vivo.[110] Furthermore, migration of osteoclast precursor cells to the bone surface was inhibited, reducing bone resorption.[110] These data were confirmed by in vivo studies that showed saracatinib decreased the formation of osteolytic lesions from tumor cells[111] and showed antitumor activity by blocking proliferation and invasion in both in vitro and in vivo prostate cancer models.[112,113]

These preclinical data supported further clinical investigations of Src inhibitors (mainly dasatinib) in CRPC.

Clinical data

Dasatinib was assessed in a phase II trial enrolling chemotherapy-naive men with CRPC. End points included changes in PSA responses, bone scans, measurable disease, and also markers of bone metabolism, namely urinary N-telopeptide (uNTX) and bone alkaline phosphatase, which are markers of osteoblastic and osteoclastic activity, respectively. Forty-seven patients were enrolled and received dasatinib dosed at either 100 mg or 70 mg twice daily.[114] Dasatinib was generally well tolerated and treatment-related adverse events were moderate. Lack of progression was achieved in 20 (43%) patients at week 12. Only 3 patients (6%) had a PSA decline greater than or equal to 50%. Of 41 evaluable patients, 21 (51%) had greater than or equal to 40% reduction in urinary N-telopeptide by week 12. Of 15 patients with increased urinary N-telopeptide at baseline, 8 (53%) normalized on study. Of 40 evaluable patients, 24 (60%) had reduction in bone alkaline phosphatase at week 12. In an expansion of phase II study evaluating safety and efficacy of 100 mg once-daily dasatinib, a lack of disease progression was observed in 21 of 48 patients (44%) at week

12 and in 8 (17%) at week 24. Urine N-telopeptide was reduced by greater than or equal to 40% from baseline in 22 (51%) of 43 patients, and bone alkaline phosphatase was decreased in 26 (59%) of 44 patients. The most common treatment-related adverse events (≥20%) were fatigue, nausea, diarrhea, headache, and anorexia.[115]

Promising activity was also reported in phase 1/2 combining dasatinib with docetaxel in men with chemonaive CRPC. Combination dasatinib and docetaxel therapy was generally well tolerated. Thirteen of 46 patients (28%) had a grade 3 to 4 toxicity. Durable 50% PSA declines occurred in 26 of 46 patients (57%). Of 30 patients with measurable disease, 18 (60%) had a PR and 14 patients (30%) had disappearance of a lesion on bone scan. Regarding bone marker evaluations, 33 of 38 (87%) and 26 of 34 (76%) had decreases in urinary N-telopeptide or bone-specific alkaline phosphatase levels, respectively.[116] A large, international, randomized, phase III trial has been conducted investigating dasatinib in combination with docetaxel in chemonaive patients with mCRPC and is now closed for inclusions and the results are pending. Dasatinib was also assessed in the postdocetaxel state but was poorly tolerated and had limited efficacy in a phase 2 clinical trial.[117]

Saracatinib has also been investigated in phase 1/2 trials in PCa. The phase I clinical trial reported a good safety profile with some clinical activity in various solid tumors and a maximal tolerated dose of 175 mg once daily.[118] The most common events greater than or equal to grade 3 were anemia, diarrhea, and asthenia. Tumor Src activity was reduced following saracatinib treatment. In a phase 2 trial of 28 patients with mCRPC, saracatinib was well tolerated and although 5 of 28 patients had PSA decline, no bone effects were reported in this trial. Saracatinib is currently in a randomized phase II trial evaluation in patients with CRPC previously treated with docetaxel.

SUMMARY

Many pathways involved in cell survival or bone metastases, in addition to the AR pathway, are currently being targeted in late-stage clinical trials supported by strong a biologic rationale and pre-clinical data. In the coming years, the interactions between basic and clinical researchers will be critical for designing new combinations for improving maximum inhibition of CRPC progression.

REFERENCES

1. La Vecchia C, Bosetti C, Lucchini F, et al. Cancer mortality in Europe, 2000–2004, and an overview of trends since 1975. Ann Oncol 2010;21:1323–60.
2. Jemal A, Siegel R, Xu J, et al. Cancer statistics. CA Cancer J Clin 2010;60:277–300.
3. Nelson WG, De Marzo AM, Isaacs WB. Prostate cancer. N Engl J Med 2003;349:366–81.
4. Attard G, Sarker D, Reid A, et al. Improving the outcome of patients with castration-resistant prostate cancer through rational drug development. Br J Cancer 2006;95:767–74.
5. Chen Y, Clegg NJ, Scher HI. Anti-androgens and androgen-depleting therapies in prostate cancer: new agents for an established target. Lancet Oncol 2009;10:981–91.
6. Attard G, Reid AH, Yap TA, et al. Phase I clinical trial of a selective inhibitor of CYP17, abiraterone acetate, confirms that castration-resistant prostate cancer commonly remains hormone driven. J Clin Oncol 2008;26:4563–71.
7. Scher HI, Beer TM, Higano CS, et al. Antitumour activity of MDV3100 in castration-resistant prostate cancer: a phase 1–2 study. Lancet 2010;375:1437–46.
8. Hanahan D, Weinberg RA. Hallmarks of cancer: the next generation. Cell 2011;144:646–74.
9. Kavallaris M. Microtubules and resistance to tubulin-binding agents. Nat Rev Cancer 2010;10: 194–204.
10. Darshan MS, Loftus MS, Thadani-Mulero M, et al. Taxane-induced blockade to nuclear accumulation of the androgen receptor predicts clinical responses in metastatic prostate cancer. Cancer Res 2011;71:6019–29.
11. Zhu ML, Horbinski CM, Garzotto M, et al. Tubulin-targeting chemotherapy impairs androgen receptor activity in prostate cancer. Cancer Res 2010;70: 7992–8002.
12. Petrylak DP, Tangen CM, Hussain MH, et al. Docetaxel and estramustine compared with mitoxantrone and prednisone for advanced refractory prostate cancer. N Engl J Med 2004;351: 1513–20.
13. Tannock IF, de Wit R, Berry WR, et al. Docetaxel plus prednisone or mitoxantrone plus prednisone for advanced prostate cancer. N Engl J Med 2004;351:1502–12.
14. Seruga B, Tannock IF. Chemotherapy-based treatment for castration-resistant prostate cancer. J Clin Oncol 2011;29:3686–94.
15. Marín-Aguilera M, Codony-Servat J, Kalko SG, et al. Identification of docetaxel resistance genes in castration-resistant prostate cancer. Mol Cancer Ther 2012;11:329–39.
16. Al Nakouzi N, Gaudin C, Delbruel L, et al. Molecular determinants of docetaxel-resistance in prostate cancer cells. AACR Meeting Abstracts 2009; 2009:2944.
17. Mita AC, Denis LJ, Rowinsky EK, et al. Phase I and pharmacokinetic study of XRP6258 (RPR 116258A), a novel taxane, administered as a 1-hour infusion

every 3 weeks in patients with advanced solid tumors. Clin Cancer Res 2009;15:723–30.

18. Pivot X, Koralewski P, Hidalgo JL, et al. A multicenter phase II study of XRP6258 administered as a 1-h I.V. infusion every 3 weeks in taxane-resistant metastatic breast cancer patients. Ann Oncol 2008;19:1547–52.

19. de Bono JS, Oudard S, Ozguroglu M, et al, TROPIC Investigators. Prednisone plus cabazitaxel or mitoxantrone for metastatic castration-resistant prostate cancer progressing after docetaxel treatment: a randomised open-label trial. Lancet 2010; 376:1147–54.

20. Lee JJ, Kelly WK. Epothilones: tubulin polymerization as a novel target for prostate cancer therapy. Nat Clin Pract Oncol 2009;6:85–92.

21. Orr GA, Verdier-Pinard P, McDaid H, et al. Mechanisms of Taxol resistance related to microtubules. Oncogene 2003;22:7280–95.

22. Altmann KH, Wartmann M, O'Reilly T. Epothilones and related structures–a new class of microtubule inhibitors with potent in vivo antitumor activity. Biochim Biophys Acta 2000;1470:M79–91.

23. O'Reilly T, McSheehy PM, Wenger F, et al. Patupilone (epothilone B, EPO906) inhibits growth and metastasis of experimental prostate tumors in vivo. Prostate 2005;65:231–40.

24. Chou TC, Dong H, Zhang X, et al. Therapeutic cure against human tumor xenografts in nude mice by a microtubule stabilization agent, fludelone, via parenteral or oral route. Cancer Res 2005;65:9445–54.

25. Pivot X, Dufresne A, Villanueva C. Efficacy and safety of ixabepilone, a novel epothilone analogue. Clin Breast Cancer 2007;7:543–9.

26. Hoffmann J, Vitale I, Buchmann B, et al. Improved cellular pharmacokinetics and pharmacodynamics underlie the wide anticancer activity of sagopilone. Cancer Res 2008;68:5301–8.

27. Galsky MD, Small EJ, Oh WK, et al. Multi-national randomized phase II trial of the epothilone B analog ixabepilone (BMS-247550) with or without estramustine phosphate in patients with progressive castrate metastatic prostate cancer. J Clin Oncol 2005;23:1439–46.

28. Hussain M, Tangen CM, Lara PN, et al. Ixabepilone (epothilone B analogue BMS-247550) is active in chemotherapy-naïve patients with hormone-refractory prostate cancer: a Southwest Oncology Group Trial S0111. J Clin Oncol 2005; 23:8724–9.

29. Rosenberg JE, Ryan CJ, Weinberg VK, et al. Phase I study of ixabepilone, mitoxantrone, and prednisone in patients with metastatic castration-resistant prostate cancer previously treated with docetaxel-based therapy: a study of the department of defense prostate cancer clinical trials consortium. J Clin Oncol 2009;27:2772–8.

30. Rosenberg JE, Weinberg VK, Kelly WK, et al. Activity of second-line chemotherapy in docetaxel-refractory hormone-refractory prostate cancer patients: randomized phase 2 study of ixabepilone or mitoxantrone and prednisone. Cancer 2007;110: 556–63.

31. Harzstark AL, Rosenberg JE, Weinberg VK, et al. Ixabepilone, mitoxantrone, and prednisone for metastatic castration-resistant prostate cancer after docetaxel-based therapy: a phase 2 study of the department of defense prostate cancer clinical trials consortium. Cancer 2011;117: 2419–25.

32. Chi KN, Beardsley E, Eigl BJ, et al. A phase 2 study of patupilone in patients with metastatic castration-resistant prostate cancer previously treated with docetaxel: Canadian Urologic Oncology Group study P07a. Ann Oncol 2012;23:53–8.

33. Graff J, Smith DC, Neerkonch L, et al. Phase II study of sagopilone (ZK-EPO) plus prednisone as first-line chemotherapy in patients with metastatic androgen-independent prostate cancer (AIPC) [abstract]. J Clin Oncol 2008;26(May 20 Suppl): 5141.

34. Bryant HE, Schultz N, Thomas HD, et al. Specific killing of BRCA2-deficient tumours with inhibitors of poly(ADP-ribose) polymerase. Nature 2005; 434:913–7.

35. Farmer H, McCabe N, Lord CJ, et al. Targeting the DNA repair defect in BRCA mutant cells as a therapeutic strategy. Nature 2005;434:917–21.

36. Gelmon KA, Tischkowitz M, Mackay H, et al. Olaparib in patients with recurrent high-grade serous or poorly differentiated ovarian carcinoma or triple-negative breast cancer: a phase 2, multicentre, open-label, non-randomised study. Lancet Oncol 2011;12:852–61.

37. Olaussen KA, Dunant A, Fouret P, et al. DNA repair by ERCC1 in non-small-cell lung cancer and cisplatin-based adjuvant chemotherapy. N Engl J Med 2006;355:983–91.

38. Kamal NS, Soria JC, Mendiboure J, et al, International Adjuvant Lung Trial-Bio Investigators. MutS homologue 2 and the long-term benefit of adjuvant chemotherapy in lung cancer. Clin Cancer Res 2010;16:1206–15.

39. Bellmunt J, Paz-Ares L, Cuello M, et al. ERCC1 as a novel prognostic marker in advanced bladder cancer patients receiving cisplatin-based chemotherapy. Ann Oncol 2007;18:522–8.

40. Kote-Jarai Z, Leongamornlert D, Saunders E, et al. BRCA2 is a moderate penetrance gene contributing to young-onset prostate cancer: implications for genetic testing in prostate cancer patients. Br J Cancer 2011;105:1230–4.

41. Gallagher DJ, Gaudet MM, Pal P, et al. Germline BRCA mutations denote a clinicopathologic subset

of prostate cancer. Clin Cancer Res 2010;16: 2115–21.

42. Nakabayashi M, Sartor O, Jacobus S, et al. Response to docetaxel/carboplatin-based chemotherapy as first- and second-line therapy in patients with metastatic hormone-refractory prostate cancer. BJU Int 2008;101:308–12.

43. Ross RW, Beer TM, Jacobus S, et al, Prostate Cancer Clinical Trials Consortium. A phase 2 study of carboplatin plus docetaxel in men with metastatic hormone-refractory prostate cancer who are refractory to docetaxel. Cancer 2008;112:521–6.

44. Sternberg CN, Petrylak DP, Sartor O, et al. Multinational, double-blind, phase III study of prednisone and either satraplatin or placebo in patients with castrate-refractory prostate cancer progressing after prior chemotherapy: the SPARC trial. J Clin Oncol 2009;27:5431–8.

45. Loriot Y, Massard C, Gross-Goupil M, et al. Combining carboplatin and etoposide in docetaxel-pretreated patients with castration-resistant prostate cancer: a prospective study evaluating also neuroendocrine features. Ann Oncol 2009;20:703–8.

46. Gallagher DJ, Cronin AM, Milowsky MI, et al. Germline BRCA mutation does not prevent response to taxane-based therapy for the treatment of castration-resistant prostate cancer. BJU Int 2012; 109:713–9.

47. Tomlins SA, Rhodes DR, Perner S, et al. Recurrent fusion of TMPRSS2 and ETS transcription factor genes in prostate cancer. Science 2005;310:644–8.

48. King JC, Xu J, Wongvipat J, et al. Cooperativity of TMPRSS2-ERG with PI3-kinase pathway activation in prostate oncogenesis. Nat Genet 2009;41: 524–6.

49. Haffner MC, Aryee MJ, Toubaji A, et al. Androgen-induced TOP2B-mediated double-strand breaks and prostate cancer gene rearrangements. Nat Genet 2010;42:668–75.

50. Brenner JC, Ateeq B, Li Y, et al. Mechanistic rationale for inhibition of poly(ADP-ribose) polymerase in ETS gene fusion-positive prostate cancer. Cancer Cell 2011;19:664–78.

51. Fong PC, Boss DS, Yap TA, et al. Inhibition of poly(ADP-ribose) polymerase in tumors from BRCA mutation carriers. N Engl J Med 2009;361:123–34.

52. Hussain M, Carducci MA, Slovin SF, et al. Pilot study of veliparib (ABT-888) with temozolomide (TMZ) in patients (pts) with metastatic castration-resistant prostate cancer (mCRPC) [abstract: 224]. J Clin Oncol 2012;30(Suppl 5).

53. Galluzzi L, Larochette N, Zamzami N, et al. Mitochondria as therapeutic targets for cancer chemotherapy. Oncogene 2006;25:4812–30.

54. McDonnell TJ, Troncoso P, Brisbay SM, et al. Expression of the protooncogene bcl-2 in the prostate and its association with emergence of

androgen-independent prostate cancer. Cancer Res 1992;52:6940–4.

55. Banerjee D. Technology evaluation: G-3139. Curr Opin Mol Ther 1999;1:404–8.

56. Benimetskaya L, Miller P, Benimetsky S, et al. Inhibition of potentially anti-apoptotic proteins by antisense protein kinase C-alpha (Isis 3521) and antisense bcl-2 (G3139) phosphorothioate oligodeoxynucleotides: relationship to the decreased viability of T24 bladder and PC3 prostate cancer cells. Mol Pharmacol 2001;60:1296–307.

57. Oltersdorf T, Elmore SW, Shoemaker AR, et al. An inhibitor of Bcl-2 family proteins induces regression of solid tumours. Nature 2005;435:677–81.

58. Bray K, Chen HY, Karp CM, et al. Bcl-2 modulation to activate apoptosis in prostate cancer. Mol Cancer Res 2009;7:1487–96.

59. Tolcher AW, Kuhn J, Schwartz G, et al. A phase I pharmacokinetic and biological correlative study of oblimersen sodium (Genasense, g3139), an antisense oligonucleotide to the bcl-2 mRNA, and of docetaxel in patients with hormone-refractory prostate cancer. Clin Cancer Res 2004;10:5048–57.

60. Sternberg CN, Dumez H, Van Poppel H, et al. Docetaxel plus oblimersen sodium (Bcl-2 antisense oligonucleotide): an EORTC multicenter, randomized phase II study in patients with castration-resistant prostate cancer. Ann Oncol 2009;20: 1264–9.

61. Liu G, Kelly WK, Wilding G, et al. An open-label, multicenter, phase I/II study of single-agent AT-101 in men with castrate-resistant prostate cancer. Clin Cancer Res 2009;15:3172–6.

62. Sonpavde G, Matveev V, Burke JM, et al. Randomized phase II trial of docetaxel plus prednisone in combination with placebo or AT-101, an oral small molecule Bcl-2 family antagonist, as first-line therapy for metastatic castration-resistant prostate cancer. Ann Oncol 2012;23:1803–8.

63. Rocchi P, So A, Kojima S, et al. Heat shock protein 27 increases after androgen ablation and plays a cytoprotective role in hormone-refractory prostate cancer. Cancer Res 2004;64: 6595–602.

64. Miyake H, Nelson C, Rennie PS, et al. Testosterone-repressed prostate message-2 is an antiapoptotic gene involved in progression to androgen independence in prostate cancer. Cancer Res 2000; 60:170–6.

65. Gleave M, Miyake H, Zangemeister-Wittke U, et al. Antisense therapy: current status in prostate cancer and other malignancies. Cancer Metastasis Rev 2002;21:79–92.

66. Zellweger T, Miyake H, July LV, et al. Chemosensitization of human renal cell cancer using antisense oligonucleotides targeting the antiapoptotic gene clusterin. Neoplasia 2001;3:360–7.

67. Carver JA, Rekas A, Thorn DC, et al. Small heat-shock proteins and clusterin: intra- and extra-cellular molecular chaperones with a common mechanism of action and function? IUBMB Life 2003;55:661–8.

68. Nizard P, Tetley S, Le Drean Y, et al. Stress-induced retrotranslocation of clusterin/ApoJ into the cytosol. Traffic 2007;8:554–65.

69. Steinberg J, Oyasu R, Lang S, et al. Intracellular levels of SGP-2 (clusterin) correlate with tumor grade in prostate cancer. Clin Cancer Res 1997;3:1707–11.

70. July LV, Akbari M, Zellweger T, et al. Clusterin expression is significantly enhanced in prostate cancer cells following androgen withdrawal therapy. Prostate 2002;50:179–88.

71. Song H, Zhang B, Watson MA, et al. Loss of Nkx3.1 leads to the activation of discrete downstream target genes during prostate tumorigenesis. Onco-gene 2009;28:3307–19.

72. Sowery RD, Hadaschik BA, So AI, et al. Clusterin knockdown using the antisense oligonucleotide OGX-011 re-sensitizes docetaxel-refractory pros-tate cancer PC-3 cells to chemotherapy. BJU Int 2008;102:389–97.

73. Gleave M, Miyake H. Use of antisense oligonucleo-tides targeting the cytoprotective gene, clusterin, to enhance androgen- and chemo-sensitivity in prostate cancer. World J Urol 2005;23:38–46.

74. Chi KN, Eisenhauer E, Fazli L, et al. A phase I pharmacokinetic and pharmacodynamic study of OGX-011, a 2′-methoxyethyl antisense oligonucle-otide to clusterin, in patients with localized prostate cancer. J Natl Cancer Inst 2005;97:1287–96.

75. Chi KN, Siu LL, Hirte H, et al. A phase I study of OGX-011, a 2′-methoxyethyl phosphorothioate antisense to clusterin, in combination with docetax-el in patients with advanced cancer. Clin Cancer Res 2008;14:833–9.

76. Scher HI, Halabi S, Tannock I, et al. Design and end points of clinical trials for patients with pro-gressive prostate cancer and castrate levels of testosterone: recommendations of the Prostate Cancer Clinical Trials Working Group. J Clin Oncol 2008;26:1148–59.

77. Chi KN, Hotte SJ, Yu EY, et al. Randomized phase II study of docetaxel and prednisone with or without OGX-011 in patients with metastatic castration-resistant prostate cancer. J Clin Oncol 2010;28:4247–54.

78. Saad F, Hotte S, North S. Randomized phase II trial of custirsen (OGX-011) in combination with docetaxel or mitoxantrone as second-line therapy in patients with metastatic castrate-resistant prostate cancer pro-gressing after first-line docetaxel: CUOG trial P-06c. Clin Cancer Res 2011;17:5765–73.

79. Zoubeidi A, Zardan A, Beraldi E, et al. Cooperative interactions between androgen receptor (AR) and heat-shock protein 27 facilitate AR transcriptional activity. Cancer Res 2007;67:10455–65.

80. Zoubeidi A, Zardan A, Wiedmann RM, et al. Hsp27 promotes insulin-like growth factor-I survival signaling in prostate cancer via p90Rsk-dependent phosphorylation and inactivation of BAD [Erratum appears in Cancer Res 2011;71:5054]. Cancer Res 2010;70:2307–17.

81. Kato K, Tokuda H, Mizutani J, et al. Role of HSP27 in tumor necrosis factor-α-stimulated interleukin-6 synthesis in osteoblasts. Int J Mol Med 2011;28: 887–93.

82. Cornford PA, Dodson AR, Parsons KF, et al. Heat shock protein expression independently predicts clinical outcome in prostate cancer. Cancer Res 2000;60:7099.

83. Rocchi P, Jugpal P, So A, et al. Small interference RNA targeting heat-shock protein 27 inhibits the growth of prostatic cell lines and induces apoptosis via caspase-3 activation in vitro. BJU Int 2006;98:1082–9.

84. Andrieu C, Taieb D, Baylot V, et al. Heat shock protein 27 confers resistance to androgen ablation and chemotherapy in prostate cancer cells through eIF4E. Oncogene 2010;29:1883–96.

85. Hotte SJ, Yu EY, Hirte HY, et al. Phase I trial of OGX-427, a 2′methoxyethyl antisense oligonucleo-tide (ASO), against heat shock protein 27 (Hsp27): final results [abstract: 3077]. J Clin Oncol 2010; 28(Suppl):15s.

86. Chi KN, Hotte SJ, Ellard S, et al. A randomized phase II study of OGX-427 plus prednisone versus predni-sone alone in patients with chemotherapy-naive metastatic castration-resistant prostate cancer [abstract: 121]. J Clin Oncol 2012;30(Suppl 5).

87. Cecchi F, Rabe DC, Bottaro DP. Targeting the HGF/Met signalling pathway in cancer. Eur J Cancer 2010;46:1260–70.

88. Davies G, Watkins G, Mason MD, et al. Targeting the HGF/SF receptor c-met using a hammerhead ribozyme transgene reduces in vitro invasion and migration in prostate cancer cells. Prostate 2004; 60:317–24.

89. Verras M, Lee J, Xue H, et al. The androgen receptor negatively regulates the expression of c-Met: impli-cations for a novel mechanism of prostate cancer progression. Cancer Res 2007;67:967–75.

90. Humphrey PA, Zhu X, Zarnegar R, et al. Hepato-cyte growth factor and its receptor (c-MET) in pros-tatic carcinoma. Am J Pathol 1995;147:386–96.

91. Gupta A, Karakiewicz PI, Roehrborn CG, et al. Predic-tive value of plasma hepatocyte growth factor/scatter factor levels in patients with clinically localized pros-tate cancer. Clin Cancer Res 2008;14:7385–90.

92. Yasuda K, Nagakawa O, Akashi T, et al. Serum active hepatocyte growth factor (AHGF) in benign prostatic disease and prostate cancer. Prostate 2009;69:346–51.

93. Dai Y, Siemann DW. BMS-777607, a small-molecule met kinase inhibitor, suppresses hepatocyte growth factor-stimulated prostate cancer metastatic phenotype in vitro. Mol Cancer Ther 2010;9:1554–61.

94. Yakes FM, Chen J, Tan J, et al. Cabozantinib (XL184), a novel MET and VEGFR2 inhibitor, simultaneously suppresses metastasis, angiogenesis, and tumor growth. Mol Cancer Ther 2011;10:2298–308.

95. Tu WH, Zhu C, Clark C, et al. Efficacy of c-Met inhibitor for advanced prostate cancer. BMC Cancer 2010;10:556.

96. Salgia R, Hong S, Sherman S, et al. A phase 1 dose-escalation study of the safety and pharmacokinetics (PK) of XL184, a VEGFR and MET kinase inhibitor, administered orally to patients (pts) with advanced malignancies. AACR-NCI-EORTC International Conference: Molecular Targets and Cancer Therapeutics. San Francisco, October 22–26, 2007, A152.

97. Hussain M, Smith MR, Sweeney C, et al. Cabozantinib (XL184) in metastatic castration-resistant prostate cancer (mCRPC): results from a phase II randomized discontinuation trial [abstract: 4516]. J Clin Oncol 2011;29(Suppl).

98. Saylor PJ, Lee RJ, Smith MR. Emerging therapies to prevent skeletal morbidity in men with prostate cancer. J Clin Oncol 2011;29:3705–14.

99. Asim M, Siddiqui IA, Hafeez BB, et al. Src kinase potentiates androgen receptor transactivation function and invasion of androgen-independent prostate cancer C4-2 cells. Oncogene 2008;27:3596–604.

100. Cai H, Babic I, Wei X, et al. Invasive prostate carcinoma driven by c-Src and androgen receptor synergy. Cancer Res 2011;71:862–72.

101. Efstathiou E, Titus MA, Tsavachidou D, et al. MDV3100 effects on androgen receptor (AR) signaling and bone marrow testosterone concentration modulation: a preliminary report [abstract: 4501]. J Clin Oncol 2011;29(Suppl).

102. Rice L, Lepler S, Pampo C, et al. Impact of the SRC inhibitor dasatinib on the metastatic phenotype of human prostate cancer cells. Clin Exp Metastasis 2012;29:133–42.

103. Cai H, Smith DA, Memarzadeh S, et al. Differential transformation capacity of Src family kinases during the initiation of prostate cancer. Proc Natl Acad Sci U S A 2011;108:6579–84.

104. Lombardo LJ, Lee FY, Chen P, et al. Discovery of N-(2-chloro-6-methyl- phenyl)-2-(6-(4-(2-hydroxyethyl)-piperazin-1-yl)-2-methylpyrimidin-4-ylamino)thiazole-5-carboxamide (BMS-354825), a dual Src/Abl kinase inhibitor with potent antitumor activity in preclinical assays. J Med Chem 2004;47:6658–61.

105. Tatarov O, Mitchell TJ, Seywright M, et al. SRC family kinase activity is up-regulated in hormone-refractory prostate cancer. Clin Cancer Res 2009;15:3540–9.

106. Park SI, Zhang J, Phillips KA, et al. Targeting SRC family kinases inhibits growth and lymph node metastases of prostate cancer in an orthotopic nude mouse model. Cancer Res 2008;68:3323–33.

107. Koreckij T, Nguyen H, Brown LG, et al. Targeting SRC family kinases inhibits growth and lymph node metastases of prostate cancer in an orthotopic nude mouse model. Br J Cancer 2009;101:263–8.

108. Dayyani F, Parikh N, Song JH, et al. Effect of dual inhibition of the Src and insulin-like growth factor-1 receptor (IGF-1R) pathways on antitumor effects in prostate cancer (PCa) [abstract: e15004]. J Clin Oncol 2011;29(Suppl).

109. Hennequin LF, Allen J, Breed J, et al. N-(5-chloro-1, 3-benzodioxol-4-yl)-7-[2-(4-methylpiperazin-1-yl) ethoxy]-5-(tetrahydro-2H-pyran-4-yloxy)quinazolin-4-amine, a novel, highly selective, orally available, dual-specific c-Src/Abl kinase inhibitor. J Med Chem 2006;49:6465–88.

110. de Vries TJ, Mullender MG, van Duin MA, et al. The Src inhibitor AZD0530 reversibly inhibits the formation and activity of human osteoclasts. Mol Cancer Res 2009;7:476–88.

111. Yang JC, Bai L, Yap S, et al. Effect of the specific Src family kinase inhibitor saracatinib on osteolytic lesions using the PC-3 bone model. Mol Cancer Ther 2010;9:1629–37.

112. Yang JC, Ok JH, Busby JE, et al. Aberrant activation of androgen receptor in a new neuropeptide autocrine model of androgen-insensitive prostate cancer. Cancer Res 2009;69:151–60.

113. Chang YM, Bai L, Liu S, et al. Src family kinase oncogenic potential and pathways in prostate cancer as revealed by AZD0530. Oncogene 2008;27:6365–75.

114. Yu EY, Wilding G, Posadas E, et al. Phase II study of dasatinib in patients with metastatic castration-resistant prostate cancer. Clin Cancer Res 2009;15:7421–8.

115. Yu EY, Massard C, Gross ME, et al. Once-daily dasatinib: expansion of phase II study evaluating safety and efficacy of dasatinib in patients with metastatic castration-resistant prostate cancer. Urology 2011;77:1166–71.

116. Araujo JC, Mathew P, Armstrong AJ, et al. Dasatinib combined with docetaxel for castration-resistant prostate cancer: results from a phase 1-2 study. Cancer 2012;118:63–71.

117. Twardowski, Chen C, Kraft AS, et al. A phase II trial of dasatinib in subjects with hormone-refractory prostate cancer previously treated with chemotherapy [abstract: 4575]. J Clin Oncol 2011;29(Suppl).

118. Baselga J, Cervantes A, Martinelli E, et al. Phase I safety, pharmacokinetics, and inhibition of SRC activity study of saracatinib in patients with solid tumors. Clin Cancer Res 2010;16:4876–83.

Bone-Targeted Agents
Preventing Skeletal Complications in Prostate Cancer

Alicia K. Morgans, MD*, Matthew R. Smith, MD, PhD

KEYWORDS

- Prostate cancer • Skeletal complications • Bone • Side effects of therapy • Skeletal related events
- ADT

KEY POINTS

- Skeletal complications from metastases and androgen deprivation therapy are common in prostate cancer survivors.
- New pharmacologic approaches to preventing skeletal related events and other complications in this population are being employed.
- In addition to palliating pain caused by bone metastases in prostate cancer, the well-tolerated radiopharmaceutical Alpharadin appears to prolong life.

NORMAL BONE PHYSIOLOGY

Healthy bone is perpetually in a state of turnover, striking a delicate balance between bone resorption by osteoclasts and bone formation by osteoblasts. Estrogen plays an important role in the regulation of this balance through estrogen receptors on osteoblasts and osteoclasts.[1] In low estrogen states, the balance favors bone resorption rather than formation. Low estrogen levels are likely one of the most significant contributors to the decline of bone mineral density (BMD) in hypogonadal states.

Additional regulatory signaling occurs via the receptor activator of nuclear factor-κB ligand (RANKL) system.[2] RANKL, a member of the tumor necrosis factor superfamily of proteins, is produced by osteoblasts and bone marrow stromal cells. It binds to RANK receptors on osteoclasts and osteoclast precursors to induce differentiation, activation, and survival of osteoclasts. The activation of RANK ultimately causes increased osteoclast activity and bone resorption. The action of osteoprotegerin (OPG), a protein produced by osteoblasts and other stromal tissues, decreases osteoclast activity by OPG binding RANKL, preventing the RANK/RANKL interaction. Relative levels of OPG and RANKL are thought to play a pivotal role in determining the degree to which bone resorption and formation occur.[3]

PATHOPHYSIOLOGY OF BONE METASTASES

Bone lesions in prostate cancer appear osteoblastic radiographically, but both osteoblast and osteoclast activity is upregulated.[4–6] Osteoclast activity is enhanced by several mechanisms, including marrow stromal and tumor secretion of stimulatory proteins that act on nearby osteoclasts. Stromal cells produce RANKL and macrophage colony-stimulating factor (M-CSF) receptor, both of which stimulate osteoclast differentiation and activation.[7] Tumor cells also promote osteoclast activity by producing M-CSF and parathyroid hormone–related protein.[7] It has also been proposed that osteoclast activation may be explained almost entirely by the effect of androgen deprivation therapy (ADT), one of the most common treatments for recurrent or metastatic prostate cancer.[8] The mechanism of osteoblast activity promotion is

Department of Hematology/Oncology, Massachusetts General Hospital Cancer Center, 55 Fruit Street, Boston, MA 02114, USA
* Corresponding author.
E-mail address: alicia.morgans@vanderbilt.edu

Urol Clin N Am 39 (2012) 533–546
http://dx.doi.org/10.1016/j.ucl.2012.07.009
0094-0143/12/$ – see front matter © 2012 Elsevier Inc. All rights reserved.

less well defined, but is presumed to be driven by stromal and tumor secretion of osteoblasts-stimulating factors, such as insulinlike growth factor, bone-morphogenic proteins, transforming growth factor-beta, fibroblast growth factors, and others.[9]

CLINICAL COMPLICATIONS OF BONE METASTASES

The most common site of metastatic disease in advanced prostate cancer is bone, especially the bones of the axial skeleton, pelvis, and long bones. Spread to bone occurs via hematogenous dissemination. The biology of bone metastases is complex. Multiple factors appear to contribute to the bone tropism in prostate cancer, including blood flow in the bone marrow, expression of adhesive molecules on cancer cells that bind them to the bone matrix and stroma, and a rich supply of growth factors in the bone microenvironment.[10–12] There is also a significant amount of reciprocal signaling between osteoblasts, osteoclasts, fibroblasts, and other cells of the bone microenvironment and prostate cancer cells through the secretion of cytokines, proteases, and growth factors that promote prostate cancer cell survival and growth.[13]

Both pathologic fractures directly related to metastatic lesions and treatment-related benign osteoporotic fractures occur commonly in men with prostate cancer. Up to 22% of men with metastatic castrate-resistant prostate cancer (CRPC) experience pathologic fractures during the course of their disease because of weakened bone integrity in the area of metastasis.[14] Benign osteoporotic fractures occur owing to the treatment-related decline of BMD that can result in osteoporosis and increase an individual's risk of fracture.[15,16] Several large retrospective database analyses of men with nonmetastatic prostate cancer demonstrated that men treated with ADT have a significantly higher rate of fracture that those who were not, and the risk increases over time as BMD falls.[17,18]

Bone metastases are also associated with the development of additional skeletal complications. Both pain and weakness can develop from bone or nerve involvement with metastases. Hypocalcemia and subsequent secondary hyperparathyroidism occur owing to increased osteoblast activity in metastatic deposits.

TREATMENT-RELATED OSTEOPOROSIS

ADT, via bilateral orchiectomies or through administration of gonadotropin-releasing hormone (GnRH) agonists or antagonists, is the cornerstone of systemic treatment for prostate cancer. The goal of ADT is to dramatically lower serum testosterone, typically lower than 20 ng/dL, or less than 5% of baseline values. Because of peripheral aromatization of testosterone to estradiol, reducing serum testosterone causes estradiol levels to fall. Estradiol levels decline to lower than 20% of baseline values, reaching levels as low as or lower than those of postmenopausal women.

ADT is widely used, both in subgroups of men with prostate cancer who clearly have improved overall survival with ADT, and in those in whom a survival benefit has not been demonstrated. One group that appears to benefit from treatment with ADT is men with metastatic disease who have an improved overall survival and quality of life with treatment. Men undergoing treatment with radiation for high-risk localized disease or locally advanced prostate cancer experience prolonged survival with the addition of ADT.[19] Finally, there is evidence that men who have positive lymph nodes after radical prostatectomy have improved overall survival when treated with ADT.[20] Although there is no evidence of improved overall survival in men with a prostate-specific antigen (PSA)-only relapse, this population is frequently treated with ADT alone or in combination with salvage radiation.[19]

The major causes of osteoporosis in men are use of steroids, alcohol use, or hypogonadism.[21] The intended therapeutic effect of ADT is marked hypogonadism. Consistent with the important role of gonadal steroids in normal bone metabolism in men, ADT decreases BMD and is associated with greater fracture risk. Within 6 to 9 months of initiating ADT, BMD falls.[22–24] BMD continues to decline during treatment at a rate of 2% to 3% per year.[22–25] This is substantially faster than typical age-related decline in men of 0.5% to 1.0%.

ADT is also associated with an increased fracture rate.[17,18] Within 5 years of initiating therapy with ADT, the incidence of fracture approaches 20%.[17] Several large retrospective analyses found that men treated with ADT experience a 21% to 45% relative increase in fracture risk as compared with men not treated with ADT.[17,18,26] Additionally, a Surveillance Epidemiology and End Results (SEER) Medicare analysis of more than 50,000 men with prostate cancer found a fracture rate of 19.4% in men treated with ADT, whereas the rate of fracture in men not undergoing treatment was 12.6% ($P<.001$).[17] A second analysis of Medicare data from the same year included 4000 men with nonmetastatic prostate cancer and reported a relative risk of fracture of 1.21 among men treated with ADT as compared with those who were not (95% confidence interval [CI], 1.14–1.29, $P<.01$).[18]

MECHANISMS OF TREATMENT-RELATED BONE LOSS

ADT decreases BMD through several mechanisms. Both testosterone and estrogen are important for maintaining normal bone homeostasis, and ADT causes a significant decline in both testosterone and estrogen. When serum testosterone is low, less testosterone is available to undergo peripheral aromatization to estradiol. Low estrogen states are associated with increased bone resorption. In healthy men, studies demonstrate a decline in BMD when estradiol levels are low, and an inverse relationship between fracture risk and estradiol levels.[27–29]

ADT also affects the rate of bone turnover and skeletal sensitivity to parathyroid hormone. Serum markers of osteoblast activity, like bone-specific alkaline phosphatase and osteocalcin, and markers of osteoclast activity, such as N-telopeptide, increase in men treated with ADT.[24] These markers generally increase within 6 to 12 weeks of initiating therapy with ADT, and plateau approximately 6 months after starting therapy. ADT also increases skeletal sensitivity to parathyroid hormone.[30]

OSTEOCLAST-TARGETED THERAPY

Two osteoclast-targeted therapies have been studied in men with prostate cancer. Bisphosphonates are used to prevent skeletal-related events (SREs) in metastatic CRPC. SREs are a group of skeletal complications associated with malignancy. The term typically encompasses the following outcomes: pathologic fractures, cord compression, and the use of surgery or radiation to treat unstable or painful metastatic lesions in bone. Some studies also include the development of hypercalcemia or hypocalcemia in the definition. Denosumab, a fully humanized monoclonal antibody targeting RANKL, has been approved to prevent SREs in metastatic solid tumors, including CRPC, and to increase BMD in men at risk for ADT-associated bone loss.

Bisphosphonates

Bisphosphonates prevent bone resorption through several mechanisms, including decreased osteoclast differentiation and survival and increased osteoblast survival.[31] Bisphosphonate molecules are structurally similar to native pyrophosphate molecules that normally adhere to hydroxyapatite crystal-binding sites. The molecules attach to binding sites located in areas of bone resorption, reducing osteoclast activity by preventing their adherence to the bone surface and the formation of the ruffled border. Bisphosphonates impair osteoclast progenitor differentiation and survival via their effects on osteoblasts.[31]

Bisphosphonates vary by the R2 group attached to their common structural backbone. The R2 group determines the potency of the molecule, with nitrogen-containing bisphosphonates like pamidronate, alendronate, and zoledronic acid being significantly more potent than simple bisphosphonates like clodronate and etidronate, which are non-nitrogenous. Among the nitrogen-containing bisphosphonates, those that contain secondary or tertiary amino groups, such as zoledronic acid, are significantly more potent than other compounds.[32] Zoledronic acid is estimated to be at least 100 times more potent than pamidronate and more than 1000 times as potent as etidronate in vitro.[32]

Several bisphosphonates are currently used in patients with cancer. Indications include hypercalcemia, low BMD, and metastatic lesions in bone. As early as the 1990s, evidence demonstrated that pamidronate decreased the risk of skeletal complications in individuals with metastatic breast cancer and multiple myeloma.[33,34] Pamidronate was subsequently approved for use in these populations in 1995. Zoledronic acid was approved to prevent skeletal complications in multiple myeloma and in any solid tumor with bone metastases in 2002.[14,35,36] The study that specifically led to its approval in metastatic prostate cancer, Zometa 039, demonstrated a reduction in SRE as compared with placebo.[14]

Denosumab

As described previously, bone exists in state of continuous remodeling, striking a balance between osteoclast resorption and osteoblast formation of new bone. The RANKL/RANK system plays a key role in achieving this balance. Currently, the only available therapy that targets this system is denosumab, a fully human monoclonal antibody directed at RANKL. The drug mimics the action of OPG by binding RANKL and reducing osteoclast action. It has a half-life of more than 30 days, does not accumulate in bone, like bisphosphonates, and can be used in patients with renal insufficiency.[37] Similar to bisphosphonates, treatment with denosumab carries a small risk of developing osteonecrosis of the jaw.[38]

Denosumab has been studied to prevent the development of osteoporosis and reduce the risk of fracture in postmenopausal women.[39,40] In the fracture-prevention trial, 7868 postmenopausal women with osteoporosis were randomized to receive placebo or twice-yearly denosumab. Women in the denosumab group developed fewer new vertebral fractures, nonvertebral fractures, and hip fractures than those in the placebo group during the 36-month follow-up period (relative decreased risk of vertebral fractures 68%, nonvertebral fractures 20%, and hip fractures 40%).[41] Denosumab was approved by the Food and Drug Administration (FDA) to treat postmenopausal women with osteoporosis based on this study.

Denosumab was also studied in women with breast cancer who were being treated with aromatase inhibitors.[42] Aromatase inhibitors are associated with a decline in BMD in women owing to the inhibition of peripheral tissue estrogen production. A recent study demonstrated that denosumab prevents the loss of BMD at the lumbar spine in women with breast cancer being treated with aromatase inhibitors as compared with placebo (BMD increased by 5.5% and 7.6% at 12 and 24 months, respectively [$P<.0001$ at both time points]).

CLINICAL USES OF OSTEOCLAST-TARGETED THERAPIES IN PROSTATE CANCER
Prevention of Therapy-related Fragility Fractures

Several medications have been evaluated for prevention of fragility fractures, the most clinically relevant end point in this population (**Table 1**). Denosumab, the fully human monoclonal antibody against RANKL, has been approved to prevent treatment-related fragility fractures in men treated with ADT.[43] Toremifene, a selective estrogen

receptor modulator (SERM) has been studied in this setting, but has not been approved for use because of an unacceptable risk-benefit ratio.[44] Multiple bisphosphonates, including alendronate, pamidronate, zoledronic acid, and neridronate, have been evaluated to prevent a decline in BMD, but those studies were not powered to evaluate fracture prevention.[15,45–49]

The National Comprehensive Cancer Network and National Osteoporosis Foundation (NOF) created guidelines for the treatment of secondary osteoporosis associated with ADT and fracture prevention. These guidelines suggest that all men older than 50 years who are being treated with ADT should be treated with calcium (1200 mg per day) and vitamin D (1000 IU per day). They also recommend additional pharmacologic therapy for fracture prevention for any individual with a 10-year probability of hip fracture of 3% or more or a 20-year probability of major osteoporotic fracture of 20% or more.

An individual's 10-year probability of fracture depends on multiple factors besides BMD.[50,51] BMD is routinely used as a surrogate end point for fracture in clinical trials, but most fractures occur in men whose BMD is not in the osteoporotic range. A man's risk of fracture increases by approximately 30-fold between the ages of 50 and 90, and the decline of BMD with age accounts for only a 4-fold increase in risk of fracture.[50] To address this,

Table 1
Bone-targeted therapies evaluated for the prevention of therapy-related fragility fractures

Study	N	Study Population	Arms	Outcome
Denosumab Halt 138[43]	1468	Men with nonmetastatic prostate cancer being treated with a GnRH agonist and at high risk of fracture.	Denosumab 60 mg subcutaneously every 6 mo vs placebo for 3 y	Denosumab was associated with a significant increase in BMD ($P<.001$) and a decrease in the incidence of vertebral fractures (RR 0.38 as compared with placebo, $P = .006$).
Toremifene protocol G300203[44]	1294	Men with nonmetastatic prostate cancer being treated with ADT who were at high risk of fracture.	Toremifene 80 mg orally daily vs placebo	Toremifene was associated with a 50% reduction in the relative risk of new vertebral fracture and an increase in bone mineral density ($P = .05$). Elevated risk of thromboembolic events in the toremifene arm.

Abbreviations: ADT, androgen deprivation therapy; BMD, bone mineral density; GnRH, gonadotropin-releasing hormone; RR, relative risk.

the NOF recommends using the World Health Organization (WHO)/Fracture Risk Assessment (FRAX) computer-based tool to calculate the 10-year probability of hip or major osteoporotic fracture.[52] This population-specific assessment is based on various easily obtained clinical factors in addition to BMD, and it can be calculated without BMD data if that is not available.

In clinical practice, more individuals meet criteria for pharmacologic management of therapy-related osteoporosis than would be expected based on the WHO definition of osteoporosis alone (T-score of <–2.5 alone). One recent study applied FRAX to 363 patients with nonmetastatic prostate cancer being treated with ADT in an academic practice.[53] In that cohort, 51.2% met criteria for pharmacologic treatment. Age played a major role in the risk stratification, with 3.3% of men younger than 70 years and 99.8% of men 80 years or older meeting criteria.[53]

Denosumab HALT 138

Denosumab was studied in a phase 3, multicenter, double-blind, randomized-controlled trial evaluating whether it could prevent osteoporosis and reduce the rate of fracture in men treated with ADT (see **Table 1**).[43] Men in the study were treated with a GnRH agonist for nonmetastatic hormone-sensitive prostate cancer, and were at high risk of fracture based on low baseline BMD, age older than 70 years, or previous fragility fracture. A total of 1468 subjects were randomized to receive denosumab or placebo subcutaneously every 6 months, and BMD was evaluated at 24 and 36 months. The primary end point in the study was the change in lumbar spine BMD, and incidence of new vertebral fracture was included as a secondary end point.

The trial found that there was both an increase in BMD and a decrease in the rate of clinical fracture in men treated with denosumab as compared with placebo.[43] At 24 months, there was a 5.6% increase in lumbar spine BMD in the group treated with denosumab as compared with a 1.0% decrease in BMD in the placebo group ($P<.001$). Significant differences in BMD were evident in some patients as soon as 1 month after treatment. At 36 months, the denosumab group had significantly fewer vertebral fractures, with an incidence of 1.5% in the denosumab group and 3.9% in the placebo group (relative risk 0.38, $P = .006$).

Subgroup analyses revealed that denosumab improved BMD at all skeletal sites in all subgroups.[54] The men with the most pronounced improvement in BMD were those with the highest markers of bone turnover (serum C-telopeptide and tartrate-resistant alkaline phosphatase). Adverse events were not significantly different between the 2 groups.

Based on the results of this trial, denosumab was recently approved by the FDA for fracture prevention in men receiving ADT.

Toremifene Protocol G300203

Selective estrogen receptor modulators (SERMs), including raloxifene and toremifene, have been studied to prevent therapy-related fragility fractures in men treated with ADT, but are not approved for use in men with prostate cancer.[44,55]

Toremifene was evaluated in a recently reported multicenter, international phase III study of 1294 men with nonmetastatic prostate cancer who were being treated with ADT (see **Table 1**).[44] Men were at high risk of fracture owing to low BMD or age older than 70 years. Subjects were randomized to receive oral toremifene daily or placebo, and they were followed for 2 years. The primary end point in the study was development of new vertebral fractures, and BMD was assessed as a secondary end point. This study revealed that toremifene was associated with a relative risk reduction of 50.0% in the incidence of new vertebral fractures, with a fracture incidence of 2.5% in the toremifene group versus 4.9% in the placebo group (95% CI –1.5 to 75.0, $P = .05$). Notably, toremifene was also associated with a higher rate of venous thromboembolic events than placebo, and has not been approved for fracture prevention in men receiving ADT (2.6% vs 1.1%, respectively).[44]

METASTATIC CASTRATION-RESISTANT PROSTATE CANCER

There have been 3 contemporary randomized controlled trials of bisphosphonates to prevent skeletal complications in patients with CRPC and bone metastases (**Table 2**). Zoledronic acid is the only bisphosphonate approved to prevent skeletal-related events in men with metastatic prostate cancer. In a recent global randomized-controlled trial, denosumab was superior to zoledronic acid for prevention of SREs in men with CRPC and bone metastases and is approved to prevent SREs in this setting.

Zometa 039

The Zometa 039 trial provided the basis for the FDA approval of zoledronic acid for the prevention of SRE in CRPC with bone metastases. The study included 643 men with CRPC and asymptomatic or minimally symptomatic bone metastases (see **Table 2**).[14] Subjects were randomized to receive

Table 2
Randomized-controlled trials of bone-targeted therapies in prostate cancer with bone metastases

Study	N	Study Population	Arms	Outcome
Zometa 039[14]	643	Men with CRPC and symptomatic or minimally symptomatic bone metastases	Zoledronic acid 4 mg IV every 3 wk vs Placebo	Zoledronic acid was associated with significantly fewer SRE (33.2% vs 44.2%) and a trend toward improved overall survival.
CGP 032/INT 05[57]	350	Men with CRPC and symptomatic bone metastases	Pamidronate 90 mg IV every 3 wk or placebo	No difference in self-reported pain score, analgesic use, or SREs.
NCIC CTG PR.6[58]	209	Men with CRPC and symptomatic bone metastases	Clodronate 1500 mg IV every 3 wk or placebo	No difference in palliative response, overall quality of life, overall survival, duration of response, or symptomatic disease progression.
Denosumab protocol 20050103[38]	1901	Men with CRPC	Denosumab 120 mg subcutaneously or zoledronic acid 4 mg IV every 4 wk	Denosumab prolonged the median time to first on-study SRE by 3.6 mo (met both noninferior and superiority end points). No difference in overall survival or adverse events (including osteonecrosis of the jaw).
MRC PR05[59,60]	311	Men with castration-sensitive prostate cancer with bone metastases	Clodronate 2080 mg orally daily vs placebo	Trend toward improved progression-free and overall survival with clodronate on initial analysis, and significantly prolonged overall survival at 8-y analysis.
CALGB/CTSU	680[a]	Men with castration-sensitive prostate cancer with bone metastases	Zoledronic acid 4 mg IV every 4 weeks or placebo	Endpoints are SRE and prostate cancer death. Study is ongoing.

Abbreviations: CRPC, castrate-resistant prostate cancer; IV, intravenous; SRE, skeletal-related event.
[a] Target accrual.

4 mg intravenous (IV) zoledronic acid, 8 mg IV zoledronic acid, or placebo every 3 weeks for 15 months, in addition to treatment with ADT and any other therapy provided by their treating physician. The primary end point was the proportion of patients having at least 1 SRE, defined as pathologic bone fracture, spinal cord compression, surgery to bone, radiation to bone, or change in antineoplastic therapy to treat bone pain.

Because of an unacceptable number of grade 3 elevations in creatinine in the 8-mg zoledronic acid arm, changes were made in zoledronic acid dosing and administration. All participants in the 8-mg zoledronic acid group were switched to 4-mg dosing for the remainder of the trial, and creatinine was assessed before each dose. In addition, the infusion period of zoledronic acid was lengthened from 5 minutes to 15 minutes. Following these changes, the frequency of adverse renal events was similar between the zoledronic acid and placebo arms. At the conclusion of the study, only the 4-mg zoledronic acid and placebo data were compared in the primary efficacy analysis.

At the study's conclusion, a significantly smaller proportion of men in the 4-mg zoledronic acid arm experienced SRE than in the placebo arm (33.2% vs 44.2%; $P = .021$).[56] The median time to first SRE was shorter in the placebo arm than in the 4-mg zoledronic acid arm (321 day vs not reached; $P = .009$). Urinary markers of bone resorption were lower in the zoledronic acid arms than the placebo arm ($P = .011$ for both doses of zoledronic acid vs placebo). There was no significant difference in overall survival between the zoledronic acid and placebo groups.

CGP 032 and INT 05

CGP 032 and INT 05 evaluated the effectiveness of IV pamidronate for pain reduction in men with CRPC and symptomatic bone metastases (see **Table 2**).[57] Both trials were similarly designed multicenter, randomized, placebo-controlled trials, which allowed their results to be pooled and reported together. Between the 2 trials, 350 men with CRPC and painful bone metastases were randomized to receive pamidronate (90 mg IV) or placebo every 3 weeks for 27 weeks. The primary end point was change from baseline self-reported pain score, and secondary end points included analgesic use and the proportion of patients with an SRE (defined as pathologic fracture, radiation or surgery to bone, spinal cord compression, or hypercalcemia). Serum and urinary markers of bone turnover were also assessed.

At the conclusion of the studies, the pooled results were unable to demonstrate a difference between the pamidronate and placebo arms in self-reported pain score, analgesic use, proportion of patients with an SRE, or overall survival.[57] Urinary markers of bone turnover were significantly lower in the pamidronate group.

There are several possible reasons for the lack of apparent efficacy of pamidronate in these studies while zoledronic acid demonstrated efficacy in SRE prevention. First, pamidronate is significantly less potent than zoledronic acid, being approximately 100 times less potent than zoledronic acid in vitro. In vivo pamidronate decreases urinary N-teleopeptide, a marker of bone turnover, by approximately 50%, whereas zoledronic acid decreases biomarkers of osteoclast activity by 70% to 80%.[14] Additional reasons for the difference in outcome between these studies and the Zometa 039 trial include a patient population with more advanced disease (symptomatic bone metastases vs asymptomatic metastases) and less precise study end points.

National Cancer Institute of Canada Clinical Trials Group PR.6

Clodronate was evaluated in National Cancer Institute of Canada Clinical Trials Group PR.6 study to determine its ability to palliate bone pain in men with CRPC and symptomatic bone metastases (see **Table 2**).[58] The study included 209 men treated with mitoxantrone (12 mg/m^2 IV every 3 weeks) and prednisone (5 mg orally twice daily) who were randomized to receive clodronate 1500 mg IV or placebo every 3 weeks. The primary end point was palliative response determined by a reduction in patient-reported pain intensity index to zero or by 2 points, or a decrease in analgesic use by 50%, without an increase in either. Secondary end points included duration of response, symptomatic disease progression-free survival, and overall quality of life.

Clodronate did not increase the palliative response of men with CRPC and symptomatic metastatic bone lesions when compared with placebo (46% response vs 39% response in clodronate and placebo, respectively; $P = .54$). When compared with placebo, clodronate was equivalent in its effect on overall quality of life, overall survival, duration of response, and symptomatic disease progression-free survival. A subgroup analysis indicated that clodronate may provide some benefit as compared with placebo for pain palliation in men with severe pain, but the investigators note that additional evidence will be necessary to confirm this conclusion.

Denosumab Protocol 20050103

Denosumab was compared with zoledronic acid in an international, phase III, randomized, controlled trial to evaluate its ability to prevent SRE in men with CRPC (see **Table 2**).[38] The trial included 1901 men who were randomized to receive denosumab (120 mg subcutaneously every 4 weeks) or zoledronic acid (4 mg IV every 4 weeks). The primary end point was time to first on-study SRE, defined as pathologic fracture, radiation to bone, surgery to bone, or spinal cord compression. The study aimed to demonstrate noninferiority of denosumab as compared with zoledronic acid. Secondary objectives were to assess for superiority of denosumab and compare drug safety profiles.

After a median follow-up of 12.2 months for men treated with denosumab and 11.2 months for men receiving zoledronic acid, denosumab prolonged the median time to first on-study SRE by 3.6 months as compared with zoledronic acid (hazard ratio [HR] 0.82, 95% CI 0.71–0.95; P = .0002 for noninferiority; P = .008 for superiority).[38] Overall survival was similar between the denosumab and zoledronic acid groups. The safety profiles were also similar. Compared with zoledronic acid, denosumab was associated with similar rates of osteonecrosis of the jaw (1% vs 2%; P = .09) and higher rates of hypocalcemia (6% vs 13%; P<.001). Denosumab was approved by the FDA for use in individuals with metastatic solid tumors, including prostate cancer, for the prevention of SREs.

METASTATIC CASTRATION-SENSITIVE PROSTATE CANCER
Bisphosphonates

Several studies have evaluated the use of bisphosphonates in men with hormonally sensitive metastatic prostate cancer. Initial data from one study evaluating clodronate for the prevention of symptomatic skeletal disease progression or prostate cancer death was negative. Long-term data from that study demonstrating an improved overall survival with clodronate has not yet been incorporated into widespread clinical practice. A second study in this population, CALGB/CTSU (cancer and leukemia group B/cancer trials support unit) 90202, is investigating the use of zoledronic acid in this setting and is ongoing.

Medical Research Council PR05

The Medical Research Council (MRC) PR05 study evaluated clodronate in men with metastatic prostate cancer who were initiating or continued to be responsive to initial treatment with ADT (see Table 2). In the study, 311 men were randomized to clodronate (2080 mg orally daily) or placebo in addition to continuing treatment with primary ADT.[59] The primary study end point was bone progression-free survival defined as time to either symptomatic disease progression or prostate cancer death. Compared with placebo, clodronate did not significantly improve bone progression-free survival (HR 0.79; 95% CI 0.61–1.02; P = .066). Treatment with clodronate was associated with longer overall survival, a secondary end point of the study (8-year overall survival, 22% vs 14%; HR 0.77; 95% CI 0.60–0.98; P = .032).[60]

CALGB/CTSU 90202

A second study investigating the use of bisphosphonates in men with hormonally responsive metastatic prostate cancer is the ongoing CALGB/CTSU 90202 (NCT00079001) trial (see Table 2). The study aims to randomize 680 men with castrate-sensitive disease and skeletal metastases to receive zoledronic acid (4 mg IV every 4 weeks) or placebo. End points include SRE and prostate cancer death. Because it is FDA approved for prevention of SRE in metastatic castrate-resistant disease, patients cross over to zoledronic acid when they develop castrate-resistant disease or experience an SRE. This study remains open to enrollment.

PREVENTION OF BONE METASTASES

Several osteoclast-targeted therapies have been evaluated to prevent metastases in men with high-risk or locally advanced disease. Two bisphosphonates, clodronate and zoledronic acid, were studied in randomized, placebo-controlled trials. In MRC PR04, clodronate failed to significantly prolong bone-metastasis–free survival. A trial evaluating the ability of zoledronic acid to prolong time to first metastasis, Zometa 704, did not reach its accrual goal and was therefore not evaluable. The Zometa European Study (ZEUS) is an ongoing European randomized-controlled trial evaluating the efficacy of zoledronic acid in metastasis prevention in men with high-risk prostate cancer. In contrast, a recently reported randomized, placebo-controlled, phase III trial demonstrated that denosumab prolonged bone-metastasis–free survival when compared with placebo.

MRC PR04

Clodronate was evaluated in a randomized, double-blind, placebo-controlled trial for the prevention of symptomatic bone metastases in the MRC PR04 study (Table 3). The trial enrolled 508 men with locally advanced prostate cancer (T2-T4, N0, N+, or NX, M0) who were considered to be at high risk of developing metastases.[61] Men were randomized to 5 years of treatment with clodronate (2080 mg orally per day) or placebo, and most received treatment of their prostate cancer consistent with standard of care at the time (external beam radiation, external beam radiation and hormonal therapy, or primary hormonal therapy). The primary end point was bone-metastasis–free survival, a composite end point that included development of symptomatic bone metastasis or death from prostate cancer. After median follow-up of 118 months and 148 primary end point events, there was no difference in bone-metastasis–free survival or overall survival between the 2 groups. There was a trend toward men in the placebo arm experiencing fewer events than those in the clodronate arm, although this

Table 3
Bone-targeted therapies evaluated for metastasis prevention in nonmetastatic prostate cancer

Study	N	Study Population	Arms	Outcome
MRC PR04[61]	508	Men with locally advanced prostate cancer at high risk of developing metastases.	Clodronate 2080 mg orally daily vs placebo for 5 y	No difference in bone-metastasis–free survival or overall survival.
Zometa 704[62]	398	Men with CRPC and rising PSA without radiographic evidence of metastatic disease.	Zoledronic acid 4 mg IV every 4 wk vs placebo	Poor accrual and low event rate caused early closure of the trial and impairs analysis of study results.
ZEUS[63]	1300	Men with high-risk localized castrate-sensitive prostate cancer	Zoledronic acid 4 mg IV every 3 mo or placebo for 48 mo	Target accrual complete, data acquisition and analysis ongoing.
Denosumab protocol 20050147[64]	1435	Men with nonmetastatic CRPC at high risk of developing metastatic disease	Denosumab 120 mg subcutaneously every 4 wk vs placebo.	Denosumab prolonged median bone-metastasis–free survival by 4.2 mo as compared with placebo. No difference in overall survival between groups.

Abbreviations: CRPC, castrate-resistant prostate cancer; IV, intravenous; PSA, prostate-specific antigen.

did not reach significance (HR 1.22, 95% CI 0.88–1.68; P = .23). Excluding PSA level, after 226 events, men in the clodronate arm had shorter time to disease progression than those in the placebo arm (HR 1.31, 95% CI 1.01–1.70; P = .041). Overall survival at 5 years was similar between the 2 groups at 78%. Despite evidence of a survival advantage in the castrate-sensitive metastatic setting after long-term follow-up, there was no difference in overall survival after long-term follow-up in this population with locally advanced castrate-sensitive disease.[60]

Zometa 704

Zometa 704 was a randomized-controlled trial evaluating the ability of zoledronic acid to prolong time to first metastasis in men with CRPC and a rising PSA but no radiographic evidence of metastatic disease (see **Table 3**).[62] Men were randomized to receive zoledronic acid (4 mg IV every 4 weeks) or placebo. The primary end point was time to first metastatic bone lesion, and subjects were evaluated by bone scan every 4 months.

Although planned accrual was 991, the trial was closed after only 398 men had enrolled owing to a low event rate. Analysis of the available data found no difference in time to first metastasis between zoledronic acid and placebo, although

the low event rate and early study termination precludes reliable conclusions about efficacy of zoledronic acid in this setting.

ZEUS

ZEUS is an ongoing randomized, controlled, open-label study evaluating the ability of zoledronic acid to prevent bone metastases in a high-risk population (see **Table 3**).[63] Subjects have high-risk localized castrate-sensitive prostate cancer, defined by having one of the following disease characteristics: PSA of 20 ng/mL or higher, lymph-node–positive disease, or Gleason score of 8 to 10. Subjects were randomized to receive zoledronic acid (4 mg IV every 3 months for 48 months) or placebo, and additional treatment was delivered per standard of care. The primary end point is the proportion of men who develop at least 1 bone metastasis during a 48-month study period. Target accrual of 1300 men has been met and the study is ongoing.

Denosumab Protocol 20050147

Denosumab has been evaluated for its activity in metastasis prevention in a recently reported international, phase III, double-blind, randomized-controlled trial, Denosumab Protocol 20050147 (see **Table 3**). This study randomized 1435 men with nonmetastatic CRPC at high risk of developing metastatic disease to receive denosumab (120 mg subcutaneously every 4 weeks) or placebo.[64,65] High risk was defined as PSA of 8.0 μg/L or higher, PSA doubling time of 10 months or less, or both. The primary end point of the trial was bone-metastasis–free survival, which included time to first bone metastasis (symptomatic or asymptomatic) or death from any cause. Overall survival was a secondary end point.

Denosumab prolonged median bone-metastasis–free survival by 4.2 months as compared with placebo (29.5 months [95% CI 25.4–33.3] versus 25.2 months [95% CI 22.2–29.5], respectively).[64] Additionally, denosumab delayed time to first bone metastasis when compared with placebo (median 33.2 months [95% CI 29.5–38.0] vs 29.5 months [95% CI 22.4–33.1], respectively). Overall survival was equivalent between groups (median overall survival of 43.9 months with denosumab and 44.8 months with placebo [HR 1.01, 95% CI 0.85–1.20; P = .91]). Notable adverse events included hypocalcemia and osteonecrosis of the jaw in 2% and 5% of men receiving denosumab, respectively. Hypocalcemia occurred in fewer than 1% of men receiving placebo, and there were no episodes of osteonecrosis of the jaw.

RADIOISOTOPES

Both alpha-emitting and beta-emitting radioisotopes have been studied for pain palliation in men with prostate cancer and painful bone metastases. Two beta-emitting radioisotopes, Strontium-89 and Samarium-153, have been approved for bone metastasis pain palliation in men with prostate cancer. Radium-223, an alpha-emitting radioisotope, has also been studied for palliation of bone pain in men with metastatic prostate cancer. In a recently reported international, phase III, randomized, placebo-controlled trial, radium-223 prolonged overall survival in men with CRPC and painful bone metastases.

Strontium-89 and Samarium-153

Strontium-89 and Samarium-153 are beta-emitting radioisotopes that have been approved for use in men with CRPC and painful bone metastases. They act by honing to tissues surrounding osteoblastic lesions to deliver high-energy radiation therapy locally. They are especially useful for treating multifocal lesions that are not easily targeted in a single radiation field or for the palliation of tissues that have previously received maximum doses of external beam radiation.

Several clinical trials have evaluated the efficacy of strontium-89 for pain palliation in men with CRPC and bone metastases. A British study included 284 men treated with strontium-89 or conventional focal or hemibody external beam radiation therapy.[65] Pain control was similar between the groups at 3 months, although bone marrow suppression was more common in the strontium-89 group. A phase III, randomized, controlled Canadian trial included 126 men with hormone-resistant prostate cancer and painful bone metastases who were randomized to receive strontium-89 or placebo after initial treatment with focal external beam radiation.[66] Overall survival was similar between the 2 groups, but men treated with strontium-89 had improved quality-of-life scores and more frequently discontinued pain medications at 3 months than those treated with placebo. In contrast, a European Organization for Research and Treatment of Cancer study randomized 203 men to receive local field external beam radiation or strontium-89.[67] There was no difference between the groups in pain relief, but overall survival was significantly higher in the external beam group (median overall survival 11 vs 7 months, P = .046).

Samarium-153 has also been studied in phase III, randomized, placebo-controlled studies in men with prostate cancer. In the first, 118 individuals with bone metastases from various solid tumors were randomized to 0.5 mCi/kg or 1.0 mCi/kg of samarium-153 or placebo.[68] Patients with prostate cancer made up 68% of the group. During the first 4 weeks of the study, the high dose of samarium-153 was associated with significantly less pain than placebo. There was no difference between groups in overall survival. A second study randomized 152 men with CRPC to receive samarium-153 or placebo.[69] Men receiving samarium-153 had significantly lower analgesic use at 3 and 4 weeks during the study.

Complications from beta radioisotopes occur because of the effects of radiation on the tissue surrounding metastatic lesions. The most common adverse effect is myelosuppression, and blood counts should be monitored at least once every 2 weeks during treatment. Additional complications include severe pain flare in fewer than 10% of men, and acute leukemia has rarely been associated with strontium-89.[70,71]

Alpharadin in Symptomatic Prostate Cancer

Radium-223 is an alpha-emitting radioisotope that is currently being evaluated in the Alpharadin in Symptomatic Prostate Cancer trial, an international, randomized, controlled, phase III study. The trial included 922 men with CRPC and 2 or more symptomatic bone metastases but no visceral metastases who had received docetaxel or were unfit to receive it.[72] They were randomized to radium-223 (50 kBq/kg) or placebo. The primary end point of the study was overall survival, and secondary end points included time to first SRE, time to PSA progression, and total alkaline phosphatase normalization.

After 314 events from 809 randomized patients were collected, a planned interim analysis was performed. Because radium-223 was associated with a significant improvement in overall survival as compared with placebo, the trial was closed immediately (median survival 14.0 vs 11.2 months, HR 0.695, P = .002).[72] Radium-223 also prolonged time to first SRE (13.6 months vs 8.4 months for radium-223 and placebo, respectively). The most common complications associated with radium-223 versus placebo include anemia (27% vs 27%), bone pain (43% vs 58%), and nausea (34% vs 32%). This medication is not yet approved for use in men with CRPC and symptomatic bone metastases in the United States.

SUMMARY

In prostate cancer, both metastatic lesions and the effects of hormonal therapy can have negative effects on the skeletal system. Multiple therapies have been developed to target bone-related complications for men at various stages of the disease. Evidence supports the use of osteoclast-inhibiting therapies in men treated with ADT to prevent therapy-related fragility fractures. There is also evidence that osteoclast-inhibiting therapies are beneficial in preventing SREs in men with CRPC. More recently, phase III data demonstrate that using denosumab in men with CRPC can prevent the development of metastases. Finally, radium-223 prolongs overall survival in men with CRPC and skeletal metastases after treatment with docetaxel. The spectrum of bone-targeted therapies for the skeletal complications of prostate cancer continues to evolve, providing numerous novel options in our arsenal against bone complications in this disease.

REFERENCES

1. Eriksen EF, Colvard DS, Berg NJ, et al. Evidence of estrogen receptors in normal human osteoblast-like cells. Science 1988;241(4861):84–6.
2. Boyce BF, Xing L. Biology of RANK, RANKL, and osteoprotegerin. Arthritis Res Ther 2007;9(Suppl 1):S1.
3. Hofbauer LC, Schoppet M. Clinical implications of the osteoprotegerin/RANKL/RANK system for bone and vascular diseases. JAMA 2004;292(4):490–5.
4. Berruti A, Dogliotti L, Bitossi R, et al. Incidence of skeletal complications in patients with bone metastatic prostate cancer and hormone refractory disease: predictive role of bone resorption and formation markers evaluated at baseline. J Urol 2000;164:1248–53.
5. Clarke NW, McClure J, George NJ. Osteoblast function and osteomalacia in metastatic prostate cancer. Eur Urol 1993;24:286–90.
6. Clarke NW, McClure J, George NJ. Monomorphic evidence for bone resorption and replacement in prostate cancer. Br J Urol 1991;68:74–80.
7. Guise TA, Mundy GR. Cancer and bone. Endocr Rev 1998;19(1):18–54.
8. Micahelson MD, Marujo RM, Smith MR. Contribution of androgen deprivation therapy to elevated osteoclast activity in men with metastatic prostate cancer. Clin Cancer Res 2004;10(8):2705–8.
9. Logothetis CJ, Lin SH. Osteoblasts in prostate cancer metastasis to bone. Nat Rev Cancer 2005; 5(1):21–8.
10. Roodman GD. Mechanisms of bone metastasis. N Engl J Med 2004;350:1655–64.
11. Kahn D, Weiner GJ, Ben-Haim S, et al. Positron emission tomographic measurement of bone marrow blood flow to the pelvis and lumbar vertebrae in young normal adults. Blood 1994;83:958–63.
12. Hauschka PV, Mavrakos AE, Iafrati MD, et al. Growth factors in bone matrix: isolation of multiple types by affinity chromatography on heparin-Sepharose. J Biol Chem 1986;261:12665–74.
13. Mundy GR. Metastasis to bone: causes, consequences and therapeutic opportunities. Nat Rev Cancer 2002;2:584–93.
14. Saad F, Gleason DM, Murray R, et al. Randomized, placebo-controlled trial of zoledronic acid in patients with hormone-refractory metastatic prostate carcinoma. J Natl Cancer Inst 2002;94:1458–68.
15. Smith MR, McGovern FJ, Zietman AL, et al. Pamidronate to prevent bone loss during androgen-deprivation therapy for prostate cancer. N Engl J Med 2001;345(13):948–55.
16. Mittan D, Shuko L, Miller E, et al. Bone loss following hypogonadism in men with prostate cancer treated with GnRH analogs. J Clin Endocrinol Metab 2002; 87(8):3656–61.
17. Shahinian VB, Kuo YF, Freeman JL, et al. Risk of fracture after androgen deprivation for prostate cancer. N Engl J Med 2005;352(2):154–64.
18. Smith MR, Lee WC, Brandman J, et al. Gonadotropin-releasing hormone agonists and fracture risk: a claims-based cohort study of men with nonmetastatic prostate cancer. J Clin Oncol 2005; 23(31):7897–903.
19. Sharifi N, Gulley JL, Dahut WL. Androgen deprivation therapy for prostate cancer. JAMA 2005;294(2):238–44.
20. Messing EM, Manola J, Sarosdy M, et al. Immediate hormonal therapy compared with observation after

radical prostatectomy and pelvic lymphadenectomy in men with node-positive prostate cancer. N Engl J Med 1999;341(24):1781–8.

21. Bilezikian JP. Osteoporosis in men. J Clin Endocrinol Metab 1999;84(10):3431–4.

22. Berruti A, Dogliotti L, Terrone C, et al. Changes in bone mineral density, lean body mass and fat content as measured by dual energy X-ray absorptiometry in patients with prostate cancer without apparent bone metastases given androgen deprivation therapy. J Urol 2002;167(6):2361–7.

23. Daniell HW, Dunn SR, Ferguson DW, et al. Progressive osteoporosis during androgen deprivation therapy for prostate cancer. J Urol 2000;163(1):181–6.

24. Maillefert JF, Sibiliam J, Michel F, et al. Bone mineral density in men treated with synthetic gonadotropin-releasing hormone agonists for prostatic carcinoma. J Urol 1999;161(4):1219–22.

25. Diamond TH, Thornley SW, Sekel R, et al. Hip fracture in elderly men: prognostic factors and outcomes. Med J Aust 1997;167(8):412–5.

26. Smith MR, Boyce SP, Moyneur E, et al. Risk of clinical fractures after gonadotropin-releasing hormone agonist therapy for prostate cancer. J Urol 2006;175(1):136–9.

27. Slemenda CW, Longcope C, Zhou L, et al. Sex steroids and bone mass in older men. Positive associations with serum estrogens and negative associations with androgens. J Clin Invest 1997;100(7):1755–9.

28. Khosla S, Melton LJ 3rd, Atkinson EJ, et al. Relationship of serum sex steroid levels and bone turnover markers with bone mineral density in men and women: a key role for bioavailable estrogen. J Clin Endocrinol Metab 1998;83(7):2266–74.

29. Greendale GA, Edelstein S, Barrett-Connor E. Endogenous sex steroids and bone mineral density in older women and men: the Rancho Bernardo Study. J Bone Miner Res 1997;12(11):1833–43.

30. Leder BZ, Smith MR, Fallon MA, et al. Effects of gonadal steroid suppression on skeletal sensitivity to parathyroid hormone in men. J Clin Endocrinol Metab 2001;86(2):511–6.

31. Rogers MJ, Watts DJ, Russel RG. Overview of bisphosphonates. Cancer 1997;80:1652–60.

32. Lee RJ, Saylor PJ, Smith MR. Treatment and prevention of bone complications from prostate cancer. Bone 2011;48:88–95.

33. Berenson JR, Lichtenstein A, Porter L, et al. The myeloma Aredia Study G. Efficacy of pamidronate in reducing skeletal events in patients with advanced multiple myeloma. N Engl J Med 1996;334:488–93.

34. Hortobagyi GN, Theriault RL, Porter L, et al. The Protocol 19 Aredia Breast Cancer Study G. Efficacy of pamidronate in reducing skeletal complications in patients with breast cancer and lytic bone metastases. N Engl J Med 1996;335:1785–92.

35. Rosen LS, Gordon D, Kaminski M, et al. Long-term efficacy and safety of zoledronic acid compared with pamidronate disodium in the treatment of skeletal complications in patients with advanced multiple myeloma or breast carcinoma. Cancer 2003;98:1735–44.

36. Rosen LS, Gordon D, Tchekmedyian S, et al. Zoledronic acid versus placebo in the treatment of skeletal metastases in patients with lung cancer and other solid tumors: a phase III, double-blind, randomized trial—The Zoledronic Acid Lung Cancer and Other Solid Tumors Study Group. J Clin Oncol 2003;21:3150–7.

37. Lee RJ, Saylor PJ, Smith MR. Contemporary therapeutic approaches targeting bone complications in prostate cancer. Clin Genitourin Cancer 2010;8(1):29–36.

38. Fizazi K, Carducci M, Smith M, et al. Denosumab versus zoledronic acid for treatment of bone metastases in men with castration-resistant prostate cancer: a randomised, double-blind study. Lancet 2011;377(9768):813–22.

39. McClung MR, Lewiecki EM, Cohen SB, et al. Denosumab in postmenopausal women with low bone mineral density. N Engl J Med 2006;354(8):821–31.

40. Miller PD, Bolognese MA, Lewiecki EM, et al. Effect of denosumab on bone density and turnover in postmenopausal women with low bone mass after long-term continued, discontinued, and restarting of therapy: a randomized blinded phase 2 clinical trial. Bone 2008;43(2):222–9.

41. Cummings SR, San Martin J, McClung MR, et al. Denosumab for prevention of fractures in postmenopausal women with osteoporosis. N Engl J Med 2009;361(8):756–65.

42. Ellis GK, Bone HG, Chlebowski R, et al. Randomized trial of denosumab in patients receiving adjuvant aromatase inhibitors for nonmetastatic breast cancer. J Clin Oncol 2008;26(30):4875–82.

43. Smith MR, Egerdie B, Hernandez Toriz N, et al. Denosumab in men receiving androgen-deprivation therapy for prostate cancer. N Engl J Med 2009;361(8):745–55.

44. Smith MR, Malkowicz SB, Chu F, et al. Toremifene increases bone mineral density in men receiving androgen deprivation therapy for prostate cancer: interim analysis of a multicenter phase 3 clinical study. J Urol 2008;179:152–5.

45. Greenspan SL, Nelson JB, Trump DL, et al. Effect of once-weekly oral alendronate on bone loss in men receiving androgen deprivation therapy for prostate cancer. Ann Intern Med 2007;146:416–24.

46. Diamond TH, Winters J, Smith A, et al. The antiosteoporotic efficacy of intravenous pamidronate in

men with prostate carcinoma receiving combined androgen blockade. Cancer 2001;92:1444–50.

47. Smith MR, Eastham J, Gleason DM, et al. Randomized controlled trial of zoledronic acid to prevent bone loss in men receiving androgen deprivation therapy for nonmetastatic prostate cancer. J Urol 2003;169:2008–12.

48. Michaelson MD, Kaufman DS, Lee H, et al. Randomized controlled trial of annual zoledronic acid to prevent gonadotropin-releasing hormone agonist-induced bone loss in men with prostate cancer. J Clin Oncol 2007;25:1038–42.

49. Morabito N, Gaudio A, Lasco A, et al. Neridronate prevents bone loss in patients receiving androgen deprivation therapy for prostate cancer. J Bone Miner Res 2004;19:1766–70.

50. Seeman E, Bianchi G, Khosla S, et al. Bone fragility in men—where are we? Osteoporos Int 2006;17(11):1577–83.

51. Kanis JA, Johnell O, Oden A, et al. FRAX and the assessment of fracture probability in men and women from the UK. Osteoporos Int 2008;19(4):385–97.

52. Watts NB, Lewiecki EM, Miller PD, et al. National Osteoporosis Foundation 2008 Clinician's Guide to Prevention and Treatment of Osteoporosis and the World Health Organization Fracture Risk Assessment Tool (FRAX): what they mean to the bone densitometrist and bone technologist. J Clin Densitom 2008;11(4):473–7.

53. Saylor PK, Kaufman DS, Michaelson MD, et al. Application of a fracture risk algorithm to men treated with androgen deprivation therapy for prostate cancer. J Urol 2010;183:2200–5.

54. Smith MR, Saad F, Egerdie B, et al. Effects of denosumab on bone mineral density in men receiving androgen deprivation therapy for prostate cancer. J Urol 2009;182(6):2670–5.

55. Smith MR, Fallon MA, Lee H, et al. Raloxifene to prevent gonadotropin releasing hormone agonist-induced bone loss in men with prostate cancer: a randomized controlled trial. J Clin Endocrinol Metab 2004;89:3841–6.

56. Saad F, Gleason DM, Murray R, et al. Long-term efficacy of zoledronic acid for the prevention of skeletal complications in patients with metastatic hormone refractory prostate cancer. J Natl Cancer Inst 2004;96:879–82.

57. Small EJ, Smith MR, Seaman JJ, et al. Combined analysis of two multicenter, randomized, placebo-controlled studies of pamidronate disodium for the palliation of bone pain in men with metastatic prostate cancer. J Clin Oncol 2003;21:4277–84.

58. Ernst DS, Tannock IF, Winquist EW, et al. Randomized, double-blind, controlled trial of mitoxantrone/prednisone and clodronate versus mitoxantrone/prednisone and placebo in patients with hormone-refractory prostate cancer and pain. J Clin Oncol 2003;21:3335–42.

59. Dearnaley DP, Sydes MR, Mason MD, et al. A double-blind, placebo-controlled, randomized trial of oral sodium clodronate for metastatic prostate cancer (MRC PR05 trial). J Natl Cancer Inst 2003;95:1300–11.

60. Dearnaley DP, Mason MD, Parmar MK, et al. Adjuvant therapy with oral sodium clodronate in locally advanced and metastatic prostate cancer: long-term overall survival results from the MRC PR04 and PR05 randomised controlled trials. Lancet Oncol 2009;10:872–6.

61. Mason MD, Sydes MR, Glaholm J, et al. Oral sodium clodronate for nonmetastatic prostate cancer—results of a randomized double-blind placebo-controlled trial: Medical Research Council PR04 (ISRCTN61384873). J Natl Cancer Inst 2007;99:765–76.

62. Smith MR, Kabbinavar F, Saad F, et al. Natural history of rising serum prostate specific antigen in men with castrate nonmetastatic prostate cancer. J Clin Oncol 2005;23:2918–25.

63. Wirth M, Tammela T, DeBruyne F, et al. Effectiveness of zoledronic acid for the prevention of bone metastases in high-risk prostate cancer patients. A randomised, open label, multicenter study of the European Association of Urology (EAU) in Cooperation with the Scandinavian Prostate Cancer Group (SPCG) and the Arbeitsgemeinschaft Urologische Onkologie (AUO). A report of the ZEUS study. 2008 Genitourinary Cancers Symposium [abstract no: 184]. Genitourinary Cancer Symposium. American Society of Clinical Oncology. San Francisco, February 14–16, 2008.

64. Smith M, Saad F, Coleman R, et al. Denosumab and bone-metastasis-free survival in men with castration-resistant prostate cancer: results of a phase 3, randomised, placebo-controlled trial. Lancet 2011;379(9810):39–46.

65. Quilty PM, Kirk D, Bolger JJ, et al. A comparison of the palliative effects of strontium-89 and external beam radiotherapy in metastatic prostate cancer. Radiother Oncol 1994;31:33.

66. Porter AT, McEwan AJ, Powe JE, et al. Results of a randomized phase-III trial to evaluate the efficacy of strontium-89 adjuvant to local field external beam irradiation in the management of endocrine resistant metastatic prostate cancer. Int J Radiat Oncol Biol Phys 1993;25:805.

67. Oosterhof GO, Roberts JT, de Reijke TM, et al. Strontium(89) chloride versus palliative local field radiotherapy in patients with hormonal escaped prostate cancer: a phase III study of the European Organisation for Research and Treatment of Cancer, Genitourinary Group. Eur Urol 2003;44:519.

68. Serafini AN, Houston SJ, Resche I, et al. Palliation of pain associated with metastatic bone cancer using samarium-153 lexidronam: a double-blind placebo-controlled clinical trial. J Clin Oncol 1998;16:1574.

69. Sartor O, Reid RH, Hoskin PJ, et al. Samarium-153-Lexidronam complex for treatment of painful bone metastases in hormone-refractory prostate cancer. Urology 2004;63:940.

70. Farhanghi M, Holmes RA, Volkert WA, et al. Samarium-153-EDTMP: pharmacokinetic, toxicity and pain response using an escalating dose schedule in treatment of metastatic bone cancer. J Nucl Med 1992;33:1451.

71. Kossman SE, Weiss MA. Acute myelogenous leukemia after exposure to strontium-89 for the treatment of adenocarcinoma of the prostate. Cancer 2000;88:620.

72. Parker C, Heinrich D, O'Sullivan JM, et al. Overall survival benefit and safety profile of radium-223 chloride, a first-in- class alpha-pharmaceutical: Results from a phase III randomized trial (ALSYMPCA) in patients with castration-resistant prostate cancer (CRPC) with bone metastases [abstract: 8]. Oral Abstract Session A.

Targeting Angiogenesis as a Promising Modality for the Treatment of Prostate Cancer

Jianqing Lin, MD*, William K. Kelly, DO

KEYWORDS

- Antiangiogenic therapy • Prostate cancer • Angiogenesis • Treatment

KEY POINTS

- Vascular endothelial growth factors (VEGF) and their receptors are key players for angiogenesis in prostate cancer.
- Promising early phase clinical trials using a VEGF-specific antibody for the treatment of prostate cancer did not translate an overall survival benefit in a recently reported phase III study.
- Despite increased toxicity, targeting angiogenesis in combination with systemic therapy is logical for a future trial design.
- Results from a few ongoing phase III studies are eagerly awaited.
- Better patient selection and a biomarker-driven study will likely lead the success of antiangiogenic therapy in prostate cancer.

INTRODUCTION: ANGIOGENESIS AND CANCER

Angiogenesis, or the process of new blood vessel formation, is necessary during cancer progression.[1,2] Tumor angiogenesis is recognized as one of the hallmarks of malignancy and is regarded as a prerequisite for local tumor growth and expansion.[1,2] Although tumor cells may live in an avascular state at a microscopic-sized population either as in situ tumors or as a microcylinder of tumor cells enveloping a preexisting microvessel, further growth or expansion of tumor mass critically depends on recruitment of new vessels, or angiogenic switch.[3–5] The classical angiogenic switch and features of tumor endothelium and vessel structure is summarized in **Box 1**.[3–6] Induction of the angiogenic switch depends on angiogenic balance, which is orchestrated by a variety of activators and inhibitors (see **Box 1**). The proangiogenic gene expression is increased by physiologic stimuli, such as hypoxia, which results from increased tissue mass, and is also determined by tumor cells. The main components involved in this angiogenic switch are (1) tumor cells that are genetically unstable and manifested by oncogene activation or tumor-suppressor mutation/inactivation, (2) proangiogenesis factors released from tumor cells, and (3) endothelial cells (ECs) that are genetically stable and regulated by proangiogenesis factors. Therapies involving targeting one of these 3 components are of tremendous interests to control cancer and improve survival.

VASCULAR ENDOTHELIAL GROWTH FACTORS AND THEIR RECEPTOR SIGNALING PATHWAYS

Proangiogenesis factors activate endothelial-cell proliferation and migration. They are mainly tumor-derived receptor tyrosine kinase ligands, such as vascular endothelial growth factor (VEGF), fibroblast growth factors (FGFs), platelet-derived

Department of Medical Oncology, Jefferson Kimmel Cancer Center, Thomas Jefferson University, Suite 700, 1025 Walnut Street, Philadelphia, PA 19107, USA
* Corresponding author.
E-mail address: Jianqing.lin@jefferson.edu

Urol Clin N Am 39 (2012) 547–560
http://dx.doi.org/10.1016/j.ucl.2012.07.010
0094-0143/12/$ – see front matter © 2012 Elsevier Inc. All rights reserved.

urologic.theclinics.com

> **Box 1**
> **The classical angiogenic switch and features of tumor endothelium and vessel structure**
>
> - The angiogenic switch is a discrete step in tumor development that can occur at different stages in the tumor progression depending on the nature of the tumor and its microenvironment.
>   - It has to occur to ensure exponential tumor growth.
>   - It continues as long as the tumor grows.
>   - It begins with perivascular detachment and vessel dilation, followed by angiogenic sprouting, new vessel formation and maturation, and the recruitment of perivascular cells.
>   - It is comprised of cancer cells, proangiogenesis factors, endothelial cells (endothelial progenitor cells in bone marrow or peripheral blood), and pericytes (proangiogenic monocytes and pericyte precursors).
>   - It is *off* when the effect of proangiogenic molecules (eg, vascular endothelial growth factors, fibroblast growth factors, platelet-derived growth factor β (PDGFB), epidermal growth factors, lysophosphatidic acid (LPA), and so forth) is balanced by antiangiogenic molecules (thrombospondin-1, angiostatin, endostatin, canstatin, tumstatin, and so forth) and is *on* when the net balance is tipped in favor of angiogenesis.
> - Tumor vascular endothelium is phenotypically different from that of normal vessels and it is characterized by increased fenestration and leakiness, aberrant architecture with arteriovenous shunts, multiple loops, and fan and spiral motifs. It has high vascular permeability without functional lymphatics. It has nonuniform surface markers with delayed maturation.[5,6]

growth factors (PDGF), and epidermal growth factors (EGF), but can be of other origins.

VEGF (also called VEGF-A), originally known as vascular permeability factor, is one of the most potent and well-characterized proangiogenic proteins. **Fig. 1** illustrates the family of VEGF molecules and receptors (adapted from Alfiky and Kelly,[7] also see review[8]). VEGF receptor 2 (VEGFR-2) is the major VEGF signaling receptor that mediates sprouting angiogenesis (called kinase-insert domain–containing receptor [KDR] in humans and fetal liver kinase 1 [flk-1] in mice). The role of VEGFR-1 in sprouting angiogenesis is much less clear. The binding of VEGF to VEGFR-2 leads to

a cascade of different signaling pathways (examples of which are shown in the **Fig. 1.**), resulting in the upregulation of genes involved in mediating the proliferation and migration of ECs and promoting their survival and vascular permeability. For example, the binding of VEGF to VEGFR-2 leads to dimerization of the receptor, followed by intracellular activation of the phospholipase Cγ (PLCγ)–protein kinase C(PKC)–Raf kinase-MAP/ERK kinase (MEK) mitogen-activated protein kinase (MAPK) pathway and subsequent initiation of DNA synthesis and cell growth, whereas the activation of the phosphatidylinositol 3′–kinase (PI3K)–serine/threonine protein kinase B (Akt) pathway leads to increased endothelial-cell survival. The activation of Src oncogene can lead to actin cytoskeleton changes and the induction of cell migration. The binding of VEGF-C to VEGFR-3 mediates lymphangiogenesis. The understanding of principal molecular pathways for angiogenesis and the role of angiogenesis in cancer progression has resulted in robust research investigation in antiangiogenesis therapy for cancer.

ANTIANGIOGENIC THERAPY VERSUS CYTOTOXIC CHEMOTHERAPY

The scientific basis of antiangiogenic therapy for cancer rests on 2 general principles: (1) tumor growth is angiogenesis dependent and (2) antiangiogenic therapy targets the genetically stable microvascular ECs.[4] This therapeutic approach was originally thought to be superior to cytotoxic chemotherapy because drug resistance would be less of an issue. **Table 1** summarizes the difference between antiangiogenesis therapy and cytotoxic chemotherapy. Antiangiogenesis is the mainstay treatment of recurrent or metastatic renal cell carcinoma and is able to improve the efficacy of chemotherapy for metastatic colorectal cancer, lung cancer, and glioblastoma multiforme (reviewed in[9,10]). To date, no antiangiogenic agents have been approved for use in prostate cancer (PCa), although extensive studies on angiogenesis in PCa have revealed that angiogenesis plays a role in the progression of PCa.

RATIONAL OF TARGETING ANGIOGENESIS FOR PCA: ROLE OF HYPOXIA-INDUCED FACTOR-1α AND VEGF IN PCA CARCINOGENESIS AND PROGRESSION

By directly measuring Po_2 from the pathologically involved side of the prostate, as well as from a region of normal stromal muscle for comparison, Movsas and colleagues[11] found that hypoxic regions existed in primary human PCa and

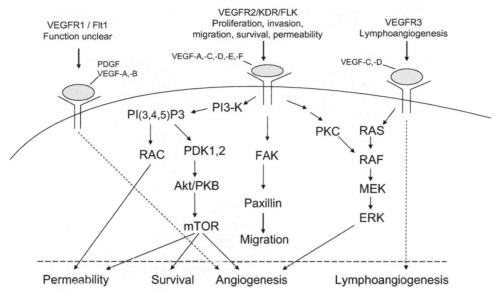

Fig. 1. VEGFs and their receptor family signaling pathway. VEGF-A is the main growth factor derived from tumor cells. VEGFR-2 dimerization and phosphorylation are activated by its binding to its ligands, and the downstream multiple signaling molecules are activated. These signaling molecules are potentially the targets for antiangiogenic therapy. ERK, extracellular-signal-regulated kinase; FAK, Focal adhesion kinase; FLK, Fetal Liver Kinase 1; FLT, fms-like tyrosine kinase; KDR, kinase insert domain receptor; MEK, MAP/ERK kinase; mTOR, mammalian target of rapamycin; PI3K, phosphatidylinositol 3-kinase; PDK, 3-phosphoinositide dependent protein kinase; PKC, protein kinase C; PI, phosphatidylinositol; RAF, serine/threonine-protein kinase encoded by Raf-1; RAS, GTPase encoded by oncogene Ras.

increasing levels of hypoxia were associated with higher clinical stages. Hypoxia-induced factor-1α (HIF-1α), a key player for angiogenesis, was found overexpressed in many common human cancers and their metastases, including PCa.[12] The significance of HIF-1α in PCa pathogenesis, crosstalk between HIF-1α and androgen receptor (AR) was reviewed by Lin and colleagues.[13] Microvessel density has been used as a surrogate histologic measure of angiogenesis within a tumor. It has been shown to correlate strongly with metastasis potential, Gleason score, and a negative clinical prognosis in PCa.[14,15]

Fig. 2 illustrates the interplay among hypoxia, HIF-1α, growth factor signaling/autocrine loop, and AR in PCa.[16,17] Collectively, HIF-1α has emerged as an important transcription factor in PCa biology and is essential in the early stages of

Table 1
Differences between antiangiogenesis and cytotoxic chemotherapy

Target	Angiogenesis Inhibitors	Chemotherapeutic Agents
	Dividing ECs (genetically stable)	Cancer cells (genetically unstable), possible dividing ECs in spouting vessels; endothelial progenitor cells in bone marrow or peripheral blood
Onset	Delayed	Immediate
Therapeutic index	Greater, so less toxic	Limited because of side effects (ie, myelosuppression, and so forth)
Effect	Cytostatic → stabilization of disease	Cytotoxic or cytostatic → regression of disease or stabilization
Tumor regression	Usually no	Yes
Maintenance therapy	Likely needed	Usually not needed but proved to be beneficial in some cases
Resistance development	Yes	Yes

Abbreviation: ECs, endothelial cells.

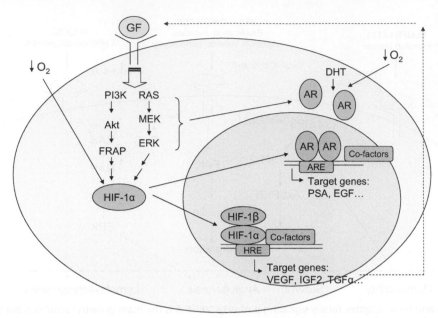

Fig. 2. Crosstalk between HIF-1α and androgen receptor in PCa cells. There are hypoxia-mediated and non–hypoxia-mediated HIF-1α upregulation pathways.[13] Non–hypoxia-mediated HIF-1α upregulation is typically mediated by growth factors (GF). GF binding to its cognate receptor tyrosine kinase activates the phosphatidylinositol 3-kinase (PI3K) and mitogen-activated protein kinase (MAPK) pathways through RAS/MEK/ERK. PI3K activates the downstream serine/threonine kinase Akt and FKBP-rapamycin-associated protein (FRAP)/mammalian target of rapamycin (mTOR). In the MAPK pathway, the extracellular-signal-regulated kinase (ERK) is activated by the upstream MAP/ERK kinase (MEK). The growth-factor signaling increases gene expression, including HIF-1. The target genes of HIF-1 include VEGF, insulin-like growth factor-2 (IGF2), and transforming growth factor-α (TGFα), and so forth, which are autocrine or paracrine growth factors enhancing HIF-1α expression. Alternatively, hypoxia can activate HIF-1α and initiate autocrine signaling. AR can be activated by GF-mediated signaling independent of its ligand dihydrotestosterone (DHT). EGF is one of AR's target genes enhancing autocrine signaling loop. Hypoxia and HIF-1 greatly potentiate the AR response to its ligand. ARE, androgen receptor element; FKBP, FK506 binding protein; HRE, hypoxia-response element; PSA, prostate-specific antigen. RAS, GTPase encoded by oncogene Ras.

prostate carcinogenesis as well as in the transition from the castrate-sensitive (androgen dependent) into the castrate-resistant (androgen independent) stage.[18] Therapeutic actions of antiandrogens or androgen deprivation therapy (ADT) in PCa actually include the inhibition of HIF-1 function.[17] Intratumoral upregulation of HIF-1 contributes to castration resistance by sensitizing AR to a very low concentration of ligand available in the environment. Thus, the inhibition of HIF-1 pathways, which is achieved by many antiangiogenic agents, is able to target AR signaling and provide a therapeutic benefit in the management of PCa.[19]

VEGF is expressed by a variety of human solid tumors, including PCa.[20,21] VEGF plays a critical role in the pathogenesis and progression of human PCa.[14,22] In human PCa cells, the expression of VEGF receptors (Flk-1/KDR) correlates with poorly differentiated tumors and poor prognosis.[22] VEGF is present in both localized and metastatic prostate tumors, and increasing the plasma concentration of VEGF correlates with metastatic

disease progression.[23–25] In patients with metastatic castration-resistant PCa cancer (mCRPC), both plasma and urine VEGF levels are independent predictors of overall survival (OS).[26,27] These data supported the role of VEGF in PCa progression and the hypothesis that inhibition of VEGF may enhance current therapies in advanced PCa.

ANTIANGIOGENIC AGENTS IN CLINICAL DEVELOPMENT FOR TREATMENT OF PCA

Angiogenesis inhibitors in clinical trials include (1) agents that directly inhibit ECs, (2) agents that block activators of angiogenesis, and (3) agents that block extracellular matrix breakdown. The extracellular matrix of tumors is a complex network of heparan sulfate proteoglycans (HSPGs), collagen, laminin, and fibronectin. Heparanase is one of the antiangiogenesis targets because it is a ubiquitous endoglycosidase that specifically cleaves HSPGs facilitating angiogenesis through growth factor release and metastasis by enhancing cell invasion, migration, intravasation, and extravasation.[28,29] In PCa, many agents were studied in the preclinical and clinical setting with the hope that either single antiangiogenic agent or in combination with other agents can suppress PCa growth and help patients live longer. **Table 2** lists the most known agents in clinical development for PCa.[28,30–42]

Table 2
Selected antiangiogenic agents in clinical development for PCa

Mechanisms and Drugs	Cellular Targets/Mechanisms	Clinical Phase of Development (Reference)
Anti-VEGF agents		
Bevacizumab	Humanized IgG monoclonal antibody to all the isoforms of VEGF	III, with docetaxel ± bevacizumab, mCRPC, completed, reported[30]
Aflibercept (VEGF-trap)	Fusion protein of the human extracellular domains of VEGFR-1 and VEGFR-2 and the Fc portion of human IgG; binds to both VEGF-A and PlGF with a higher affinity than monoclonal antibodies	III, docetaxel ± aflibercept, mCRPC, completed, (NCT00519285)
Small molecular tyrosine kinase inhibitors		
Sunitinib (SU11248)	Inhibits the VEGFR, PDGFR, Flt-3, C-kit, CSF-1R, and RET receptor tyrosine kinases	III, mCRPC with prednisone[31] II, mCRPC, with docetaxel[32]
Sorafenib (BAY 43–9006)	Raf kinase (B-Raf, C-Raf) inhibits VEGFR (VEGFR-2 and VEGFR-3), PDGFR, and C-kit	II, mCRPC, after docetaxel[33] II, mCRPC single agent[34,35]
Cabozantinib	MET, VEGFR2, C-RET, and C-KIT	III, mCRPC (NCT01522443)
AZD2171/cediranib	VEGFR2&3, FGFR, PDGFR	II, NCT00436956
Antiangiogenesis and immunomodulatory agents		
Thalidomide	Not fully understood	II, mCRPC[36–39]
Lenalidomide	Modulation of integrins and immunomodulatory and antiinflammatory effects, tumor microenvironment	III, mCRPC, on hold (NCT00988208)
Others		
Tasquinimod	Upregulates the expression of thrombospondin-1, downregulates HIF-1α and VEGF[40]	III, mCRPC (NCT01234311)
Enzastaurin	Serine/threonine kinase inhibitor of the beta isoform of protein kinase C	II, mCRPC[41]
17-allylamino-17-demethoxygeldanamycin	Inhibitors of HSP90 and promotes degradation of HIF-1α	II, mCRPC (NCT00118092)
EMD 121 974 (cilengitide, NSC 707 544)	$\alpha_v\beta_3$ and $\alpha_v\beta_5$ integrin receptor antagonist; inhibits ECs proliferation, migration, adhesion, and ultimately survival	II, nonmetastatic mCRPC[42]
PI-88	Extracellular matrix, inhibitor of angiogenesis and heparanase activity	I/II, mCRPC[28]

Abbreviations: CSF1R, colony stimulating factor 1 receptor; EC, endothelial cell; Flt-3, fms-like tyrosine kinase-3; HSP, heat shock protein; IgG, immunoglobulin G; PlGF, placental growth factor.

RATIONAL OF TARGETING ANGIOGENESIS IN COMBINATION WITH SYSTEMIC THERAPY

Cancer is driven by an extremely complicated network of signaling proteins. A mutual stimulation occurs between the stroma (ie, angiogenesis) and tumor parenchyma that sustains tumor growth, invasion, and metastasis. Therefore, the tumor cell and vascular system should be considered a functional unit regarding tumor growth. Targeting both tumor cells and angiogenesis is likely more effective than just targeting one of the tumor entities because antiangiogenic and cytotoxic agents work independently on different cellular targets. Preclinical evidence suggests that combining an antiangiogenic agent with a conventional cytotoxic agent or radiation therapy may have an additive or even synergistic antitumor effect.[43] Although the exact mechanism of the additive or synergistic effect is not known, antiangiogenic therapy has been shown to reduce interstitial fluid pressure (IFP). In tumors, there is increased IFP, which forms a barrier to transcapillary transport and is an obstacle for the delivery of therapeutic agents to the tumor site.[44] When IFP is reduced by antiangiogenic therapy, the tissue diffusion of chemotherapy is improved. In addition, conventional cytotoxic chemotherapy drugs can inhibit tumor cell proliferation or may inhibit the growth of several normal host cell types that contribute to angiogenesis pathway. Chemotherapy targets include the following: (1) bone marrow–derived proangiogenic cells that adhere to the walls of new blood vessels and further stimulate their growth by paracrine mechanisms, (2) circulating/cycling ECs present in sprouting blood vessel capillaries, and (3) authentic bone marrow–derived circulating endothelial progenitor cells that can incorporate into the lumen of growing vessels and differentiate into ECs.[45] Chemotherapy also suppresses or reduces the secretion of soluble tumor-derived growth factors and soluble endothelial growth factors, which is the key component of angiogenesis.[46]

Because multiple signaling pathways are involved in angiogenesis and more than one pathway is often dysregulated in human tumors, blocking a single pathway may not be highly effective and/or can lead to resistance when the tumor cells develop other angiogenesis mechanisms. By combining antiangiogenic agents with each other or with other modalities used in the treatment of cancer, the limitations of each therapeutic approach may be overcome, leading to enhanced efficacy with diminished toxicity and potentially overcome or delay drug resistance.

In PCa, a unique systemic therapy for advanced PCa is ADT. ADT is initiated in patients who develop metastatic disease or in patients receiving radiation therapy. In mice bearing LNCaP tumors, castration resulted in a rapid decrease in VEGF mRNA expression as well as markedly reduced tumor neovascularization. This finding is also true in vitro and in vivo in another androgen-responsive cell line CWR22Rv1.[47] The reversal of neovascularization was also demonstrated after hormone withdrawal as an early event in human PCa response to ADT.[48] It was discussed previously that androgen activates the HIF-1 signaling pathway in androgen-sensitive LNCaP cells.[17] HIF-1 helps maintain survival for PCa cells in an androgen-deprivation environment. EGF and other growth factors are mediators of this crosstalk. Agents inhibiting the HIF-1 signaling pathway can potentially sensitize PCa to ADT and are the logical choice for combining them with AR signaling inhibitors.

In this review, the authors focus on the key combination studies performed in the past several years in the treatment of PCa and hope to understand more about the complex antiangiogenic strategies for PCa treatment and shed light for future trial designs.

RECENT KEY CLINICAL TRIALS WITH ANTIANGIOGENIC AGENTS IN PCA
Bevacizumab: VEGF-Targeting Monoclonal Antibody

The use of monoclonal antibodies targeting the VEGF pathway has been a significant addition to cancer therapy.[49] Although the mechanism of action of these antibodies is still under study, the anti-VEGF antibody bevacizumab has been approved for the treatment of various solid cancers, including colorectal and lung cancer, glioblastoma, and renal cell carcinoma. Bevacizumab is being tested in other clinical settings, such as adjuvant therapy; maintenance therapy; and in combination with both chemotherapy and other targeted agents, such as the EGFR kinase inhibitor erlotinib.[50–54] In PCa, bevacizumab was studied in the neoadjuvant setting (in combination with docetaxel); in biochemically relapsed patients with low disease burden (in combination with active immune therapy sipuleucel-T); and in patients with mCRPC with or without previous chemotherapy (in combination with docetaxel or other agents) (Table 3).[39,55–58] Based on the preclinical data on the role of VEGF in PCa and the preliminary studies in patients showing that the combination of bevacizumab with docetaxel was safe and had encouraging clinical outcomes, a randomized placebo controlled phase III study with standard docetaxel and prednisone with and without bevacizumab was performed.

Table 3
Bevacizumab in PCa

Regimen	Phase	N	Population	Clinical Benefit	References
Docetaxel (70 mg/m² q3 wk × 6) plus bevacizumab (15 mg/m² q3 wk × 5)	II	41	High-risk localized, neoadjuvant	No CR, 29% reduction in tumor volume	Ross et al[55]
Sipuleucel-T q2 wk × 3 plus bevacizumab (10 mg/kg) q2 wk	II	22	increasing PSA after local treatment	PSADT 6.9 →12.7 mo	Rini et al[56]
Bevacizumab (10 mg/kg) and docetaxel (60 mg/m²) every 3 wk	II	20	mCRPC, docetaxel treated	Active and well tolerated	Di Lorenzo et al[57]
Docetaxel 75 mg/m² and bevacizumab 15 mg/kg q3 wk plus oral thalidomide 200 mg/d and prednisone 10 mg/d	II	60	mCRPC	PSA response ≥50% in 90% of patients	Ning et al[39]
Estramustine 280 mg tid on day 1–5, Docetaxel 70 mg/m² and 15 mg/kg Bevacizumab on day 2 q3 wk	II	79	mCRPC	PSA response ≥50% in 75% of patients	Picus et al[58]

Abbreviation: CR, complete response; PSA, prostate-specific antigen; PSADT: PSA doubling time.

A total of 1050 patients with chemotherapy-naive progressive mCRPC were randomly assigned to receive docetaxel plus prednisone (DP) with either bevacizumab 15 mg/kg (every 3 weeks) or placebo.[30] The primary end point was OS. There was no significant difference in the median OS for patients who were administered DP plus bevacizumab (22.6 months) compared with patients treated with DP (21.5 months) (P = .181). The median progression-free survival (PFS) was superior in the DP plus bevacizumab arm (9.9 vs 7.5 months, P = .001) as was the proportion of patients with overall response (OR) in measurable disease by response evaluation criteria in solid tumors (RECIST) (49.4% vs 35.5%, P = .0013). Grade 3 or greater treatment-related toxicity was more common with DP plus bevacizumab (75.4% vs 56.2%, P≤.001) as was the number of treatment-related deaths (4.0% vs 1.2%, P = .005), which were mostly related to infectious complications.

The study showed that there was no significant clinical benefit for adding bevacizumab to docetaxel and prednisone and the primary end point was not met. Why PFS improvement did not translate into improved OS is not known, but perhaps the longer duration of exposure of bevacizumab therapy beyond progression would make a difference in the outcome. However, this study was not designed to evaluate the role of maintenance bevacizumab therapy. Although patients were allowed to continue on single-modality bevacizumab or placebo treatment if the docetaxel therapy was not tolerated, few patients and physicians elected to continue monotherapy with bevacizumab or placebo. The role of maintenance bevacizumab therapy in a relatively slow growing tumor, such as PCa, needs to be examined because the phenomenon of rapid tumor regrowth or rebound is not uncommonly observed in patients with anti-angiogenesis therapy.[59] Although it is not clear if this phenomenon also exists in patients with mCRPC, nonsustained antiangiogenesis and regrowth may diminish the benefit from initial bevacizumab treatment.

Exploratory subset analysis suggested that patients with markers of high tumor burden or more advanced disease (low hemoglobin, increased serum alkaline phosphatase, or high lactate dehydrogenase) as well as patients with low testosterone levels (<20 ng/dL) had an improved OS with the addition of bevacizumab to docetaxel and prednisone. So another question to ask is whether there are any biologic differences between these patients and others with low disease burden. Can we assume that these cancers are growing faster but less dependent on androgen or simply because

AR machinery is not so active? A fast-growing tumor may be more prone to hypoxia and be more dependent on angiogenesis than a slow-growing tumor and low disease burden. Another question is how to identify these patients who may benefit from this combination therapy. Relevant biomarker analysis is ongoing, which is evaluating the role of circulating VEGF levels, circulating endothelial progenitors, docetaxel pharmacogenomics,[60] VEGF, and VEGFR gene polymorphism.[61]

Thalidomide-Containing Combinational Trials

Thalidomide was removed from market in the 1960s and it was found that the birth defects of the limbs could be caused by its inhibition of blood vessel growth in the limb buds of a developing fetus.[62] It was proposed that the antiangiogenic activity may be the result of its metabolites.[62,63] The mechanism of thalidomide (and metabolites) is not fully understood yet but its immunomodulatory and antiinflammatory effects likely contribute to its antiangiogenic effects.[10] It also has an effect on components of the tumor microenvironment, which has more importance for advanced malignancy.[64]

In a randomized phase II combination study, 75 patients with mCRPC received weekly docetaxel,

$30 \ mg/m^2$ for 3 weeks of a 4-week cycle with or without thalidomide 200 mg daily (**Table 4**).[36–39] Median OS was initially reported to be 14.7 months for docetaxel monotherapy and 28.9 months in the combination arm. Updated results demonstrated an OS of 25.9 months on the thalidomide arm and 14.7 months for the docetaxel monotherapy arm ($P = .0407$). One finding of concern was the high thromboembolic incidence in the combination group. However, there was no thrombosis in the subsequent patients after the initiation of prophylactic anticoagulation with low-molecular-weight heparin. There was no increased hematologic toxicity in the combination group, which was encouraging. This trial is the first randomized trial demonstrating that an antiangiogenesis agent may potentially be associated with an improved survival benefit in patients with mCRPC. However, the study was not designed to have sufficient patients to evaluate survival as a main end point.

Based on the hypothesis that combining the mechanistically different antiangiogenic agents may be more effective, a phase II trial combining thalidomide and bevacizumab with Taxotere in chemotherapy naive mCRPC was performed. Enoxaparin was used for thrombosis prevention. Ninety percent of the patients receiving the combination therapy had a Prostate-specific antigen

Table 4
Thalidomide combination in mCRPC

Regimen	Phase	N	Population	Clinical Benefit	References
Thalidomide (200 mg/d) Docetaxel (30 mg/m² day 1, 8, 15, q28 d) Enoxaparin (40 mg SC/d)	II	75	Docetaxel naive	OS of 25.9 mo in thalidomide group vs OS of 14.7 mo in control group ($P = .0407$)	Dahut et al,[36] Figg et al[37]
Thalidomide (200 mg/d) Docetaxel (30 mg/m² day 1, 8, 15 q28 d) Estramustine (tid day 1–3, 8–10, 15–17, q28 d)	II	20	Docetaxel naive	Median PFS 7.2 mo	Figg et al[38]
Thalidomide (200 mg/d) Docetaxel (75 mg/m² q3 wk) Bevacizumab (15 mg/kg q3 wk) Prednisone (10 mg/d)	II	60	Docetaxel naive	PSA response >50% in 88% of patients; PFS 18.2 mo; OS 28.2 mo	Ning et al[39]

Abbreviation: SC, subcutaneously.

(PSA) decline of more than 50%, and 88% achieved a PSA decline of more than 30% within the first 3 months of treatment. The median time to progression was 18.3 months, and the median OS was 28.2 months. Among the 33 patients with measurable disease, there were 2 confirmed complete responses and 19 confirmed partial responses, with an overall response rate of 64%. But the toxicity was also significant. A total of 18.3% of patients developed grade 2 osteonecrosis of the jaw. All of the patients developed grade 3 or 4 neutropenia, with 5 out of 60 patients (8%) developing febrile neutropenia. Significant grade 3 or 4 nonhematologic toxicities included syncope (17%), gastrointestinal perforation or fistula (7%), thrombosis (7%), and grade 3 bleeding (3%). There was one treatment-related death caused by myocardial infarction that was complicated by the development of grade 4 aortic dissection. This study proved the hypothesis that combined antiangiogenic therapy does work and may represent a new approach in the treatment of mCRPC. Because of the increased morbidity of this regimen, further phase III studies were not pursued. Instead of thalidomide, a phase II study to evaluate the toxicity and efficacy of the less-toxic lenalidomide (in combination with bevacizumab, docetaxel, and prednisone) was recently presented.[65] Among 45 patients with chemotherapy-naive mCRPC who completed 2 or more cycles of treatment, 39 (86.7%) and 30 (66.7%) had PSA declines of 50% or more and 75% or more, respectively. Of 29 patients with measurable disease, the overall response rate (RR) was 79.3%. Grade 3 or more toxicity was still significant with neutropenia (51%), febrile neutropenia (9%), anemia (19%), thrombocytopenia (11%), weight loss (2%), and hypertension (6%). There was a high incidence of osteonecrosis of the jaw (34%), which was higher than the similar study using thalidomide (18.3%). Venous thromboembolism (VTE) was not an issue in this phase II study because prophylactic enoxaparin was given daily. However, enoxaparin was not given to patients in the phase 3 study to evaluate the efficacy and safety of docetaxel and prednisone with or without lenalidomide (clinicaltrials.gov identifier: NCT00988208). The study was discontinued because of increased VTE incidence in the treatment arm.

Combinational Trials Involving Multi-Tyrosine Kinase Inhibitors

Combinatorial therapies with antiangiogenic agents are not limited to those including cytotoxic chemotherapy. Several preclinical studies and clinical trials are exploring the combination of various angiogenesis inhibitors with other targeted therapies, such as EGFR or human epidermal growth factor receptor 2 (Her2) inhibitors (cetuximab, erlotinib, and trastuzumab)[51,66–68] or proteasome inhibitors (bortezomib).[69] The advantage of the multi-tyrosine kinase inhibitors is that they affect multiple key signaling molecules in tumor angiogenesis. Although it is generally considered that these small molecular inhibitors target ECs, the malignant cells and surrounding stromal cells are also targeted. Autocrine and paracrine proangiogenic factors are inhibited, and the angiogenic switch may be turned off.

Sunitinib malate is an oral inhibitor of the tyrosine kinases of VEGFRs, platelet-derived growth factor receptor (PDGFRs), tyrosine-protein kinase (KIT or CD117), fms-like tyrosine kinase-3, colony stimulating factor 1 receptor (CSF-1R), and receptor tyrosine kinases encoded by proto-oncogene (c-RET). In combination with ADT, sunitinib (37.5 mg daily) was studied in the neoadjuvant setting. One out of 44 patients achieved a pathologic complete remission (pCR) in patients with high-risk localized PCa.[70] Based on the signal of potential activities from phase II trials in mCRPC,[33,71] a phase III trial of sunitinib with prednisone versus prednisone and placebo in men with progressive mCRPC after docetaxel-based chemotherapy was conducted.[31] Full publication is awaited. In this multicenter double-blind study, patients received prednisone 5 mg twice a day and either sunitinib 37.5 mg or placebo on a continuous once-daily dosing schedule. A total of 873 men were randomized to receive sunitinib (n = 584) or placebo (n = 289). The study was stopped for futility at the second interim analysis by the data monitoring committee. Similar to bevacizumab in combination with docetaxel in the Cancer and Leukemia Group B (CALGB) 90401 study, sunitinib improved median PFS (5.6 months vs 3.7 months, hazard ratio 0.76, $P = .0077$) but did not improve OS (13.1 months vs 12.8 months, $P = .58$) in the second-line therapy for mCRPC. No new or unexpected safety issues were identified.

Another phase I/II study combining sunitinib with docetaxel-based chemotherapy was completed.[32] The PSA response rate was 56.4% (95% confidence interval 42.3–69.7). Only 12 (22%) patients completed the study (16 cycles) and 43 (78%) discontinued (for disease progression or adverse events). The most frequent treatment-related grade 3/4 adverse events were neutropenia (53%; 15% with febrile neutropenia) and fatigue/asthenia (16%). Among 33 assessable patients, 14 (42.4%) had confirmed a partial response. Median PFS and OS were 12.6 and 21.7 months, respectively. It was concluded that this combination was moderately well tolerated with a promising response rate and survival benefit, justifying further investigation in mCRPC.

Another promising multi-tyrosine kinase inhibitor is Cabozantinib, a dual inhibitor of hepatocyte growth factor receptor (HGFR,MET) and VEGFR2. Cabozantinib is an inhibitor of MET and VEGFR2 as well as C-RET and C-KIT kinase. MET signaling promotes tumor growth, invasion, and metastasis and is upregulated in advanced PCa (**Box 2**).[72–74] A randomized discontinuation study was performed, and intriguing but promising results were reported in 2011 by the American Society of Clinical Oncology. Accrual was halted at 168 patients based on an observed high rate of clinical activity and patients unblinded. Bone effects were impressive: 86% (56 out of 65 patients) of patients evaluable by bone scan had complete or partial resolution of lesions on bone scan as early as week 6. Sixty-four percent of the patients had improved pain and 46% decreased or halted narcotics use. Median maximum increase in hemoglobin in patients with anemia was 2.2 g/dL (range, 0.6–3.5). Fifty-five percent of the patients had declines of 50% or more in plasma C-terminal telopeptide, a commonly used biomarker for bone turnover. Fifty-six percent of patients with elevated tissue alkaline phosphatase had declines of 50% or more. It also had activity for nonbone metastases, with an objective tumor shrinkage rate of 84%. Overall, the week 12 disease control rate (partial response [PR] + stable disease [SD]) was 71%. The side effects actually were similar to those of other tyrosine kinase inhibitors, such as sunitinib. The most common related grade 3 or 4 adverse events were fatigue (11%), hypertension (7%), and hand-foot syndrome (5%). No related grade 5 adverse events were reported. Dose reductions for adverse events occurred in 51% of patients, and discontinuations occurred in 10% of patients. It was considered a well-tolerated regimen. The clinical activity is likely true because both C-Met and VEGFR2 are key molecules in the bone metastatic microenvironment and targeting 2 molecules together may achieve the highest efficacy (**Box 2**). The clinical benefits of cabozantinib cannot simply be explained by its ability to block the bone uptake of technetium-99m methylene-diphosphonate (MDP), the tracer for bone scan. The phase III study is ongoing with the primary end point of pain response at week 12 durable since week 6 (ClinicalTrials.gov Identifier: NCT01522443).

FUTURE DIRECTIONS

Options to treat late-stage mCRPC continued to expand in the past few years because 3 agents with different mechanisms of action prolonged life and a fourth reduced the morbidity of skeletal metastases (**Box 3**). As one of the therapy modalities, antiangiogenic therapy will need to be studied further to see if it will improve the clinical benefit of these other novel agents. Combining or sequencing drugs that target the angiogenesis pathway with the next-generation AR signaling inhibitor (ARSI), bone targeted therapy, immunotherapy, or even second-line chemotherapy will need to be studied. Docetaxel was the only effective agent before 2004 and many agents were tested in combination with docetaxel for PCa treatment. With the availability of novel effective drugs for PCa, a variety of combination regimens

---

Box 2
C-Met oncogene in advanced PCa

- C-Met is a membrane-spanning tyrosine kinase.

  - It is overexpressed in primary PCa, further increased in expression in bone metastases and poorly differentiated PCa cells.

  - It is expressed in osteoblasts and osteoclasts.

- Androgen receptor downregulates C-Met in a ligand-dependent manner. ADT increases C-Met expression in tumor cells and its ligand hepatocyte growth factor/scatter factor (HGF/SF) expression in tumor and stromal cells.

  - C-Met is associated with the development of castrate-resistant state.

- The aberrant expression of C-Met and its ligand often correlates with poor prognosis in a variety of human malignancies, including PCa.

  - Activation of the HGF/C-Met pathway plays a role in the development of resistance to antiangiogenic therapy.

Data from Refs.[31,71,72]

Box 3
Recent key drug development for the treatment of mCRPC

- Androgen-androgen receptor axis targeted agents: Cyp17 inhibitor abiraterone acetate and androgen receptor-signaling inhibitor enzalutamide (MDV3100)

- Active immunotherapy: sipuleucel-T (Provenge)

- Bone-directed radioisotope: radium223

- Receptor activator of nuclear factor kappa-B ligand (RANKL) inhibitor: denosumab

- Second-line chemotherapy: cabazitaxel

can be tested. It is possible that an angiogenesis inhibitor in combination with ARSI or Inhibitors of cytochrome P450 17A1, or 17α-hydroxylase/17,20 lyase (Cyp17) inhibitor will significantly reduce the toxicity profile and possibly improve efficacy comparing that with docetaxel-containing regimens.

In addition to the combinational approach to improve treatment efficacy and delay resistance, searching for better angiogenic inhibitors in terms of potency, tolerability, safety, and efficacy is a burgeoning field in all aspects of cancer research. Agents like the dual C-Met and VEGFR2 inhibitor cabozantinib hold promise with a remarkable objective tumor response and clinical benefit. On the other side, narrowing the drug's use depending on predictive biomarkers will improve treatment efficacy. The CALGB 90401 study indicated that a better definition of specific targeted populations needs to be identified because bevacizumab seemed to benefit a particular subset of patients. During the treatment, research should also focus on using molecular, pharmacologic, biologic, and radiologic parameters to better measure or define objective responses. Incorporating novel imaging modalities, such as dynamic contrast-enhanced magnetic resonance imaging (DCE-MRI) may also help to characterize the efficacy of antiangiogenic agents.[75]

SUMMARY

Angiogenesis seems to play an important role in the progression of PCa. Combination therapy can target both endothelial and tumor cells to achieve better efficacy and delay drug resistance, but toxicity is still a concern. Challenges are multifold because many questions remain to be answered, such as patient selection, the need for maintenance therapy, and the timing of initiating antiangiogenic therapy given the long natural history of PCa. Novel agents, such as the dual MET and VEGFR2 inhibitor cabozantinib, need to be explored in biomarker-driven studies. Targeting angiogenesis remains to be a promising modality for the treatment of PCa, but further study needs to show where these agents will provide clinical benefits to patients.

REFERENCES

1. Folkman J. Tumor angiogenesis: therapeutic implications. N Engl J Med 1971;285(21):1182–6.
2. Hanahan D, Weinberg RA. The hallmarks of cancer. Cell 2000;100(1):57–70.
3. Folkman J. Angiogenesis-dependent diseases. Semin Oncol 2001;28(6):536–42.
4. Folkman J. Angiogenesis inhibitors: a new class of drugs. Cancer Biol Ther 2003;2(4 Suppl 1):S127–33.
5. Bergers G, Benjamin LE. Tumorigenesis and the angiogenic switch. Nat Rev Cancer 2003;3(6):401–10.
6. Carmeliet P, Jain RK. Angiogenesis in cancer and other diseases. Nature 2000;407(6801):249–57.
7. Alfiky A, Kelly WK. Bevacizumab in advanced prostate cancer. Drug management of prostate cancer. In: Figg WD, Chau CH, Small EJ, editors. Springer; 2010. p. 207–14. ISBN: 978-1603278317.
8. Kerbel RS. Tumor angiogenesis. N Engl J Med 2008;358(19):2039–49.
9. Carmeliet P, Jain RK. Molecular mechanisms and clinical applications of angiogenesis. Nature 2011;473(7347):298–307.
10. Cook KM, Figg WD. Angiogenesis inhibitors: current strategies and future prospects. CA Cancer J Clin 2010;60(4):222–43.
11. Movsas B, Chapman JD, Horwitz EM, et al. Hypoxic regions exist in human prostate carcinoma. Urology 1999;53(1):11–8.
12. Zhong H, De Marzo AM, Laughner E, et al. Overexpression of hypoxia-inducible factor 1alpha in common human cancers and their metastases. Cancer Res 1999;59(22):5830–5.
13. Lin J, Denmeade S, Carducci MA. HIF-1alpha and calcium signaling as targets for treatment of prostate cancer by cardiac glycosides. Curr Cancer Drug Targets 2009;9(7):881–7.
14. Weidner N, Carroll PR, Flax J, et al. Tumor angiogenesis correlates with metastasis in invasive prostate carcinoma. Am J Pathol 1993;143(2):401–9.
15. Strohmeyer D, Rossing C, Strauss F, et al. Tumor angiogenesis is associated with progression after radical prostatectomy in pT2/pT3 prostate cancer. Prostate 2000;42(1):26–33.
16. Semenza GL. Targeting HIF-1 for cancer therapy. Nat Rev Cancer 2003;3(10):721–32.
17. Mabjeesh NJ, Willard MT, Frederickson CE, et al. Androgens stimulate hypoxia-inducible factor 1 activation via autocrine loop of tyrosine kinase receptor/phosphatidylinositol 3'-kinase/protein kinase B in prostate cancer cells. Clin Cancer Res 2003;9(7):2416–25.
18. Kimbro KS, Simons JW. Hypoxia-inducible factor-1 in human breast and prostate cancer. Endocr Relat Cancer 2006;13(3):739–49.
19. Boddy JL, Fox SB, Han C, et al. The androgen receptor is significantly associated with vascular endothelial growth factor and hypoxia sensing via hypoxia-inducible factors HIF-1a, HIF-2a, and the prolyl hydroxylases in human prostate cancer. Clin Cancer Res 2005;11(21):7658–63.
20. Poon RT, Fan ST, Wong J. Clinical implications of circulating angiogenic factors in cancer patients. J Clin Oncol 2001;19(4):1207–25.

21. Mao K, Badoual C, Camparo P, et al. The prognostic value of vascular endothelial growth factor (VEGF)-A and its receptor in clinically localized prostate cancer: a prospective evaluation in 100 patients undergoing radical prostatectomy. Can J Urol 2008;15(5):4257–62.

22. Ferrer FA, Miller LJ, Lindquist R, et al. Expression of vascular endothelial growth factor receptors in human prostate cancer. Urology 1999;54(3):567–72.

23. Ferrer FA, Miller LJ, Andrawis RI, et al. Vascular endothelial growth factor (VEGF) expression in human prostate cancer: in situ and in vitro expression of VEGF by human prostate cancer cells. J Urol 1997;157(6):2329–33.

24. Duque JL, Loughlin KR, Adam RM, et al. Plasma levels of vascular endothelial growth factor are increased in patients with metastatic prostate cancer. Urology 1999;54(3):523–7.

25. Duque JL, Loughlin KR, Adam RM, et al. Measurement of plasma levels of vascular endothelial growth factor in prostate cancer patients: relationship with clinical stage, Gleason score, prostate volume, and serum prostate-specific antigen. Clinics (Sao Paulo) 2006;61(5):401–8.

26. Bok RA, Halabi S, Fei DT, et al. Vascular endothelial growth factor and basic fibroblast growth factor urine levels as predictors of outcome in hormone-refractory prostate cancer patients: a cancer and leukemia group B study. Cancer Res 2001;61(6):2533–6.

27. George DJ, Halabi S, Shepard TF, et al. The prognostic significance of plasma interleukin-6 levels in patients with metastatic hormone-refractory prostate cancer: results from cancer and leukemia group B 9480. Clin Cancer Res 2005;11(5):1815–20.

28. Khasraw M, Pavlakis N, McCowatt S, et al. Multicentre phase I/II study of PI-88, a heparanase inhibitor in combination with docetaxel in patients with metastatic castrate-resistant prostate cancer. Ann Oncol 2010;21(6):1302–7.

29. Sasisekharan R, Shriver Z, Venkataraman G, et al. Roles of heparan-sulphate glycosaminoglycans in cancer. Nat Rev Cancer 2002;2(7):521–8.

30. Kelly WK, Halabi S, Carducci M, et al. Randomized, double-blind, placebo-controlled phase iii trial comparing docetaxel and prednisone with or without bevacizumab in men with metastatic castration-resistant prostate cancer: CALGB 90401. J Clin Oncol 2012;30(13):1534–40.

31. Michaelson M, Oudard S, Ou Y, et al. Randomized, placebo-controlled, phase III trial of sunitinib in combination with prednisone (SU+P) versus prednisone (P) alone in men with progressive metastatic castration-resistant prostate cancer (mCRPC). J Clin Oncol 2011;29(Suppl) [abstr 4515].

32. Zurita AJ, George DJ, Shore ND, et al. Sunitinib in combination with docetaxel and prednisone in chemotherapy-naive patients with metastatic, castration-resistant prostate cancer: a phase 1/2 clinical trial. Ann Oncol 2012;23(3):688–94.

33. Sonpavde G, Periman PO, Bernold D, et al. Sunitinib malate for metastatic castration-resistant prostate cancer following docetaxel-based chemotherapy. Ann Oncol 2010;21(2):319–24.

34. Dahut WL, Scripture C, Posadas E, et al. A phase II clinical trial of sorafenib in androgen-independent prostate cancer. Clin Cancer Res 2008;14(1):209–14.

35. Chi KN, Ellard SL, Hotte SJ, et al. A phase II study of sorafenib in patients with chemo-naive castration-resistant prostate cancer. Ann Oncol 2008;19(4):746–51.

36. Dahut WL, Gulley JL, Arlen PM, et al. Randomized phase II trial of docetaxel plus thalidomide in androgen-independent prostate cancer. J Clin Oncol 2004;22(13):2532–9.

37. Figg WD, Retter AS, Steinberg SM, et al. In reply to: inhibition of angiogenesis: thalidomide or low-molecular-weight heparin? J Clin Oncol 2005;23(9):2113.

38. Figg WD, Li H, Sissung T, et al. Pre-clinical and clinical evaluation of estramustine, docetaxel and thalidomide combination in androgen-independent prostate cancer. BJU Int 2007;99(5):1047–55.

39. Ning YM, Gulley JL, Arlen PM, et al. Phase II trial of bevacizumab, thalidomide, docetaxel, and prednisone in patients with metastatic castration-resistant prostate cancer. J Clin Oncol 2010;28(12):2070–6.

40. Olsson A, Bjork A, Vallon-Christersson J, et al. Tasquinimod (ABR-215050), a quinoline-3-carboxamide anti-angiogenic agent, modulates the expression of thrombospondin-1 in human prostate tumors. Mol Cancer 2010;9:107.

41. Dreicer R, Garcia J, Hussain M, et al. Oral enzastaurin in prostate cancer: a two-cohort phase II trial in patients with PSA progression in the non-metastatic castrate state and following docetaxel-based chemotherapy for castrate metastatic disease. Invest New Drugs 2011;29(6):1441–8.

42. Alva A, Slovin S, Daignault S, et al. Phase II study of Cilengitide (EMD 121974, NSC 707544) in patients with non-metastatic castration resistant prostate cancer, NCI-6735. A study by the DOD/PCF prostate cancer clinical trials consortium. Invest New Drugs 2012;30(2):749–57.

43. Gasparini G, Longo R, Fanelli M, et al. Combination of antiangiogenic therapy with other anticancer therapies: results, challenges, and open questions. J Clin Oncol 2005;23(6):1295–311.

44. Heldin CH, Rubin K, Pietras K, et al. High interstitial fluid pressure - an obstacle in cancer therapy. Nat Rev Cancer 2004;4(10):806–13.

45. Ferrara N, Kerbel RS. Angiogenesis as a therapeutic target. Nature 2005;438(7070):967–74.

46. Folkman J. Angiogenesis and apoptosis. Semin Cancer Biol 2003;13(2):159–67.

47. Cheng L, Zhang S, Sweeney CJ, et al. Androgen withdrawal inhibits tumor growth and is associated with decrease in angiogenesis and VEGF expression in androgen-independent CWR22Rv1 human prostate cancer model. Anticancer Res 2004;24(4): 2135–40.

48. Stewart RJ, Panigrahy D, Flynn E, et al. Vascular endothelial growth factor expression and tumor angiogenesis are regulated by androgens in hormone responsive human prostate carcinoma: evidence for androgen dependent destabilization of vascular endothelial growth factor transcripts. J Urol 2001;165(2):688–93.

49. Hsu JY, Wakelee HA. Monoclonal antibodies targeting vascular endothelial growth factor: current status and future challenges in cancer therapy. BioDrugs 2009;23(5):289–304.

50. Hainsworth JD, Spigel DR, Farley C, et al. Phase II trial of bevacizumab and erlotinib in carcinomas of unknown primary site: the Minnie Pearl Cancer Research Network. J Clin Oncol 2007;25(13): 1747–52.

51. Herbst RS, O'Neill VJ, Fehrenbacher L, et al. Phase II study of efficacy and safety of bevacizumab in combination with chemotherapy or erlotinib compared with chemotherapy alone for treatment of recurrent or refractory non small-cell lung cancer. J Clin Oncol 2007;25(30):4743–50.

52. Thomas MB, Morris JS, Chadha R, et al. Phase II trial of the combination of bevacizumab and erlotinib in patients who have advanced hepatocellular carcinoma. J Clin Oncol 2009;27(6):843–50.

53. Van Cutsem E, Vervenne WL, Bennouna J, et al. Phase III trial of bevacizumab in combination with gemcitabine and erlotinib in patients with metastatic pancreatic cancer. J Clin Oncol 2009;27(13):2231–7.

54. Lubner SJ, Mahoney MR, Kolesar JL, et al. Report of a multicenter phase II trial testing a combination of biweekly bevacizumab and daily erlotinib in patients with unresectable biliary cancer: a phase II consortium study. J Clin Oncol 2010;28(21):3491–7.

55. Ross RW, Galsky MD, Febbo P, et al. Phase 2 study of neoadjuvant docetaxel plus bevacizumab in patients with high-risk localized prostate cancer: a prostate Cancer Clinical Trials Consortium trial. Cancer 2012. [Epub ahead of print].

56. Rini BI, Weinberg V, Fong L, et al. Combination immunotherapy with prostatic acid phosphatase pulsed antigen-presenting cells (provenge) plus bevacizumab in patients with serologic progression of prostate cancer after definitive local therapy. Cancer 2006;107(1):67–74.

57. Di Lorenzo G, Figg WD, Fossa SD, et al. Combination of bevacizumab and docetaxel in docetaxel-pretreated hormone-refractory prostate cancer: a phase 2 study. Eur Urol 2008;54(5):1089–94.

58. Picus J, Halabi S, Kelly WK, et al. A phase 2 study of estramustine, docetaxel, and bevacizumab in men with castrate-resistant prostate cancer: results from Cancer and Leukemia Group B Study 90006. Cancer 2011;117(3):526–33.

59. Zuniga RM, Torcuator R, Jain R, et al. Rebound tumour progression after the cessation of bevacizumab therapy in patients with recurrent high-grade glioma. J Neurooncol 2010;99(2):237–42.

60. Freedman AN, Sansbury LB, Figg WD, et al. Cancer pharmacogenomics and pharmacoepidemiology: setting a research agenda to accelerate translation. J Natl Cancer Inst 2010;102(22): 1698–705.

61. Kim DH, Xu W, Kamel-Reid S, et al. Clinical relevance of vascular endothelial growth factor (VEGFA) and VEGF receptor (VEGFR2) gene polymorphism on the treatment outcome following imatinib therapy. Ann Oncol 2010;21(6):1179–88.

62. D'Amato RJ, Loughnan MS, Flynn E, et al. Thalidomide is an inhibitor of angiogenesis. Proc Natl Acad Sci U S A 1994;91(9):4082–5.

63. Kenyon BM, Browne F, D'Amato RJ. Effects of thalidomide and related metabolites in a mouse corneal model of neovascularization. Exp Eye Res 1997; 64(6):971–8.

64. Efstathiou E, Troncoso P, Wen S, et al. Initial modulation of the tumor microenvironment accounts for thalidomide activity in prostate cancer. Clin Cancer Res 2007;13(4):1224–31.

65. Adesunloye B, Huang X, Ning YM, et al. Phase II trial of bevacizumab and lenalidomide with docetaxel and prednisone in patients with metastatic castration-resistant prostate cancer (mCRPC). J Clin Oncol 2012;30(Suppl 5): [abstr 207].

66. Puente J, Manzano A, Martin M, et al. Breast cancer: complete response with the combination of sunitinib and trastuzumab in a patient with grade III ductal carcinoma. Anticancer Drugs 2010;21(Suppl 1): S19–22.

67. Bozec A, Sudaka A, Toussan N, et al. Combination of sunitinib, cetuximab and irradiation in an orthotopic head and neck cancer model. Ann Oncol 2009;20(10):1703–7.

68. Qvortrup C, Jensen BV, Jorgensen TL, et al. Addition of sunitinib to cetuximab and irinotecan in patients with heavily pre-treated advanced colorectal cancer. Acta Oncol 2010;49(6):833–6.

69. Yeramian A, Sorolla A, Velasco A, et al. Inhibition of activated receptor tyrosine kinases by sunitinib induces growth arrest and sensitizes melanoma cells to bortezomib by blocking Akt pathway. Int J Cancer 2012;130(4):967–78.

70. Zurita A, Ward JF, Araujo JC, et al. Presurgical sunitinib malate and androgen ablation in patients with

localized prostate cancer at high risk for recurrence. J Clin Oncol 2008;26(Suppl): [abstr 16004].

71. Dror Michaelson M, Regan MM, Oh WK, et al. Phase II study of sunitinib in men with advanced prostate cancer. Ann Oncol 2009;20(5):913–20.

72. Verras M, Lee J, Xue H, et al. The androgen receptor negatively regulates the expression of c-Met: implications for a novel mechanism of prostate cancer progression. Cancer Res 2007;67(3):967–75.

73. Varkaris A, Corn PG, Gaur S, et al. The role of HGF/c-Met signaling in prostate cancer progression and c-Met inhibitors in clinical trials. Expert Opin Investig Drugs 2011;20(12):1677–84.

74. Bottaro DP, Rubin JS, Faletto DL, et al. Identification of the hepatocyte growth factor receptor as the c-met proto-oncogene product. Science 1991; 251(4995):802–4.

75. Oto A, Yang C, Kayhan A, et al. Diffusion-weighted and dynamic contrast-enhanced MRI of prostate cancer: correlation of quantitative MR parameters with Gleason score and tumor angiogenesis. AJR Am J Roentgenol 2011;197(6):1382–90.

Advanced Clinical States in Prostate Cancer

Heather H. Cheng, MD, PhD[a,b,*], Daniel W. Lin, MD[c],
Evan Y. Yu, MD[a,b]

KEYWORDS

- Clinical states • Prostate cancer • Androgen deprivation • Prostate-specific antigen
- Castration resistant • Metastatic

KEY POINTS

- Prostate-specific antigen, imaging, and symptoms are the current criteria used to categorize advanced prostate cancer into the biochemically recurrent, metastatic castration-sensitive, nonmetastatic castration-resistant, and asymptomatic and symptomatic metastatic castration-resistant clinical disease states.
- Androgen deprivation therapy is the standard of care in castration-sensitive disease and, in selected cases, can be given on an intermittent schedule.
- The options for treatment of metastatic castration-resistant prostate cancer now include docetaxel, cabazitaxel, abiraterone, and sipuleucel-T, and multiple new agents are expected in the near future.
- Improvements in biomarkers and imaging are both anticipated and urgently needed to better categorize and stratify patients for receiving appropriate and effective treatment, particularly with expanding treatment options.

INTRODUCTION

The Prostate Cancer Working Group (PCWG1 and PCWG2) assembled consensus recommendations for prostate cancer clinical disease states with the goal of standardizing criteria not only for patient enrollment into clinical trials but also for clinically relevant endpoints.[1,2] The current paradigm of clinical disease states recommended by PCWG2 includes 5 clinical subtypes in prostate cancer based on location of disease: first, locally progressing tumors and no metastatic disease, second, rising prostate-specific antigen (PSA) and no detectable metastatic disease, third, nodal spread and no visceral disease, fourth, bone disease, and fifth, visceral disease (liver and lung).[1] Although these categories are based on location of metastatic sites and are recorded for clinical trial purposes, it is frequently the case that patients are stratified more simply by the lack of detectable metastases versus the presence of detectable metastases, regardless of whether in lymph node, bone, or viscera. Additionally, there has been no consensus prognostic difference between nodal and bone disease or, perhaps more importantly, no clear directives regarding treatment based on site of metastasis.

As previously mentioned, there are limitations to the current criteria. For example, the nonmetastatic, biochemically recurrent niche is a misnomer because it can be assumed that the sources of rising PSA are microscopic metastases falling

a Division of Medical Oncology, Department of Medicine, University of Washington, 825 Eastlake Avenue East, Seattle, WA 98109, USA; b Clinical Research Division, Fred Hutchinson Center, 1100 Fairview Avenue North, Seattle, WA 98109, USA; c Department of Urology, University of Washington, 1959 Northeast Pacific Street, Seattle, WA 98195, USA
* Corresponding author. Clinical Research Division, Fred Hutchinson Center, 1100 Fairview Avenue North, PO Box 19024, Seattle, WA 98109.
E-mail address: hhcheng@u.washington.edu

Urol Clin N Am 39 (2012) 561–571
http://dx.doi.org/10.1016/j.ucl.2012.07.011

below the limits of detection of standard imaging modalities. Thus, this clinical classification does not so much define the biology of this disease state as it reflects the limitations of current imaging technology, although there is usefulness in prognosis and treatment decision making. Similarly, there is increasing evidence that castration-resistant prostate cancer (CRPC), defined by an increasing PSA level in the setting of castrate levels of serum testosterone, remains reliant on previously unrecognized intracrine tumor androgens.[3–5] This is further validated as more potent androgen axis manipulations such as abiraterone, enzalutamide (previously known as MDV3100), and others have been proved to slow prostate cancer disease progression and improve overall survival in patients with CRPC.[6–8] Nevertheless, this designation remains clinically useful in clarifying treatment options. Similarly, the distinction between the pre-docetaxel and post-docetaxel settings that are currently used should be recognized as an artifice created by the field, albeit a necessary one, for the purpose of clinical trials and the drug approval process, instead of being of biologic significance. However, as the authors discuss, these terms may be rapidly evolving along with the landscape of the field.

NONMETASTATIC (BIOCHEMICALLY RECURRENT) CASTRATION-SENSITIVE PROSTATE CANCER

Nonmetastatic castration-sensitive disease is found in patients observed to have a rising PSA, including those who have received definitive localized therapy such as surgery and/or radiation. When following prostatectomy, one commonly accepted definition of biochemical recurrence is a PSA level of 0.2 ng/mL (or greater with a second confirmatory value)[9,10] although there are other definitions for biochemical failure after prostatectomy.[11,12] When following external beam radiation, the definition of biochemical recurrence is a PSA at least 2 ng/mL higher than the nadir PSA, as dictated by the the RTO-ASTRO Phoenix consensus conference (distinct from the American Society for Radiation Oncology criteria).[13] The PCWG2 criteria for progression of disease and clinical trial eligibility include a sequence of increasing PSA values at a minimum of 1-week intervals and a 2.0 ng/mL minimum starting value.[1] If possible, PSA doubling time (PSAdt) can be estimated if 3 or more values are available at 4 or more weeks apart.[1] If criteria are met, it is standard to assess for metastatic involvement by radiographic studies, most commonly radionuclide bone and computed tomography

scanning. When no metastases are seen on imaging, the patient is considered to have non-metastatic disease, although, to reiterate, it is assumed that the source of increasing PSA levels is microscopic metastases.

The prognosis of patients with castration-sensitive prostate cancer (CSPC) can be estimated with several different measures, including the Gleason score, lymph node involvement, time to PSA recurrence, and PSAdt.[14] Several other PSA measures have been examined, such as PSA velocity and PSA density. PSAdt has emerged as a useful measurement that can be used to define prognosis. After prostatectomy, a PSAdt of greater than 10 months is correlated with a longer time to the development of distant metastases[15] and to survival.[16] Regardless of initial therapy, if PSAdt is less than 3 months, the outcome is universally poor.[17]

The mainstay of therapy in CSPC is androgen-deprivation therapy (ADT), typically accomplished through orchiectomy or by treatment with either a gonadotropin-releasing hormone agonist or antagonist. Although ADT universally suppresses PSA after initiation, the long-term benefits of starting ADT in this early setting remain unclear, with little data to support early introduction.[18,19] Consequently, any potential benefits of introduction of ADT in this setting must be balanced with concerns for short- and long-term side effects of treatment, including bone health, metabolic effects, body morphology changes, sexual side effects, and hot flashes.[20] As a consequence, the challenge remains to distinguish the patients who may benefit from earlier introduction of ADT from those who may not.

A means of minimizing the long-term side effects and improving quality of life for men with nonmetastatic prostate cancer is the use of intermittent compared with continuous ADT.[21] This has been most recently studied in the phase III randomized trial comparing intermittent versus continuous androgen suppression for patients with PSA progression after radical therapy (NCIC CTG PR.7/SWOG JPR.7/CTSU JPR.7/UK Intercontinental Trial CRUKE/01/013), in which nearly 1400 men with increasing PSA levels were randomized to receive intermittent androgen suppression (IAD) or continuous androgen deprivation (CAD) after primary or salvage radiotherapy, where IAD was given in 8-month treatment intervals with a threshold to resume therapy when PSA level was greater than 10 ng/dL. Preliminary results were reported at the American Society of Clinical Oncology (ASCO) 2011 annual meeting and demonstrated noninferiority of IAD with respect to overall survival.[22] Moreover, the IAD arm had a reduction in hot flashes and improvements in quality of life measures, including less fatigue and sexual side effects compared with the CAD arm.[23] As a result, IAD is an accepted standard of care option for men with nonmetastatic castration-sensitive disease.

Bone mineral loss and resultant osteoporotic fracture are long-term morbidities of ADT and additional threats to bone health in a disease that preferentially metastasizes to the bone in its later stages. An estimate of long-term bone effects of ADT comes from the placebo control arms of the trials of toremifene and denosumab in patients with nonmetastatic CSPC.[24,25] Patients receiving CAD and randomized to placebo had reductions in bone mineral density of between 1% and 5% at the lumbar spine, total hip, femoral neck, and distal third of radius at 24 to 36 months.[24,25] In contrast, in a study of 56 men receiving IAD, the long-term bone mineral density was only slightly lower than baseline after a median follow-up of 5.5 years.[26] The use of bone-protective agents such as zolendronic acid and denosumab are discussed further in another article in this issue by Morgans and colleagues.

An additional benefit of IAD in the setting of biochemical recurrence is the ability to glean additional prognostic information. For example, after 9 months of induction ADT, the duration of the first off-cycle interval as defined by time to reach a specific PSA threshold can prognosticate for long-term outcomes such as castration-resistance or prostate cancer mortality.[27] More recent evidence suggests that a longer time to PSA increase during the first off-cycle of IAD and after testosterone recovery (as defined as >50 ng/dL) may be associated with longer time to castration resistance.[28]

The current challenge is to further prognosticate men with nonmetastatic, biochemically recurrent castration-sensitive disease—to discriminate between patients who will benefit from IAD and those with better prognosis who would be better served with close observation. Additionally, novel agents currently approved for later stages of disease are being investigated in earlier stages, such as sipuleucel-T.[29,30] As more trials in this setting are planned, it is increasingly important to select patients with more aggressive disease features and subsequent event rates that will be adequate to design appropriate clinical trials with novel agents. Alternatively, the ability to accurately identify those with indolent disease allows us to more confidently direct these patients toward clinical trials studying nutraceuticals and less toxic agents, such as sulforaphane, which may offer lower risk of long-term morbidity.[31]

METASTATIC CSPC

Metastatic CSPC (mCSPC), as the name suggests, is defined by the presence of detectable metastases, either nodal, visceral, or bone lesions,[1] and by responsiveness to ADT. ADT is typically achieved by surgical orchiectomy or administration of a gonadotropin-releasing hormone agonist or antagonist, but either can also be combined with an oral antiandrogen for a combined androgen blockade approach. Whether this combined approach is superior has been the subject of several meta-analyses, which were in agreement in demonstrating minor differences in favor of the combined approach, although all recommend a balanced discussion with patients about risks and benefits.[32–34] A natural question is whether combined androgen blockade could be more successful in the current era of more potent hormonal agents such as abiraterone and/or enzalutamide.

Although the hallmark of therapy is ADT, here, too, there was controversy about whether the optimal treatment schedule should be intermittent or continuous. The SWOG 9346 trial recently answered this question by randomizing men with mCSPC to continuous or intermittent ADT.[35] The results from this study were presented at the plenary session of the ASCO 2012 annual meeting and revealed that the primary endpoint of noninferiority was not met when comparing IAD with CAD.[35] In other words, this study does not provide support for IAD in this disease state, although quality of life was superior for patients on IAD.[36]

Several earlier prognostic analyses have been reported from the Southwest Oncology Group clinical trial SWOG 9346, including one reporting that the PSA level after 7 months of ADT was prognostic for survival.[37] Specifically, patients whose PSA level decreased to less than 0.2 ng/mL had a median survival of 75 months. Patients whose PSA level decreased to between 0.2 and 4 ng/mL had a median survival of 44 months, and those whose PSA level never decreased to less than 4 ng/mL had a median survival of 13 months.[37] Another analysis from SWOG 9346 showed a correlation between PSA progression (as defined by an increase of $\geq$25% greater than the nadir and an absolute increase of at least 2 or 5 ng/mL) and overall survival in more than 1000 men with castration-sensitive disease who were included in the analysis.[38]

These biomarker results from SWOG 9346 have already proved to be useful in differentiating patients by different prognoses within the overly general classification of mCSPC. For instance, the post-ADT initiation 7 months PSA endpoint of

PSA of less than 0.2 ng/mL is being used as a "go or no go" decision point in randomized phase II SWOG 0925 trial,[39] testing combined ADT versus combined ADT and cixutumumab (IMC-A12), a human IgG1 monoclonal antibody that targets the insulin-like growth factor I receptor.[40] Hints from preclinical studies provide support that this agent may offer greater benefit specifically in the castration-sensitive environment,[41] validating a surrogate endpoint before launching a larger, randomized phase III trial may prove rational.

Other areas of active investigation within this disease classification include the ongoing CHAARTED (Chemohormonal Therapy versus Androgen Ablation Randomized for Extensive Disease in Prostate Cancer) study,[42] which is designed to determine whether treatment with a combination of chemohormonal therapy, thus an early introduction of docetaxel, offers improved survival compared with ADT alone when tumors are still castration sensitive. Efforts are ongoing to move newer hormonal agents such as abiraterone (anticipated phase III trial) and the upcoming SWOG 1216 trial with orteronel (TAK 700) to this earlier disease state.

NONMETASTATIC CRPC

This disease state is defined by a sequence of increasing PSA levels at a minimum of 1-week intervals with a 2.0 ng/mL minimum starting value without detectable metastases by standard imaging modalities, commonly radionuclide bone and computed tomography scanning.[1] As in the castration-sensitive setting, the distinction between metastatic and nonmetastatic in the castration-resistant setting is largely reflective of the limits of detection rather than of biology, because it is presumed that PSA is produced by microscopic metastases. Nevertheless, this classification based on PCWG2 is used to stratify patients for treatment and clinical trials because of the lack of more robust and informative criteria.[1]

Attempts to improve treatment approaches in this stage of prostate cancer have been disappointing and largely unsuccessful because of 2 main issues: (1) the heterogeneity of patient disease progression to a detectable metastatic lesion and (2) the lack of effective therapeutic interventions and thus infrequent surveillance and limited capture of patients while they are in this "premetastatic state." Regardless, these trials have provided useful data to help prognosticate and further future clinical trial planning and design.

One trial seeking to determine whether zolendronic acid could delay/prevent development of bone metastasis was unsuccessful because of

the unanticipated low number of events.[43] Fortunately, the authors characterized the natural history of nonmetastatic CRPC by evaluating events in the placebo arm of the trial. At 2-year follow-up, the median time to first bone metastases and overall survival were not reached, emphasizing that the most of these men had more indolent disease than anticipated.[43] However, PSAdt was found to be prognostic for time to discovery of bone metastasis, and this information has been helpful in guiding the design of subsequent clinical trials for patients with this clinical disease state. For example, more than half of patients with a PSAdt of less than 6.3 months developed bone metastases or died 1.5 years after randomization.[43] The randomized control trial of atrasentan versus placebo illustrates the important point that invariable disease progression leads to high rates of attrition and underpowered statistical analyses.[44] Moreover, a major consequence of infrequent restaging studies is a high screen-fail rate for studies involving this patient population—up to a third—due to identification of metastatic sites after enrollment.[45,46]

The development of bone metastases is a major morbidity of late-stage prostate cancer; thus, agents to delay or prevent bone metastases have been the aim of several clinical trials that are discussed separately. However, a remaining issue is when and how frequently bone scans are obtained to evaluate for metastases. In the nonmetastatic castration-resistant state, there is no consensus guideline on the standard PSA threshold above which bone scans are recommended. There is a clear need to balance the benefits of early detection and intervention with the risks of increased cost and potential morbidity.

Optimal management for patients in this clinical state remains an open question. In clinical practice, the addition of secondary hormonal manipulations such as antiandrogens, ketoconazole, and estrogenic therapies have long been used in efforts to impede the androgen axis, although none have been tested in a randomized clinical trial with a primary survival endpoint. Future trials with newer agents in this population hold promise in changing the standard of care and improving survival for patients whose disease burden is limited to microscopic castration-resistant metastases.

METASTATIC CRPC

The final disease state is that of metastatic CRPC (mCRPC), which is defined by a sequence of increasing PSA values at a minimum of 1-week intervals with a 2.0 ng/mL starting value, serum testosterone less than 50 ng/dL, and the presence of detectable metastases. The greatest recent advances have been made in the treatment of patients reaching this stage of disease. As is true with other cancers, clinical trials of new agents have focused first on patients with metastatic disease because demonstrating clinical benefit is more achievable within a feasible timeline as a result of their limited prognosis. However, the prognosis for patients with mCRPC is a moving target, largely because of the US Food and Drug Administration (FDA) approval of docetaxel in 2004, followed more recently by sipuleucel-T, cabazitaxel, and abiraterone, with many new promising agents in the clinical trial pipeline. One of the greatest challenges to optimal implementation of these many treatments is parsing out biologically distinct subgroups within the still heterogeneous group of patients who have mCRPC and matching the best treatment with disease biology. Within mCRPC, there is an urgent need for better prognostic, predictive, and response biomarkers, to assist with triaging appropriate drugs and timely and accurate response evaluation. These biomarkers are ever more critical in the era of a rapidly growing armamentarium that includes biologically and molecularly targeted agents.

Currently, the prognosis for patients with mCRPC can be estimated through the use of several measures, including an earlier predictive model incorporating lactate dehydrogenase, PSA, alkaline phosphatase, Gleason score, Eastern Cooperative Oncology Group performance status, hemoglobin, and visceral disease involvement to estimate prognosis.[47] More recently, an updated nomogram has incorporated additional independent prognostic factors, including pretreatment PSAdt.[48] Other prognostic models follow the response to docetaxel because of a significant association observed between tumor response and median overall survival.[49] Additionally, a 30% or greater decline in PSA levels has been associated with a radiographic response.[50] Pain from bone metastases has also been studied in men with mCRPC, in whom worse pain interference scores have been associated with an increased risk of death,[51] and many trials now use pain measures for eligibility criterion and as major trial endpoints. Pain and quality of life measures must continue to be evaluated using validated assessment measures.[52]

Circulating tumor cells (CTCs) have garnered considerable interest as biomarkers of prognosis in disease.[53] Baseline CTCs have been shown to be associated with survival[54,55] and have been proposed as an intermediate endpoint for survival.[56] CTCs are currently under investigation in multiple large, phase III trials to further validate their utility with in hope of eventually using changes in CTCs as a meaningful surrogate endpoint for survival. Ultimately, the power of CTCs may extend beyond simple enumeration to molecular characterization. The hope is that mechanisms of tumor sensitivity and resistance to specific therapies may be elucidated with a simple tube of blood with CTCs.

None of these measures—response to docetaxel, pain interference scores, or CTCs—are yet routinely used to define distinct clinical disease states with respect to clinical practice or enrollment in clinical trials. Currently, patients with mCRPC are further divided based on whether they are asymptomatic or symptomatic (which can include, but is not limited to, pain) and whether they are have not yet undergone chemotherapy or have received chemotherapy (mainly referring to docetaxel). These latter 2 distinctions are arbitrary and simplistic and, importantly, do not reflect the biology of disease but instead the practical necessity of a minimal criteria for subdividing disease states to prioritize the growing number of treatment options.

The current armamentarium of therapeutics for mCRPC consists of several major classes: androgen ablative agents, immunotherapy, cytotoxic chemotherapy, and bone-targeted agents, including radioisotopes. In addition, novel molecularly targeted agents and antiangiogenic agents are in phase II/III testing, and results are eagerly anticipated. Each of these are discussed in further detail in other articles in this issue.

Historically, the cytotoxic chemotherapeutics have included mitoxantrone and estramustine. However, the landscape changed in 2004 when docetaxel was approved for mCRPC by the FDA following results of 2 phase III, multi-institution, randomized trials.[57,58] Cabazitaxel, another taxane, was approved for treatment of patients who received prior docetaxel in 2010 following the phase III trial of cabazitaxel plus prednisone compared to mitoxantrone plus prednisone in hormone refractory metastatic prostate cancer (TROPIC).[59] Cabazitaxel is now being directly tested as a first-line cytotoxic directly against docetaxel.[60]

Sipuleucel-T is a first-in-class, autologous dendritic cell therapeutic vaccine designed to prime the T-cell response against prostatic acid phosphatase, a prostate cancer antigen. The phase III trial of Sipuleucel-T active cellular immunotherapy treatment of metastatic prostate cancer after failing hormone therapy (IMPACT) demonstrated that at median follow-up of 34 months, patients in the sipuleucel-T arm had a 4.1-month improvement in median survival, leading to its

FDA approval in 2010.[61] Of note, a difference in radiographic progression-free survival by an independent review board was not observed,[61] highlighting the limitations of our surrogate endpoints, particularly with newer biologically driven therapies. Other immunotherapies are also being investigated for mCRPC, including ipilimumab, a monoclonal antibody recently FDA approved for metastatic melanoma,[62] and Prostvac-VF, a therapeutic PSA-targeted poxviral vaccine.[63] Phase III studies are under way to further test these immunotherapies.[64,65]

Considerable excitement surrounds the development of several new agents aimed at further blocking androgen receptor signaling at the level of the prostate cancer tumor cells—either by inhibiting androgen synthesis or by blocking the androgen receptor. Abiraterone was the first agent to be FDA approved and is part of the first group, blocking synthesis of androgen through inhibition of the steroidogenic enzymes 17,20-lyase and 17α-hydroxylase. The phase III trial of abiraterone acetate in castration-resistant prostate cancer previously treated with docetaxel-based chemotherapy (Cougar 301) was performed in patients who had been previously treated with docetaxel, and results showed that abiraterone with prednisone increased overall survival compared with placebo with prednisone.[8] The follow-up phase III trial of abiraterone acetate in chemotherapy-naive patients with metastatic castration-resistant prostate cancer (Cougar 302) was conducted to determine benefit in asymptomatic and minimally symptomatic patients with mCRPC before chemotherapy. The Independent Data Monitoring Committee unanimously recommended unblinding based on a planned interim analysis of progression-free survival, overall survival, and clinical benefit, which was reported at the ASCO 2012 annual meeting. At 43-month follow-up, neither median progression-free or overall survival in the abiraterone arm had been reached, but the hazard ratio for progression-free survival was reported as 0.43 (95% confidence interval, 0.35–0.52), and for overall survival, it was 0.75 (95% confidence interval, 0.61–0.93) in favor of abiraterone.[66] Another newer hormonal agent garnering much excitement is enzalutamide (MDV3100), which has been tested in the phase III trial of oral MDV3100 in patients with progressive castration-resistant prostate cancer previously treated with docetaxel-based chemotherapy (AFFIRM) and demonstrated a median overall survival of 18.4 months for enzalutamide versus 13.6 months in the placebo arm.[67] In addition, results are anticipated in the phase III trial of MDV3100 in chemotherapy-naive patients with progressive metastatic

prostate cancer who have failed androgen deprivation therapy (PREVAIL).[68] Close on the heels are several other agents aimed at blocking androgen synthesis including orteronel (TAK700) and ARN 509.[69]

Bone-targeted agents such as zoledronic acid and, more recently, denosumab are already in widespread clinical use to prevent skeletal-related events for patients with bone metastases.[70,71] Joining the arsenal of bone-targeting agents is ^{223}Ra-chloride, which is an alpha emitter that has a limited range compared with beta or gamma emitters, thus minimizing bone marrow toxicity.[72] In the phase III trial of alpharadin in the treatment of patients with symptomatic hormone refractory prostate cancer with skeletal metastases (ALSYMPCA), of 922 patients with prostate cancer bone metastases, ^{223}Ra significantly improved overall survival compared with placebo (median 14.0 vs 11.2 months) and demonstrated a low incidence of myelosuppression.[73]

Several molecularly targeted agents including tyrosine kinase inhibitors such as dasatinib[74–77] and, more recently, cabozantinib[78–80] are in later-stage clinical trials. In addition, the antisense molecules OGX-011 (targeting clusterin)[81,82] and OGX-427 (targeting heat shock protein 27)[83] and antiangiogenic agent tasquinimod[84–86] are also the subjects of intense study in the field.

FUTURE DISEASE STATES

The past decade has produced a dizzying array of new therapeutic options for patients with advanced prostate cancer, with more promising new agents in the pipeline **Fig. 1**. In the midst of this newfound wealth comes the challenge and responsibility of optimizing treatment algorithms now that there are more options from which to choose. To advance the field, it is imperative that clinical and laboratory investigators collaborate to identify rational sequencing and optimal combinations of currently and soon-to-be available agents. Clinical trials addressing these questions must incorporate careful dissection and cataloging of the mechanisms of treatment resistance following different sequential and combinatorial treatment schemes.

The authors are hopeful that clinical disease states will be further refined by improvements in technologies for detection such as more sensitive capture of CTCs and more sensitive imaging of metastases. Several new imaging technologies are being used in research studies and promise more sensitive detection of disease: whole body magnetic resonance imaging,[87] ^{11}C-acetate positon-emission tomography (PET),[88] ^{11}C-choline

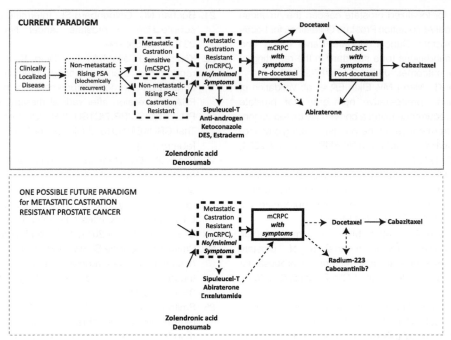

Fig. 1. Current paradigm for advanced disease states in prostate cancer, and one possible future paradigm for mCRPC.

PET,[89] fluoride PET,[90] and in combinations such as 16β-^{18}F-fluoro-5α-dihydrotestosterone PET.[91] Of these, fluoride PET[90] and whole body magnetic resonance imaging[87] are most feasible for widespread use. If these emerging modalities are validated and become more accessible at a reasonable cost, they have the potential to drive more sensitive and precise definitions of the current disease states.[92–94]

Perhaps most exciting is the emergence of cancer genomics whereby newer, faster, and ever less expensive methods such as next-generation sequencing are being applied to DNA, RNA, epigenetic DNA methylation states, and so forth.[95] Much of this foundational work is currently being done to define the genomic complexity of prostate cancer in its different stages,[96,97] the relationships to prognosis,[98] and the relationships to new candidate molecular biomarkers.[99] These new discoveries will soon pave the way for more sophisticated, biologically and molecularly defined disease classifications, allowing much more precisely tailored treatments for patients with prostate cancer in the future.

REFERENCES

1. Scher HI, Halabi S, Tannock I, et al. Design and end points of clinical trials for patients with progressive prostate cancer and castrate levels of testosterone: recommendations of the Prostate Cancer Clinical Trials Working Group. J Clin Oncol 2008;26(7): 1148–59.

2. Bubley GJ, Carducci M, Dahut W, et al. Eligibility and response guidelines for phase II clinical trials in androgen-independent prostate cancer: recommendations from the Prostate-Specific Antigen Working Group. J Clin Oncol 1999;17(11):3461–7.

3. Mohler JL, Gregory CW, Ford OH 3rd, et al. The androgen axis in recurrent prostate cancer. Clin Cancer Res 2004;10(2):440–8.

4. Titus MA, Schell MJ, Lih FB, et al. Testosterone and dihydrotestosterone tissue levels in recurrent prostate cancer. Clin Cancer Res 2005;11(13):4653–7.

5. Montgomery RB, Mostaghel EA, Vessella R, et al. Maintenance of intratumoral androgens in metastatic prostate cancer: a mechanism for castration-resistant tumor growth. Cancer Res 2008;68(11):4447–54.

6. Scher HI, Fizazi K, Saad F, et al. Effect of MDV3100, an androgen receptor signaling inhibitor (ARSI), on overall survival in patients with prostate cancer post-docetaxel: results from the phase III AFFIRM study. J Clin Oncol 2012;30(Suppl 5). LBA1.

7. Scher HI, Beer TM, Higano CS, et al. Antitumour activity of MDV3100 in castration-resistant prostate cancer: a phase 1-2 study. Lancet 2010;375(9724): 1437–46.

8. de Bono JS, Logothetis CJ, Molina A, et al. Abiraterone and increased survival in metastatic prostate cancer. N Engl J Med 2011;364(21):1995–2005.

9. Cookson MS, Aus G, Burnett AL, et al. Variation in the definition of biochemical recurrence in patients

treated for localized prostate cancer: the American Urological Association Prostate Guidelines for Localized Prostate Cancer Update Panel report and recommendations for a standard in the reporting of surgical outcomes. J Urol 2007;177(2):540–5.

10. Greene KL, Meng MV, Elkin EP, et al. Validation of the Kattan preoperative nomogram for prostate cancer recurrence using a community based cohort: results from cancer of the prostate strategic urological research endeavor (CAPSURE). J Urol 2004; 171(6 Pt 1):2255–9.

11. Amling CL, Bergstralh EJ, Blute ML, et al. Defining prostate specific antigen progression after radical prostatectomy: what is the most appropriate cut point? J Urol 2001;165(4):1146–51.

12. Stephenson AJ, Kattan MW, Eastham JA, et al. Defining biochemical recurrence of prostate cancer after radical prostatectomy: a proposal for a standardized definition. J Clin Oncol 2006;24(24): 3973–8.

13. Roach M 3rd, Hanks G, Thames H Jr, et al. Defining biochemical failure following radiotherapy with or without hormonal therapy in men with clinically localized prostate cancer: recommendations of the RTOG-ASTRO Phoenix Consensus Conference. Int J Radiat Oncol Biol Phys 2006;65(4):965–74.

14. Roach M 3rd, Lu J, Pilepich MV, et al. Predicting long-term survival, and the need for hormonal therapy: a meta-analysis of RTOG prostate cancer trials. Int J Radiat Oncol Biol Phys 2000;47(3):617–27.

15. Pound CR, Partin AW, Eisenberger MA, et al. Natural history of progression after PSA elevation following radical prostatectomy. JAMA 1999;281(17): 1591–7.

16. Freedland SJ, Humphreys EB, Mangold LA, et al. Risk of prostate cancer-specific mortality following biochemical recurrence after radical prostatectomy. JAMA 2005;294(4):433–9.

17. D'Amico AV, Moul J, Carroll PR, et al. Prostate specific antigen doubling time as a surrogate end point for prostate cancer specific mortality following radical prostatectomy or radiation therapy. J Urol 2004;172(5 Pt 2):S42–6 [discussion: S46–47].

18. Messing EM, Manola J, Sarosdy M, et al. Immediate hormonal therapy compared with observation after radical prostatectomy and pelvic lymphadenectomy in men with node-positive prostate cancer. N Engl J Med 1999;341(24):1781–8.

19. Messing EM, Manola J, Yao J, et al. Immediate versus deferred androgen deprivation treatment in patients with node-positive prostate cancer after radical prostatectomy and pelvic lymphadenectomy. Lancet Oncol 2006;7(6):472–9.

20. Casey RG, Corcoran NM, Goldenberg SL. Quality of life issues in men undergoing androgen deprivation therapy: a review. Asian J Androl 2012;14(2): 226–31.

21. Buchan NC, Goldenberg SL. Intermittent androgen suppression for prostate cancer. Nat Rev Urol 2010;7(10):552–60.

22. Klotz L, O'Callaghan CJ, Ding K. A phase III randomized trial comparing intermittent versus continuous androgen suppression for patients with PSA progression after radical therapy: NCIC CTG PR.7/SWOG JPR.7/CTSU JPR.7/UK Intercontinental Trial CRUKE/01/013. J Clin Oncol 2011;29(Suppl 7) [abstract: 3].

23. Crook JM, O'Callaghan CJ, Ding K, et al. A phase III randomized trial of intermittent versus continuous androgen suppression for PSA progression after radical therapy (NCIC CTG PR.7/SWOG JPR.7/ CTSU JPR.7/ UK Intercontinental Trial CRUKE/01/ 013). J Clin Oncol 2011;29(Suppl) [abstract: 4514].

24. Smith MR, Egerdie B, Hernandez Toriz N, et al. Denosumab in men receiving androgen-deprivation therapy for prostate cancer. N Engl J Med 2009; 361(8):745–55.

25. Smith MR, Malkowicz SB, Brawer MK, et al. Toremifene decreases vertebral fractures in men younger than 80 years receiving androgen deprivation therapy for prostate cancer. J Urol 2011;186(6):2239–44.

26. Yu EY, Kuo KF, Gulati R, et al. Long-term dynamics of bone mineral density during intermittent androgen deprivation for men with nonmetastatic, hormone-sensitive prostate cancer. J Clin Oncol 2012; 30(15):1864–70.

27. Yu EY, Gulati R, Telesca D, et al. Duration of first off-treatment interval is prognostic for time to castration resistance and death in men with biochemical relapse of prostate cancer treated on a prospective trial of intermittent androgen deprivation. J Clin Oncol 2010;28(16):2668–73.

28. Yu EY, Kuo KF, Hunter-Merrill R. Relationship of time to testosterone (T) and PSA rises during the first "off treatment" interval (1OFF) of intermittent androgen deprivation (IAD) with time to castration resistance (CRPC) and prostate cancer mortality (PCM) in men with biochemical relapse (BR). J Clin Oncol 2012;30(Suppl 5) [abstract: 99].

29. Beer TM, Bernstein GT, Corman JM, et al. Randomized trial of autologous cellular immunotherapy with sipuleucel-T in androgen-dependent prostate cancer. Clin Cancer Res 2011;17(13):4558–67.

30. Dendreon. Sequencing of Sipuleucel-T and ADT in Menwith Non-metastatic Prostate Cancer. Available at: ClinicalTrials.gov(NCT01431391). Accessed August 15, 2012.

31. Gibbs A, Schwartzman J, Deng V, et al. Sulforaphane destabilizes the androgen receptor in prostate cancer cells by inactivating histone deacetylase 6. Proc Natl Acad Sci U S A 2009;106(39):16663–8.

32. Schmitt B, Bennett C, Seidenfeld J, et al. Maximal androgen blockade for advanced prostate cancer. Cochrane Database Syst Rev 2000;(2):CD001526.

33. Schmitt B, Wilt TJ, Schellhammer PF, et al. Combined androgen blockade with nonsteroidal antiandrogens for advanced prostate cancer: a systematic review. Urology 2001;57(4):727–32.

34. Samson DJ, Seidenfeld J, Schmitt B, et al. Systematic review and meta-analysis of monotherapy compared with combined androgen blockade for patients with advanced prostate carcinoma. Cancer 2002;95(2):361–76.

35. Hussain M, Tangen CM, Higano CS, et al. Intermittent (IAD) versus continuous androgen deprivation (CAD) in hormone sensitive metastatic prostate cancer (HSM1PC) patients (pts): results of S9346 (INT-0162), an international phase III trial. J Clin Oncol 2012;(Suppl):30 [abstract: 4].

36. Moinpour C, Berry DL, Ely B, et al. Preliminary quality-of-life outcomes for SWOG-9346: intermittent androgen deprivation in patients with hormone-sensitive metastatic prostate cancer (HSM1PC)—Phase III. J Clin Oncol 2012;30(Suppl) [abstract: 4571].

37. Hussain M, Tangen CM, Higano C, et al. Absolute prostate-specific antigen value after androgen deprivation is a strong independent predictor of survival in new metastatic prostate cancer: data from Southwest Oncology Group Trial 9346 (INT-0162). J Clin Oncol 2006;24(24):3984–90.

38. Hussain M, Goldman B, Tangen C, et al. Prostate-specific antigen progression predicts overall survival in patients with metastatic prostate cancer: data from Southwest Oncology Group Trials 9346 (Intergroup Study 0162) and 9916. J Clin Oncol 2009;27(15):2450–6.

39. Southwest Oncology Group. Bicalutamide and goserelin or leuprolide acetate with or without cixutumumab in treating patients with newly diagnosed metastatic prostate cancer. Available at: Clinical Trials.gov/ct2/show/NCT01120236. Accessed August 15, 2012.

40. Rowinsky EK, Youssoufian H, Tonra JR, et al. IMC-A12, a human IgG1 monoclonal antibody to the insulin-like growth factor I receptor. Clin Cancer Res 2007;13(18 Pt 2):5549s–55s.

41. Wu JD, Odman A, Higgins LM, et al. In vivo effects of the human type I insulin-like growth factor receptor antibody A12 on androgen-dependent and androgen-independent xenograft human prostate tumors. Clin Cancer Res 2005;11(8):3065–74.

42. Eastern Cooperative Oncology Group. Androgen ablation therapy with or without chemotherapy in treating patients with metastatic prostate cancer. Available at: ClinicalTrials.gov/ct2/show/NCT00309985. Accessed August 15, 2012.

43. Smith MR, Kabbinavar F, Saad F, et al. Natural history of rising serum prostate-specific antigen in men with castrate nonmetastatic prostate cancer. J Clin Oncol 2005;23(13):2918–25.

44. Smith MR, Cook R, Lee KA, et al. Disease and host characteristics as predictors of time to first bone metastasis and death in men with progressive castration-resistant nonmetastatic prostate cancer. Cancer 2011;117(10):2077–85.

45. Smith MR, Saad F, Coleman R, et al. Denosumab and bone-metastasis-free survival in men with castration-resistant prostate cancer: results of a phase 3, randomised, placebo-controlled trial. Lancet 2012;379(9810):39–46.

46. Yu EY, Miller K, Nelson J, et al. Detection of previously unidentified metastatic disease as a leading cause of screening failure in a phase III trial of zibotentan versus placebo in patients with nonmetastatic, castration resistant prostate cancer. J Urol 2012;188(1):103–9.

47. Halabi S, Small EJ, Kantoff PW, et al. Prognostic model for predicting survival in men with hormone-refractory metastatic prostate cancer. J Clin Oncol 2003;21(7):1232–7.

48. Armstrong AJ, Garrett-Mayer ES, Yang YC, et al. A contemporary prognostic nomogram for men with hormone-refractory metastatic prostate cancer: a TAX327 study analysis. Clin Cancer Res 2007; 13(21):6396–403.

49. Armstrong AJ, Garrett-Mayer E, de Wit R, et al. Prediction of survival following first-line chemotherapy in men with castration-resistant metastatic prostate cancer. Clin Cancer Res 2010;16(1):203–11.

50. Sonpavde G, Pond GR, Berry WR, et al. The association between radiographic response and overall survival in men with metastatic castration-resistant prostate cancer receiving chemotherapy. Cancer 2011;117(17):3963–71.

51. Halabi S, Vogelzang NJ, Ou SS, et al. Progression-free survival as a predictor of overall survival in men with castrate-resistant prostate cancer. J Clin Oncol 2009;27(17):2766–71.

52. Tannock IF, Osoba D, Stockler MR, et al. Chemotherapy with mitoxantrone plus prednisone or prednisone alone for symptomatic hormone-resistant prostate cancer: a Canadian randomized trial with palliative end points. J Clin Oncol 1996;14(6):1756–64.

53. Danila DC, Fleisher M, Scher HI. Circulating tumor cells as biomarkers in prostate cancer. Clin Cancer Res 2011;17(12):3903–12.

54. Danila DC, Heller G, Gignac GA, et al. Circulating tumor cell number and prognosis in progressive castration-resistant prostate cancer. Clin Cancer Res 2007;13(23):7053–8.

55. de Bono JS, Scher HI, Montgomery RB, et al. Circulating tumor cells predict survival benefit from treatment in metastatic castration-resistant prostate cancer. Clin Cancer Res 2008;14(19):6302–9.

56. Scher HI, Jia X, de Bono JS, et al. Circulating tumour cells as prognostic markers in progressive, castration-resistant prostate cancer: a reanalysis

of IMMC38 trial data. Lancet Oncol 2009;10(3): 233–9.

57. Tannock IF, de Wit R, Berry WR, et al. Docetaxel plus prednisone or mitoxantrone plus prednisone for advanced prostate cancer. N Engl J Med 2004; 351(15):1502–12.

58. Southwest Oncology Group. Combination therapy in treating patients with advanced prostate cancer that has not responded to hormone therapy. Available at: ClinicalTrials.gov/ct2/show/NCT00004001. Accessed August 15, 2012.

59. de Bono JS, Oudard S, Ozguroglu M, et al. Prednisone plus cabazitaxel or mitoxantrone for metastatic castration-resistant prostate cancer progressing after docetaxel treatment: a randomised open-label trial. Lancet 2010;376(9747):1147–54.

60. Sanofi-Aventis. Cabazitaxel versus docetaxel both with prednisone in patients with metastatic castration resistant prostate cancer (FIRSTANA). Available at: ClinicalTrials.gov/ct2/show/NCT01308567. Accessed August 15, 2012.

61. Kantoff PW, Higano CS, Shore ND, et al. Sipuleucel-T immunotherapy for castration-resistant prostate cancer. N Engl J Med 2010;363(5):411–22.

62. OHSU Knight Cancer Institute. Ipilimumab in combination with androgen suppression therapy in treating patients with metastatic hormone-resistant prostate cancer. Available at: Clinicaltrials.gov/ct2/show/NCT01498978. Accessed August 15, 2012.

63. Kantoff PW, Schuetz TJ, Blumenstein BA, et al. Overall survival analysis of a phase II randomized controlled trial of a Poxviral-based PSA-targeted immunotherapy in metastatic castration-resistant prostate cancer. J Clin Oncol 2010;28(7):1099–105.

64. BN ImmunoTherapeutics. A phase 3 efficacy study of a recombinant vaccinia virus vaccine to treat metastatic prostate cancer (prospect). Available at: ClinicalTrials.gov/ct2/show/NCT01322490. Accessed August 15, 2012.

65. Squibb B-M. Phase 3 study of immunotherapy to treat advanced prostate cancer. Available at: ClinicalTrials.gov/ct2/show/NCT01057810. Accessed August 15, 2012.

66. Ryan CJ, Smith MR, De Bono JS, et al. Interim analysis results of COU-AA-302, a randomized, phase III study of abiraterone acetate in chemotherapy naive patients with metastatic castration-resistant prostate cancer. J Clin Oncol 2012;(Suppl) (ASCO Abstract LBA4518).

67. de Bono JS, et al. Primary, secondary, and quality-of-life endpoint results from the phase III AFFIRM study of MDV3100, an androgen receptor signaling inhibitor. J Clin Oncol 2012;(Suppl) (ASCO abstract 4519).

68. Medivation, Inc. A safety and efficacy study of oral MDV3100 in chemotherapy-naive patients with progressive metastatic prostate cancer (PREVAIL).

Available at: ClinicalTrials.gov/ct2/show/NCT01212991. Accessed August 15, 2012.

69. Clegg NJ, Wongvipat J, Joseph JD, et al. ARN-509: a novel antiandrogen for prostate cancer treatment. Cancer Res 2012;72(6):1494–503.

70. Saad F, Gleason DM, Murray R, et al. Long-term efficacy of zoledronic acid for the prevention of skeletal complications in patients with metastatic hormone-refractory prostate cancer. J Natl Cancer Inst 2004;96(11):879–82.

71. Fizazi K, Carducci M, Smith M, et al. Denosumab versus zoledronic acid for treatment of bone metastases in men with castration-resistant prostate cancer: a randomised, double-blind study. Lancet 2011;377(9768):813–22.

72. Bruland OS, Nilsson S, Fisher DR, et al. High-linear energy transfer irradiation targeted to skeletal metastases by the alpha-emitter 223Ra: adjuvant or alternative to conventional modalities? Clin Cancer Res 2006;12(20 Pt 2):6250s–7s.

73. Parker C, Heinrich D, O'Sullivan JM. Overall survival benefit and safety profile of radium-223 chloride, a first-in-class alpha-pharmaceutical: results from a phase III randomized trial (ALSYMPCA) in patients with castration-resistant prostate cancer (CRPC) with bone metastases. J Clin Oncol 2012;(Suppl 5) [abstract: 8].

74. Araujo JC, Mathew P, Armstrong AJ, et al. Dasatinib combined with docetaxel for castration-resistant prostate cancer: results from a phase 1-2 study. Cancer 2012;118(1):63–71.

75. Yu EY, Massard C, Gross ME, et al. Once-daily dasatinib: expansion of phase II study evaluating safety and efficacy of dasatinib in patients with metastatic castration-resistant prostate cancer. Urology 2011;77(5):1166–71.

76. Yu EY, Wilding G, Posadas E, et al. Phase II study of dasatinib in patients with metastatic castration-resistant prostate cancer. Clin Cancer Res 2009;15(23):7421–8.

77. Squibb BM. Randomized study comparing docetaxel plus dasatinib to docetaxel plus placebo in castration-resistant prostate cancer (READY). Available at: ClinicalTrials.gov/ct2/show/NCT00744497. Accessed August 15, 2012.

78. Hussain M. Cabozantinib (XL184) in metastatic castration-resistant prostate cancer (mCRPC): results from a phase II randomized discontinuation trial. J Clin Oncol 2011;29(Suppl) [abstract: 4516].

79. Exelixis. Study of cabozantinib (XL184) versus prednisone in men with metastatic castration-resistant prostate cancer previously treated with docetaxel and abiraterone or MDV3100 (COMET-1). Available at: ClinicalTrials.gov/ct2/show/NCT01605227. Accessed August 15, 2012.

80. Exelixis. Study of cabozantinib (XL184) versus mitoxantrone plus prednisone in men with previously treated symptomatic castration-resistant prostate

cancer (COMET-2). Available at: ClinicalTrials.gov/ct2/show/NCT01522443. Accessed August 15, 2012.

81. Teva Pharmaceutical Industries. Comparison of docetaxel/prednisone to docetaxel/prednisone in combination with OGX-011 in men with prostate cancer (SYNERGY). Available at: ClinicalTrials.gov/ct2/show/NCT01188187. Accessed August 15, 2012.

82. Chi KN, Hotte SJ, Yu EY, et al. Randomized phase II study of docetaxel and prednisone with or without OGX-011 in patients with metastatic castration-resistant prostate cancer. J Clin Oncol 2010;28(27):4247–54.

83. Chi KN. A randomized phase II study of OGX-427 plus prednisone versus prednisone alone in patients with chemotherapy-naive metastatic castration-resistant prostate cancer. J Clin Oncol 2012; 30(Suppl 5) [abstract: 121].

84. Armstrong AJ. Phase II study of tasquinimod in chemotherapy-naive patients with metastatic castrate-resistant prostate cancer (CRPC): safety and efficacy analysis including subgroups. J Clin Oncol 2011;29(Suppl 7) [abstract: 126].

85. Armstrong AJ. Tasquinimod and survival in men with metastatic castration-resistant prostate cancer: results of long-term follow-up of a randomized phase II placebo-controlled trial. J Clin Oncol 2012;30(Suppl) [abstract: 4550].

86. Active Biotech AB. A study of tasquinimod in men with metastatic castrate resistant prostate cancer. Available at: ClinicalTrials.gov/ct2/show/NCT01234311. Accessed August 15, 2012.

87. Bradley D, Hussain M, Galban C, et al. Application of the functional diffucsion map (fDM) to assess treatment response in metastatic prostate cancer (PCa). J Clin Oncol 2009 [abstract: 66].

88. Yu EY, Muzi M, Hackenbracht JA, et al. C11-acetate and F-18 FDG PET for men with prostate cancer bone metastases: relative findings and response to therapy. Clin Nucl Med 2011;36(3):192–8.

89. Fuccio C, Castellucci P, Schiavina R, et al. Role of (11)C-choline PET/CT in the re-staging of prostate cancer patients with biochemical relapse and negative results at bone scintigraphy. Eur J Radiol 2012;81(8):e893–6.

90. Kjolhede H, Ahlgren G, Almquist H, et al. Combined (18) F-fluorocholine and (18) F-fluoride positron emission tomography/computed tomography imaging for staging of high-risk prostate cancer. BJU Int 2012. [Epub ahead of print].

91. Autio KA, et al. 18F-16beta-fluoro-5alpha-dihydrotestosterone (FDHT) PET as a prognostic biomarker for survival in patients with metastatic castrate-resistant prostate cancer (mCRPC). J Clin Oncol 2012;30(Suppl) [abstract: 4517].

92. Kwee TC, Takahara T, Ochiai R, et al. Complementary roles of whole-body diffusion-weighted MRI and 18F-FDG PET: the state of the art and potential applications. J Nucl Med 2010;51(10): 1549–58.

93. Schoder H, Larson SM. Positron emission tomography for prostate, bladder, and renal cancer. Semin Nucl Med 2004;34(4):274–92.

94. Jadvar H. Prostate cancer: PET with 18F-FDG, 18F- or 11C-acetate, and 18F- or 11C-choline. J Nucl Med 2011;52(1):81–9.

95. Prensner JR, Rubin MA, Wei JT, et al. Beyond PSA: the next generation of prostate cancer biomarkers. Sci Transl Med 2012;4(127):127rv3.

96. Berger MF, Lawrence MS, Demichelis F, et al. The genomic complexity of primary human prostate cancer. Nature 2011;470(7333):214–20.

97. Tomlins SA, Laxman B, Dhanasekaran SM, et al. Distinct classes of chromosomal rearrangements create oncogenic ETS gene fusions in prostate cancer. Nature 2007;448(7153):595–9.

98. Yoshimoto M, Joshua AM, Cunha IW, et al. Absence of TMPRSS2: ERG fusions and PTEN losses in prostate cancer is associated with a favorable outcome. Mod Pathol 2008;21(12):1451–60.

99. Tomlins SA, Aubin SM, Siddiqui J, et al. Urine TMPRSS2: ERG fusion transcript stratifies prostate cancer risk in men with elevated serum PSA. Sci Transl Med 2011;3(94):94ra72.

The Experience with Cytotoxic Chemotherapy in Metastatic Castration-Resistant Prostate Cancer

Mario A. Eisenberger, MD*, Emmanuel S. Antonarakis, MD

KEYWORDS

- Cytotoxic chemotherapy • Metastatic castration-resistant prostate cancer • Docetaxel

KEY POINTS

- Docetaxel was the first chemotherapy agent to improve survival in men with metastatic castration-resistant prostate cancer (mCRPC) and is the chemotherapy drug of choice for the initial treatment of symptomatic mCRPC.
- Cabazitaxel is the second chemotherapy drug to demonstrate improved survival and is the current standard for patients with mCRPC who have progressed during or after receiving docetaxel-containing chemotherapy regimens.
- Mitoxantrone is a reasonable second- or third-line chemotherapy agent and has been shown to reduce bone pain and improve quality of life, without a demonstrable survival benefit.
- Several clinical trials are currently comparing docetaxel and cabazitaxel as first-line therapies for men with chemotherapy-naive mCRPC, but cabazitaxel is not currently recommended as first-line treatment outside of a clinical trial.

THE EXPERIENCE WITH CHEMOTHERAPY IN THE PRE-TAXANE ERA

The taxane agents (docetaxel and cabazitaxel) represent the current standard chemotherapy drugs used for the treatment of advanced castration-resistant prostate cancer (CRPC).[1–6] However, in the years preceding the Food and Drug Administration (FDA) approval of docetaxel (which occurred in 2004) and cabazitaxel (in 2010), various other chemotherapeutic drugs were being used, although none had demonstrated evidence of improved survival.[7] Importantly, the historical data reported in the literature should be evaluated in the context of when it was published. More specifically, clinical trials conducted before

the late 1980s should be evaluated separately from those reported subsequently, because of the introduction and availability of serum prostate-specific antigen (PSA) measurement in 1987. In addition, the evolving data with chemotherapy during the past 3 decades suggest that the survival of patients with metastatic castration-resistant prostate cancer (mCRPC) is substantially longer than previously described, which is probably also a reflection of lead-time effect caused by PSA-detecting treatment failure earlier in the disease process. Therefore, patients in contemporary chemotherapy trials have lesser tumor burden. In addition, the incidence and severity of critical clinical parameters associated with poor prognosis (such as anemia, renal dysfunction,

Department of Oncology, The Sidney Kimmel Comprehensive Cancer Center, The Johns Hopkins University, Baltimore, MD, USA
* Corresponding author. Bunting/Blaustein Cancer Research Building, 1650 Orleans Street, Room 1M51, Baltimore, MD.
E-mail address: eisenma@jhmi.edu

Urol Clin N Am 39 (2012) 573–581
http://dx.doi.org/10.1016/j.ucl.2012.07.012
0094-0143/12/$ – see front matter © 2012 Elsevier Inc. All rights reserved.

urologic.theclinics.com

symptoms, and impaired functional status) are much less frequent in contemporary series, which, in part, explains the differences in clinical outcomes since PSA was introduced. A historical perspective of chemotherapy development in the pre-docetaxel era is outlined later in this article.

There is modest single-agent activity with the alkylating drug, cyclophosphamide, with reported responses in only about 10% to 20% of patients based on the older literature. In more recent reports, cyclophosphamide given in standard oral doses or high intravenous doses with hematopoietic growth factors support has been reported to have a higher order of activity.[8–10] Doxorubicin, 5-fluorouracil, and cisplatin, agents all of which have demonstrable antitumor activity in other various tumor types, have shown only modest single-agent benefits in patients with mCRPC.[7] None of these agents are used with any frequency in the current era.

Estramustine phosphate is a nitrogen mustard derivative of estradiol, which has demonstrated limited single-agent activity in advanced prostate cancer.[7] This drug has been shown to exert its cytotoxic activity through microtubule inhibition[11] and binding to nuclear matrix,[12] which provided the rationale for testing this compound in combination with other agents targeting the microtubule, such as vinblastine, paclitaxel, docetaxel, and vinorelbine. However, in a prospective randomized study conducted in patients with castration-resistant disease, estramustine phosphate given at an oral dosage of 560 mg/d was not shown to be superior to placebo in terms of palliative effects or survival.[7,13] In addition, venous thromboembolic disease was a significant toxicity with this agent. It is considered that estramustine has only marginal activity in mCRPC, and because of its unfavorable therapeutic index (safety/efficacy) compared with more modern chemotherapeutics, its use in mCRPC has virtually been abandoned.

The treatment with the best response in the pre-taxane era is mitoxantrone. Mitoxantrone is a semisynthetic anthracenedione derivative that has shown modest subjective benefits with otherwise minimal evidence of objective antitumor activity or survival improvement.[3] A prospective randomized comparison of mitoxantrone plus prednisone with prednisone alone resulted in significant improvements of various quality-of-life issues including bone pain response.[4] However, survival was not significantly different between the treatment arms. This study provided the justification for the FDA approval of the combination of mitoxantrone and prednisone for the symptomatic treatment of patients with metastatic prostate cancer in 1997. In current practice,

mitoxantrone is rarely used, although it can sometimes be a reasonable agent used in third-line chemotherapy and beyond, if other life-prolonging chemotherapy drugs have already been exhausted.

TAXANES IN MCRPC

Both paclitaxel (extracted from the bark of the Pacific yew tree, *Taxus brevifolia*) and docetaxel (from the leaves of the European yew tree) disrupt microtubule function that is required for chromosome segregation at mitosis, thereby promoting apoptosis in eukaryotic cells.[14,15] Nonetheless, the exact mechanism by which these drugs act against prostate cancer cells is not entirely clear. Prostate cancers tend to have low growth fractions, as compared with many normal cells and most other cancers; yet prostate cancer cells remain sensitive to taxane drugs. One possibility is that microtubule function may be needed for other critical cell processes, such as nuclear-cytoplasmic shuttling of critical regulatory proteins essential for prostate cancer cell viability,[16] including translocation of the androgen receptor from the cytoplasm into the nucleus.

DOCETAXEL

Although paclitaxel and docetaxel showed promising activity against prostate cancer in early clinical trials, only docetaxel has been subjected to large-scale trials testing effects on survival in patients with mCRPC. Docetaxel, given intravenously every 3 weeks (75 mg/m^2) to men with prostate cancer in an initial small trial (n = 35), was associated with a 46% serum PSA response rate.[17] In a series of clinical trials featuring intravenous weekly docetaxel (35–40 mg/m^2), serum PSA response rates ranged from 41% to 64%.[18–22] The addition of estramustine (see earlier discussion) to docetaxel appeared to produce significant benefits in early studies, both for serum PSA responses (45%–74%) and for measurable disease responses (11%–57%).[23–27]

These initial promising studies conducted in the late 1990s eventually resulted in the design and execution of 2 definitive randomized phase 3 studies, known as TAX-327 and SWOG-9916. The TAX-327 study (considered the pivotal trial for FDA approval of docetaxel in prostate cancer) included 3 treatment arms: docetaxel, 75 mg/m^2, every 3 weeks plus prednisone, 10 mg/d; weekly docetaxel, 30 mg/m^2, (5 of 6 weeks) plus prednisone; and mitoxantrone, 12 mg/m^2, every 3 weeks plus prednisone.[4] A total of 1006 patients were randomized into the 3 arms. The docetaxel every-3-weeks regimen resulted in significantly superior survival and higher PSA and pain response rates compared with the mitoxantrone arm. The overall survival was 18.9 versus 16.5 months; the hazard ratio (HR) for risk of death was 0.76 (confidence interval [CI], 0.62–0.92) (**Fig. 1**). The weekly docetaxel regimen showed a trend toward survival benefit compared with mitoxantrone, but this did not reach statistical significance.[28] A significantly greater proportion of patients who were treated with the 3-weekly docetaxel regimen experienced a reduction in pain (35% vs 22%, $P = .01$), a greater than or equal to 50% reduction in PSA (45% vs 32%, $P<.001$), and an improvement in quality of life (22% vs 13%, $P = .009$) compared with patients who received mitoxantrone, which itself had previously shown a quality-of-life improvement. Grade 3/4 toxicity was infrequent, other than neutropenia (32%), but the incidence of febrile neutropenia during the entire course of chemotherapy was 3% or less.

The second study, SWOG-9916, evaluated the combination of docetaxel plus estramustine versus mitoxantrone plus prednisone. The median overall survival was superior in the group receiving the docetaxel regimen: 17.5 versus 15.6 months, HR 0.80 (CI, 0.67–0.90).[5] The patient characteristics in this trial were similar to those of the TAX-327 study, as were the survival outcomes. The incorporation of estramustine in the docetaxel regimen, however, was characterized by increased gastrointestinal and vascular toxicities (mostly thromboembolic complications).[5] Because of the high rate of venous thromboses with estramustine, prophylactic low-dose warfarin and aspirin were added to that arm, although did not reduce the incidence of thromboembolism. Similarly, 20% and 15%, respectively, of patients in the docetaxel-estramustine arm had grade 3/4 gastrointestinal and cardiovascular toxicities. Although comparisons between the docetaxel arms across these 2 seminal trials may not be entirely appropriate because of differences in treatment schedules, patient populations, and docetaxel dosing (60 mg/m^2 in SWOG-9916 and 75 mg/m^2 in TAX-327), it may be concluded that estramustine is unlikely to add significantly to the activity of single-agent docetaxel. Consequently, estramustine is not currently used in this disease.

Based on these 2 pivotal studies, docetaxel was approved by the FDA in 2004 as the first life-prolonging chemotherapy for use as front-line treatment of mCRPC. TAX-327 was designed to include 10 cycles of docetaxel at 3-week intervals, although there were no preexisting data to justify this approach. Therefore, in clinical practice, it is reasonable to administer docetaxel for a total of up to 10 doses. However, another commonly used approach has been to treat patients with a shorter number of chemotherapy cycles (usually between 5 and 7) until stabilization of disease is observed and then to hold treatment until subsequent progression (PSA progression, clinical progression, or both). This approach provides a rationale for docetaxel retreatment before moving to second-line chemotherapeutic options. Indeed, this pattern of chemotherapy administration can be viewed as intermittent docetaxel treatment. Preliminary published reports with intermittent chemotherapy indicate that this approach is feasible and has potential advantages in terms of extending disease control without increased toxicity.[29–31]

CROSSOVER FROM MITOXANTRONE TO DOCETAXEL OR VICE VERSA

The TAX-327 study did not include a crossover design allowing crossover from mitoxantrone to docetaxel and vice versa. As reported, treatment with docetaxel on the TAX-327 trial benefited all patient subgroups (pain vs no pain, ECOG performance status of 0/1 vs 2, and most other prognostic groups). Because the toxicity picture of mitoxantrone was more favorable than that of docetaxel, one consideration was whether patients could be treated initially with mitoxantrone, derive a reasonable quality-of-life benefit (delay of symptoms and pain), and then be treated with docetaxel at the time of subsequent progression. To investigate this issue, Berthold and colleagues[32]

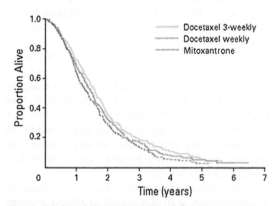

Fig. 1. Updated TAX-327 survival figures. A comparison of docetaxel plus prednisone (weekly vs 3-weekly) versus mitoxantrone plus prednisone. (*Data from* Berthold DR, Pond GR, de Wit R, et al. Survival and PSA response of patients in the TAX 327 study who crossed over to receive docetaxel after mitoxantrone or vice versa. Ann Oncol 2008;19:1749–53.)

reported retrospective data addressing the experience with crossover treatments from mitoxantrone to docetaxel and vice versa. In that analysis, 232 crossover patients were investigated, and the median survival after crossover was 10 months and did not depend on direction of crossover. Data on PSA response were available for 96 patients: PSA response ($\geq$50% reduction) occurred in 15% men receiving mitoxantrone after docetaxel and 28% of men receiving docetaxel after mitoxantrone. Median PSA progression-free survival was 3.4 months for mitoxantrone after docetaxel and 5.9 months for docetaxel after mitoxantrone. In that analysis, response to first-line chemotherapy did not predict outcome of second-line treatment. While retrospective, these data indicate that the response to second-line docetaxel (after mitoxantrone) is substantially lower than reported in the first-line setting, and although survival after crossover was similar, this only included a small number of selected patients who were considered candidates for second-line treatment. In summary, the totality of the available evidence strongly supports the use of docetaxel as the first-line treatment of choice for patients with mCRPC.

PROGNOSTIC FACTORS AND OUTCOME OF PATIENTS WITH MCRPC TREATED WITH DOCETAXEL

Armstrong and colleagues[33] evaluated TAX-327 for several prognostic covariates of interest. Among those factors evaluated with univariate analysis were age; performance status; pain at baseline; baseline levels of hemoglobin, alkaline phosphatase, and PSA; presence of visceral and/or liver metastases; pretreatment PSA doubling time; type of progression (measurable, nonmeasurable, bone scan, and PSA-only progression); number of metastatic sites; Gleason score; presence of multiple bony metastases; and prior estramustine or second-line hormonal therapy. Ten independent prognostic factors (other than treatment group) were identified to be prognostic for survival in multivariate analysis: (1) presence of liver metastases (HR, 1.66; $P = .02$); (2) number of metastatic sites (HR, 1.63 if $\geq$2 sites; $P<.01$); (3) clinically significant pain (HR, 1.48; $P<.01$); (4) Karnofsky performance status (HR, 1.39 if $\leq$70; $P = .02$); (5) type of progression (HR, 1.37 for measurable disease progression and 1.29 for bone scan progression; $P = .01$ and .02, respectively); (6) pretreatment PSA doubling time (HR, 1.19 if <55 days; $P = .07$); (7) PSA level (HR, 1.17 per log rise; $P<.01$); (8) tumor grade (HR, 1.18 for high grade; $P = .07$); (9) alkaline phosphatase

(HR, 1.27 per log rise; $P<.01$); and (10) hemoglobin (HR, 1.11 per unit decline; $P = .01$) (**Table 1**). An additional novel independent factor in this analysis was the mode of disease progression at baseline (ie, before trial enrollment), wherein men who had progression by bone scan and measurable soft tissue disease had a 1.28- and 1.40-fold increased risk of death, respectively, compared with men without these modes of progression, such as PSA-only progression ($P = .01$ and <0.01, respectively). A survival nomogram was developed to assist in the definition of the prognosis of patients based on clinical criteria, and this is outlined in **Fig. 2**.

DOCETAXEL-BASED COMBINATIONS

Based on encouraging initial reports of uncontrolled studies, various therapeutic modalities have been developed in combination with docetaxel in phase 3 trials. GVAX, a vaccine composed of prostate cancer cell lines modified to secrete granulocyte macrophage colony-stimulating factor (GM-CSF), underwent a phase 3 trial in combination with docetaxel in patients with symptomatic mCRPC. This trial, known as VITAL-2, was interrupted early because of an unexpected higher death rate in the GVAX arm. Another trial, VITAL-1, compared GVAX against docetaxel in patients with asymptomatic CRPC and found no overall survival difference either.[34]

DN-101 is a high-dose formulation of calcitriol, an activated vitamin D analogue that has antiproliferative effects against prostate cancer cells in vitro. The combination of docetaxel plus calcitriol was evaluated in a randomized phase 2 trial that suggested an improvement in overall survival, with a significant improvement in greater than or equal to 50% PSA reduction compared with docetaxel monotherapy. However, the results of a phase 3 trial (ASCENT-2) conducted in 953 men with progressive CRPC found a significantly shorter overall survival for the combination of docetaxel plus calcitriol compared with docetaxel plus prednisone (17.8 vs 20.2 months).[35] The reasons for the shorter survival were unclear but could relate to the use of the weekly schedule of docetaxel in the control arm (which was not as effective as the every-3-week schedule in the pivotal TAX-327 study).

Other compounds that have been studied in combination with docetaxel in phase 3 trials include the anti-VEGF antibody bevacizumab, aflibercept (VEGF trap), the Bcl-2 inhibitor oblimersen, the endothelin antagonists atrasentan and zibotentan, and the immunomodulatory drug lenalidomide. Unfortunately, none of these docetaxel-based combinations have been able to

Table 1
Prognostic variables of patients treated with first-line docetaxel chemotherapy on TAX-327 trial

Variable	HR (95% CI)	P Value
Chemotherapy type (vs every-3-wk docetaxel)		
Weekly docetaxel	1.12 (0.90–1.39)	0.320
Mitoxantrone	1.43 (1.16–1.77)	0.001
Liver metastases	1.66 (1.09–2.54)	0.019
Number of metastatic sites (>3 vs ≤3)	1.63 (1.23–2.15)	0.001
Pain at baseline	1.48 (1.23–1.79)	0.001
Karnofsky performance status (≤70 vs ≥80)	1.39 (1.06–1.82)	0.016
Progression type		
Measurable disease	1.37 (1.10–1.70)	0.005
Bone scan progression	1.29 (1.06–1.57)	0.010
Baseline PSA doubling time (<55 vs >55 d)	1.19 (0.99–1.42)	0.066
Baseline (log) PSA (for every unit rise in [log] PSA in ng/dL)	1.17 (1.10–1.25)	0.001
Tumor grade (Gleason ≥8 vs Gleason ≤7)	1.18 (0.99–1.42)	0.069
Alkaline phosphatase, log scale (per [log] unit rise, IU/L)	1.27 (1.15–1.39)	0.001
Hemoglobin (per unit decline, g/dL)	1.11 (1.03–1.19)	0.004

NOTE: $n = 635$ with 518 failures, excluding missing values for pain, performance status, and tumor grade at baseline. Concordance index = 0.69.

Data from Armstrong AJ, Garrett-Mayer ES, Yang YC, et al. A contemporary prognostic nomogram for men with hormone-refractory metastatic prostate cancer: a TAX327 study analysis. Clin Cancer Res 2007;13:6396–403.

demonstrate improved overall survival over the use of docetaxel alone. In some cases (eg, with docetaxel plus bevacizumab), the combination treatment significantly improved progression-free survival over docetaxel alone, but this did not translate into an overall survival benefit. Currently, there are 2 phase 3 docetaxel combination studies with results pending. These studies are investigating combinations of docetaxel with Src inhibitors (dasatinib) and the ant-apoptotic chaperone molecule custirsen.

In conclusion, although docetaxel remains the gold-standard first-line chemotherapy for mCRPC, no significant additional benefit has been realized with several docetaxel combination strategies. Although at this time the authors cannot recommend the combination of docetaxel with other targeted therapies in the context of standard clinical care, their knowledge of the biologic mechanisms involved in the progression of mCRPC has reached a level at which the discovery of more effective targeted combination approaches will probably further improve outcomes in the future.

CABAZITAXEL

Cabazitaxel is a second-generation taxane that exhibited cytotoxic activity against a broad range of cancer cell lines and tumor models with greater potency than docetaxel in multidrug-resistant tumor cells. An additional characteristic of cabazitaxel is its ability to penetrate the blood-brain barrier in vivo, which is not achievable with other taxanes.[36,37]

A phase 1 trial using this agent determined that cabazitaxel had linear pharmacokinetics similar to docetaxel and highlighted the favorable safety profile of cabazitaxel compared with docetaxel. The principal dose-limiting toxicity of cabazitaxel was neutropenia; other observed side-effects (including nausea, vomiting, diarrhea, and fatigue) were generally mild-to-moderate.[36] Twelve of the 24 patients evaluable for clinical response in the phase 1 study had stable disease for more than 4 months, and there were 2 partial responses observed in men with mCRPC, both of which had a reduction in measurable disease and significant declines in PSA levels.

The phase 3 (TROPIC) trial was a randomized, open-label, multinational trial conducted to assess whether cabazitaxel plus prednisone improved overall survival compared with mitoxantrone plus prednisone in men with mCRPC who had progressed either during or after docetaxel chemotherapy.[36] Patients aged more than or equal to 18 years with mCRPC progression despite docetaxel treatment were all given prednisone, 10 mg/d, and also randomized to receive either intravenous cabazitaxel, 25 mg/m^2,

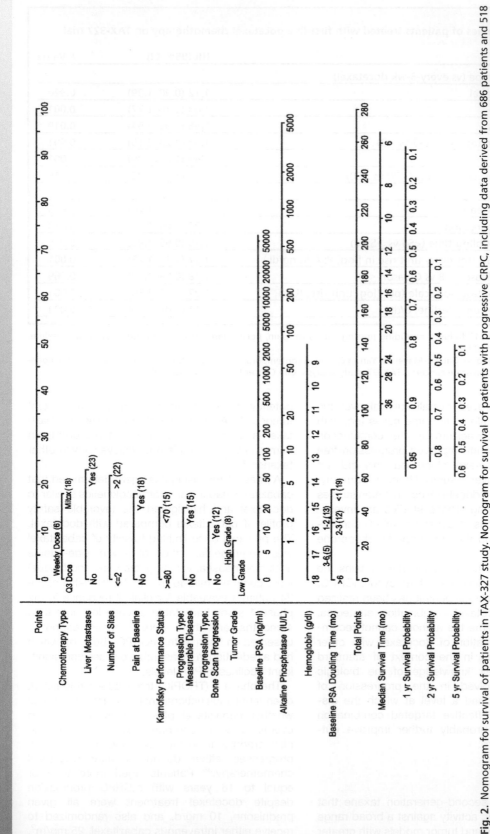

Fig. 2. Nomogram for survival of patients in TAX-327 study. Nomogram for survival of patients with progressive CRPC, including data derived from 686 patients and 518 mortality events. Note: a present pain intensity of greater than or equal to 2 and an analgesic score of greater than or equal to 10 defined in the original protocol indicate the presence of significant pain. Instructions for physician: locate the liver metastasis axis. Draw a straight line upward to the point axis to determine how many points toward survival the patient receives for the presence or absence of liver metastases. Repeat this process for each predictor variable and sum the points for each predictor. Locate this sum on the total points axis. Draw a straight line downward from the total points axis to identify the predicted median survival and the predicted 1-year, 2-year, and 5-year overall survival probabilities. Instructions to patient: "Mr. X, if we had 100 men exactly like you, we would expect <<nomogram prediction × 100>> to be alive in 1, 2, and 5 y, respectively, and we expect 50 of those to be alive after <<median survival prediction>> months." (*From* Armstrong AJ, Garrett-Mayer ES, Yang YC, et al. A contemporary prognostic nomogram for men with hormone-refractory metastatic prostate cancer: a TAX327 study analysis. Clin Cancer Res 2007;13:6396–403.)

or mitoxantrone, 12 mg/m^2, every 3 weeks for 10 cycles. A total of 755 patients were included in the study (cabazitaxel; n = 378 and mitoxantrone; n = 377). The median follow-up for both treatment groups was 12.8 months. Treatment groups were balanced with regard to demographics and baseline disease characteristics. All patients had to have evidence of disease progression with first-line docetaxel treatment. Approximately 70% of patients had progressed within 3 months of completing docetaxel treatment; almost one-third of patients had progressed while they were receiving docetaxel.

The study met its primary endpoint, demonstrating significantly improved median overall survival in patients receiving cabazitaxel (15.1 months; 95% CI, 14.1–16.3 months) compared with those who received mitoxantrone (12.7 months; 95% CI, 11.6–13.7 months). The HR for death was 0.70 (95% CI, 0.59–0.83; P<.0001). In addition to the survival benefit, cabazitaxel roughly doubled median progression-free survival compared with mitoxantrone (cabazitaxel 2.8 months vs mitoxantrone 1.4 months; P<.0001). Moreover, cabazitaxel treatment significantly improved objective response rate (RECIST criteria) more than 2-fold compared with mitoxantrone (P<.001). The PSA response rate (≥50% decline) was significantly higher in the cabazitaxel group compared with the mitoxantrone group, and patients receiving cabazitaxel also had a significantly longer median time-to-PSA-progression.[36]

Patients in the cabazitaxel and mitoxantrone groups received a median of 6 and 4 cycles of treatment, respectively. The most common adverse events experienced by patients were hematologic toxicities. There was a greater incidence of hematologic events with grade greater than or equal to 3 severity in patients who received cabazitaxel. For example, 81.7% and 7.5% of patients in the cabazitaxel group experienced grade greater than or equal to 3 neutropenia and febrile neutropenia, respectively, compared with 58% and 1.3% of patients in the mitoxantrone group. Cabazitaxel treatment also increased the incidence of nonhematologic toxicities, including diarrhea (46.6% vs 10.5% for mitoxantrone; grade ≥3 diarrhea [6.2% vs 0.3%]) and asthenia (20.5% vs 4.6% for mitoxantrone; grade ≥3 asthenia [12.4% vs 2.4%]). In addition, 5% of men on the cabazitaxel arm died from causes other than disease progression within 30 days of receiving cabazitaxel. This compares with a 1% drug-related death rate in the mitoxantrone group. The most common cause of death in patients who were treated with cabazitaxel was neutropenia, including its clinical consequences such as septicemia. However, no further deaths due to neutropenic complications occurred in the cabazitaxel group after the Independent Data Monitoring Committee communication to the TROPIC investigators about the need to strictly adhere to the study protocol regarding dose delays and modifications and managing neutropenia with GM-CSF according to American Society for Clinical Oncology guidelines.

Based on the results of the TROPIC trial, cabazitaxel was approved by the FDA in June 2010 and by the European Medicines Agency in 2011 for use in combination with prednisone for the treatment of docetaxel-pretreated mCRPC. Cabazitaxel is currently being evaluated as a first-line treatment of mCRPC in 2 separate clinical trials. The first study (designated as FIRSTANA) is a standard multiinstitutional, multinational phase 3 comparison between cabazitaxel (in 2 doses: 25 mg/m^2 and 20 mg/m^2) and standard every-3-weeks docetaxel (75 mg/m^2) in men with chemotherapy-naive mCRPC. The second study, TAXYNERGY, is a national multicenter randomized phase 2 trial to evaluate the benefit of an early switch from first-line docetaxel/prednisone to cabazitaxel/prednisone (or the opposite sequence) in men with chemotherapy-untreated mCRPC. The latter trial aims to asses PSA response after 12 weeks on study and to use this information to maintain treatment with the current taxane (if PSA reductions exceed 30%) or to switch to the alternative taxane (if PSA declines of less than 30% are observed by 12 weeks). This trial also aims to explore circulating tumor cell-based molecular markers and mechanisms of taxane resistance in men with mCRPC who have not received prior chemotherapy. Finally, in the second-line (post-docetaxel) setting, cabazitaxel is also currently being prospectively evaluated at 2 different doses (25 mg/m^2 vs 20 mg/m^2) in a multinational randomized trial (PROSELICA).

SUMMARY

In the vast majority of patients with mCRPC, docetaxel chemotherapy (at a dose of 75 mg/m^2 given intravenously every 3 weeks) remains the strong standard-of-care for first-line treatment, whereas historical drugs such as mitoxantrone and others are seldom used in the modern era. In men who have progressed during or after docetaxel-based therapy, strong evidence supports the use of cabazitaxel (at a dose of 25 mg/m^2 given intravenously every 3 weeks) in patients with adequate performance status and a reasonable life expectancy. The emergence of additional novel therapies for the management of mCRPC (such as sipuleucel-T, abiraterone, enzalutamide, and radium-223) is likely to complicate the therapeutic decision process, although these new drugs are certainly a welcome addition to the therapeutic arsenal for this disease. Considerations of patient performance status, comorbidities, disease characteristics, and patient preferences should guide these treatment decisions.

REFERENCES

1. Kantoff PW, Halabi S, Conaway M, et al. Hydrocortisone with or without mitoxantrone in men with hormone-refractory prostate cancer: results of the Cancer and Leukemia Group B 9182 study. J Clin Oncol 1999;17:2506–13.

2. Ernst DS, Tannock IF, Winquist EW, et al. Randomized, double-blind, controlled trial of mitoxantrone/prednisone and clodronate versus mitoxantrone/prednisone and placebo in patients with hormone-refractory prostate cancer and pain. J Clin Oncol 2003;21:3335–42.

3. Tannock IF, Osoba D, Stockler MR, et al. Chemotherapy with mitoxantrone plus prednisone or prednisone alone for symptomatic hormone-resistant prostate cancer: a Canadian randomized trial with palliative end points. J Clin Oncol 1996;14:175–84.

4. Tannock IF, de Wit R, Berry WR, et al. Docetaxel plus prednisone or mitoxantrone plus prednisone for advanced prostate cancer. N Engl J Med 2004;351:1502–12.

5. Petrylak DP, Tangen CM, Hussain MH, et al. Docetaxel and estramustine compared with mitoxantrone and prednisone for advanced refractory prostate cancer. N Engl J Med 2004;351:1513–20.

6. Kantoff P. Recent progress in management of advanced prostate cancer. Oncology 2005;19:631–6.

7. Eisenberger MA. Chemotherapy for prostate carcinoma. NCI Monogr 1988;7:151–63.

8. Von Roemeling R, Fisher HA, Horton J. Daily oral cyclophosphamide is effective in hormone-refractory prostate cancer: a phase-I/II pilot study [abstracts 665]. Proc Am Soc Clin Oncol 1992;11:213.

9. Smith D, Vogelzang N, Goldberg H, et al. High-dose cyclophosphamide with granulocyte-macrophage colony stimulating factor in hormone refractory prostate cancer [abstracts 666]. Proc Am Soc Clin Oncol 1992;11:213.

10. Abell F, Wilkes J, Divers L, et al. Oral cyclophosphamide for hormone-refractory prostate cancer [abstracts 646]. Proc Am Soc Clin Oncol 1995;14:213.

11. Hudes G, Einhorn L, Ross E, et al. Vinblastine versus vinblastine plus oral estramustine phosphate for patients with hormone-refractory cancer: a Hoosier Oncology Group and Fox Chase Network Phase III trial. J Clin Oncol 1999;17:3160–6.

12. Hartley AS, Kruse E. Nuclear protein matrix as a target for estramustine-induced cell death. Prostate 1986;9:387–95.

13. Iversen P, Rasmussen F. Estramustine phosphate versus placebo in hormone-refractory prostate cancer. Danish prostate cancer group study 9002 [abstracts 41]. Proc Am Urol Assoc 1995;153:239A.

14. Horwitz SB. Taxol (paclitaxel): mechanisms of action. Ann Oncol 1994;5(Suppl 6):S3–6.

15. Jordan MA, Wilson L. Microtubules as a target for anticancer drugs. Nat Rev Cancer 2004;4:253–65.

16. Mabjeesh NJ, Escuin D, LaVallee TM, et al. 2ME2 inhibits tumor growth and angiogenesis by disrupting microtubules and dysregulating HIF. Cancer Cell 2003;3:363–75.

17. Picus J, Schultz M. Docetaxel (Taxotere) as monotherapy in the treatment of hormone-refractory prostate cancer: preliminary results. Semin Oncol 1999;26(Suppl 17):14–8.

18. Beer TM, Pierce WC, Lowe BA, et al. Phase II study of weekly docetaxel in symptomatic androgen-independent prostate cancer. Ann Oncol 2001;12:1273–9.

19. Beer TM, Berry W, Wersinger EM, et al. Weekly docetaxel in elderly patients with prostate cancer: efficacy and toxicity in patients at least 70 years of age compared with patients younger than 70 years. Clin Prostate Cancer 2003;2:167–72.

20. Berry W, Dakhil S, Gregurich MA, et al. Phase II trial of single-agent weekly docetaxel in hormone-refractory, symptomatic, metastatic carcinoma of the prostate. Semin Oncol 2001;28(Suppl 15):8–15.

21. Ferrero JM, Foa C, Thezenas S, et al. A weekly schedule of docetaxel for metastatic hormone-refractory prostate cancer. Oncology 2004;66:281–7.

22. Gravis G, Bladou F, Salem N, et al. Weekly administration of docetaxel for symptomatic metastatic hormone-refractory prostate carcinoma. Cancer 2003;98:1627–34.

23. Savarese D, Taplin ME, Halabi S, et al. A phase II study of docetaxel (Taxotere), estramustine, and low-dose hydrocortisone in men with hormone-refractory prostate cancer: preliminary results of cancer and leukemia group B Trial 9780. Semin Oncol 1999;26(Suppl 17):39–44.

24. Petrylak DP, Macarthur RB, O'Connor J, et al. Phase I trial of docetaxel with estramustine in androgen-independent prostate cancer. J Clin Oncol 1999;17:958–67.

25. Oudard S, Banu E, Beuzeboc P, et al. Multicenter randomized phase II study of two schedules of docetaxel, estramustine, and prednisone versus mitoxantrone plus prednisone in patients with metastatic hormone-refractory prostate cancer. J Clin Oncol 2005;23:3343–51.

26. Kreis W, Budman DR, Fetten J, et al. Phase I trial of the combination of daily estramustine phosphate and intermittent docetaxel in patients with metastatic hormone refractory prostate carcinoma. Ann Oncol 1999;10:33–8.

27. Sinibaldi VJ, Carducci MA, Moore-Cooper S, et al. Phase II evaluation of docetaxel plus one-day oral estramustine phosphate in the treatment of patients with androgen independent prostate carcinoma. Cancer 2002;94:1457–65.

28. Berthold DR, Pond GR, Soban F, et al. Docetaxel plus prednisone or mitoxantrone plus prednisone for advanced prostate cancer: updated survival in the TAX 327 study. J Clin Oncol 2008;26:242–5.

29. Beer TM, Garzotto M, Henner WD, et al. Intermittent chemotherapy in metastatic androgen-independent prostate cancer. Br J Cancer 2003;89:968–70.

30. Meulenbeld HJ, Hamberg P, de Wit R. Chemotherapy in patients with castration-resistant prostate cancer. Eur J Cancer 2009;45:161–71.

31. De Wit R. Chemotherapy in hormono refractory prostate cancer. BJU Int 2008;101:11–5.

32. Berthold DR, Pond GR, de Wit R, et al. Survial and PSA response of patients in the TAX 327 study who crossed over to receive doctaxel after mitoxantrone or vive versa. Ann Oncol 2008;19: 1749–53.

33. Armstrong AJ, Garrett-Mayer ES, Yang YC, et al. A contemporary prognostic nomogram for men with hormone-refractory metastatic prostate cancer: a TAX327 study analysis. Clin Cancer Res 2007;13: 6396–403.

34. Small E, Demkow T, Gerritsen WR, et al. A phase III trial of GVAX immunotherapy for prostate cancer in combination with docetaxel versus docetaxel plus prednisone in symptomatic, castration-resistant prostate cancer (CRPC). Genitourinary Cancers Symposium 2009. Orlando (FL): American society of clinical oncology; 2009.

35. Beer TM, Ryan CW, Venner PM, et al. ASCENT Investigators. Intermittent chemotherapy in patients with metastatic androgen-independent prostate cancer: results from ASCENT, a double-blinded, randomized comparison of high-dose calcitriol plus docetaxel with placebo plus docetaxel. Cancer 2008;112:326–30.

36. De Bono JS, Oudard S, Ozguroglu M, et al. Prednisone plus cabazitaxel or mitoxantrone for metastatic castration-resistant prostate cancer progressing after docetaxel treatment: a randomised open label trial. Lancet 2010;376:1147–54.

37. Smith TJ, Khatcherossian J, Lyman GH, et al. 2006 update of recommendations for the use of white blood cell growth factors: an evidence-based clinical practice guideline. J Clin Oncol 2006;24:3187–205.

Management of Docetaxel Failures in Metastatic Castrate-Resistant Prostate Cancer

Sumanta K. Pal, MD[a], Brian Lewis, MD[b],
Oliver Sartor, MD[b,c,d],*

KEYWORDS

- Sipuleucel-T • Cabazitaxel • Abiraterone • mCRPC

KEY POINTS

- Multiple new agents are available for metastatic castrate resistant prostate cancer.
- Abiraterone and cabazitaxel are FDA approved in the post-docetaxel space.
- Sipuleucel-T is FDA approved for patients with metastatic CRPC that have minimal or no symptoms.
- MDV-3100 and radium-223 are two additional agents that have also reported positive phase 3 trials for metastatic CRPC.
- No comparative trials have been conducted between any of these newer agents, leaving clinicians with many questions.

INTRODUCTION

In 1941, Huggins and colleagues[1,2] noted the dramatic effects of surgical castration in the treatment of metastatic prostate cancer. This landmark development revolutionized the therapy of the disease, and over time, pharmacologic methods of castration were developed as an alternative to surgical methods.[3] Huggins recognized early on that "despite regressions of great magnitude, it is obvious that there are many failures of endocrine therapy to control the disease."[4] Though this disease state has undergone several nomenclature changes (including androgen-independent prostate cancer and hormone refractory prostate cancer), today we refer to this disease state as castration-resistant prostate cancer (CRPC), which may or not be metastatic. The onset of the metastatic CRPC (mCRPC) occurs at a median of about 9 years after androgen-deprivation therapy (ADT) for patients initially treated for nonmetastatic disease or 1 to 3 years after ADT for patients initially treated for metastatic disease.[5,6]

For decades, clinical trials failed to show a definitive advantage with novel therapies for mCRPC.[7,8] Two pivotal trials examining docetaxel-based regimens were the first to demonstrate an overall survival benefit in patients with mCRPC. In the TAX 327 trial, patients were randomized to receive either mitoxantrone-prednisone or docetaxel-prednisone in one of two schedules.[9] Ultimately, docetaxel at a dose of 75 mg/m^2 intravenously

Funding sources: Dr Pal: NIH Loan Repayment Plan (LRP) and NIH K12 2K12CA001727-16A1.
Conflicts of interest: Dr Pal: Sanofi (Speakers Bureau), Dr Lewis: None, Dr Sartor: Consultant: Sanofi, Algeta, Bayer, Medivation, Takeda, JNJ. Investigator: Sanofi, Bayer, Algeta, Takeda.
[a] Department of Medical Oncology & Experimental Therapeutics, City of Hope Comprehensive Cancer Center, 1500 East Duarte Road, Duarte, CA 91010, USA; [b] Department of Medicine, Tulane University School of Medicine, 1430 Tulane Avenue, SL-42, New Orleans, LA 70112, USA; [c] Department of Urology, Tulane University School of Medicine, 1430 Tulane Avenue, SL-42, New Orleans, LA 70112, USA; [d] Tulane Cancer Center, Tulane Medical School, 1430 Tulane Avenue, SL-42, New Orleans, LA 70112, USA
* Corresponding author. Tulane Cancer Center, Tulane Medical School, 1430 Tulane Avenue, SL-42, New Orleans, LA 70112.
E-mail address: osartor@tulane.edu

Urol Clin N Am 39 (2012) 583–591
http://dx.doi.org/10.1016/j.ucl.2012.07.013
0094-0143/12/$ – see front matter © 2012 Elsevier Inc. All rights reserved.

(IV) every 3 weeks with prednisone daily led to a survival advantage over standard mitoxantrone-prednisone therapy (18.9 months vs 16.5 months, P = .009). In Southwest Oncology Group (SWOG) trial, 9916 patients were randomized to receive either docetaxel-estramusine or mitoxantrone-prednisone.[10] Again, a survival advantage was noted with docetaxel-based therapy (17.5 months vs 15.6 months, P = .02). The cumulative data from these studies led to the approval of docetaxel-prednisone–based therapy for mCRPC on May 19, 2004.[11]

In the ensuing years, several different approaches were taken to build on the success of docetaxel in patients with mCRPC. One approach was to explore combinations of novel therapies with docetaxel. Unfortunately, to date, these studies have proven somewhat disappointing.[12–19] A second approach to the patient with mCRPC has been to explore the efficacy of novel therapies either before or after docetaxel therapy. These efforts have thus far proven to be more fruitful than explorations of combination therapy.[20] To date, the bulk of progress has been made in the postdocetaxel space, in which agents such as cabazitaxel, abiraterone, MDV3100, and radium-223 have demonstrated statistically significant benefits in overall survival.[21–24] Thus far, cabazitaxel-prednisone and abiraterone-prednisone are FDA approved. Although some agents (ie, abiraterone, radium-223) may ultimately straddle predocetaxel and postdocetaxel spaces,[25] this article focuses on the current postdocetaxel strategies. The clinical data related to each agent is reviewed in detail to provide the physician with a framework with which to approach the docetaxel-refractory patient.

CABAZITAXEL

Structurally, docetaxel and the novel taxane cabazitaxel are similar, with two hydroxyl side chains (docetaxel) substituted for two methoxy groups (cabazitaxel) (**Fig. 1**).[26] Both exert their preclinical activity through inhibition of microtubule disassembly, akin to other taxanes.[27–29] However, early in its development, the preclinical activity of cabazitaxel was noted to be distinct from docetaxel. In a variety of cell lines (including P388 [lymphoblastic leukemia], HL60 [promyelocytic leukemia], and Calc18 [breast adenocarcinoma] models), cabazitaxel was noted to inhibit growth at relatively low concentrations, with mean inhibitory concentration[27–29] in the range of 3 to 29 nM.[30] The antitumor activity of cabazitaxel was maintained in cell lines that were resistant to other standard taxanes as well. In murine xenograft models of prostate cancer (including the hormone-

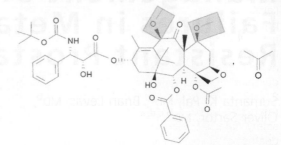

Fig. 1. Structure of cabazitaxel. Highlighted are two entities in the cabazitaxel chemical structure that differ from docetaxel: the two methoxy groups of cabazitaxel are substituted with hydroxyl side chains in docetaxel.

resistant DU145 cell line), near complete tumor regressions were observed.[31,32]

The encouraging preclinical data for cabazitaxel led to initiation of a phase I clinical trial.[33] In this study, 25 patients with advanced solid tumors were treated with doses of cabazitaxel ranging from 10 to 25 mg/m^2. Eight patients with advanced prostate cancer were enrolled on the study, representing the largest subgroup based on tumor type. Pharmacokinetic data from this study indicated a triphasic model of elimination ($t_{1/2}$ = 2.5 minutes, 1.3 hours, and 77.3 hours for the three phases, respectively). Notably, the recommended phase II dose emerging from the study was 20 mg/m^2, given dose-limiting toxicities of febrile neutropenia and grade 4 neutropenia occurring at a dose of 25 mg/m^2. Two patients attained a partial response in this phase I effort—both patients with advanced prostate cancer who had received prior mitoxantrone and docetaxel.

A separate phase I study examined doses of cabazitaxel ranging from 10 to 30 mg/m^2 IV every 3 weeks; the recommended phase II dose in this effort was 25 mg/m^2.[34] Akin to the previously noted phase I study, the most frequent toxicities were neutropenia, febrile neutropenia, diarrhea, and infection. This study helped establish the extent of ex vivo plasma protein binding (approximately 92%); cabazitaxel showed high binding to both lipoproteins and albumin. The intrapatient variability of the area under the curve between 0 to 48 hours (AUC_{0-48}) was also ascertained in this study and was estimated to be approximately 27%.

A phase II exploration of cabazitaxel in heavily pretreated breast cancer used a phase II dose of 20 mg/m^2 as a starting dose but allowed escalation to 25 mg/m^2 provided tolerance of the initial dose level.[35] Although originally designed as a three-arm, randomized phase II study evaluating both cabazitaxel and a distinct novel taxane (larotaxel),[36] the trial design was modified owing to poor accrual to include just one arm. Patients may have received prior taxane in either the adjuvant or metastatic setting. With a total of 67 patients, the overall response rate was 14%, and the median duration of response was 7.6 months (range, 2.6–18.7 months). Although two complete responses were observed, several concerning safety signals were seen in this study, with two deaths due to nonhematologic toxicity noted within 30 days of study treatment.

A rather unique element of the clinical development of cabazitaxel is its evolution from phase I to phase III assessment in prostate cancer—there was no phase II evaluation of the drug outside of the setting of breast cancer. The phase III TROPIC study built on the preclinical efficacy of cabazitaxel seen in preclinical models of hormone-resistant prostate cancer and the responses seen in the phase I assessment.[24] In this study, 775 patients with docetaxel refractory disease were randomized to receive either cabazitaxel at 25 mg/m^2 IV every 3weeks with prednisone or mitoxantrone with prednisone. The definition of docetaxel-refractory disease used employed in TROPIC included either (1) response evaluation criteria in solid tumors–based progression, or (2) two consecutive prostate-specific antigen (PSA) rises at least 1 week apart. Patients were initially permitted to enroll with any prior docetaxel exposure, but the study was later modified to include patients who had at least a cumulative docetaxel dose of 225 mg/m^2.[37,38]

The study met its primary end point, demonstrating a significant improvement in median overall survival from 12.7 months with mitoxantrone-prednisone to 15.1 months with cabazitaxel-prednisone ($P<.001$).[24] Furthermore, progression-free survival was improved with cabazitaxel-based therapy (2.8 months vs 1.4 months, $P<.0001$). Pain relief, as assessed by the McGill-Melzack pain questionnaire, was not distinct between arms. The positive survival advantage led to the FDA approval of cabazitaxel on June 17, 2010.[39] Interestingly, post hoc analyses show that this survival advantage actually extends to the overall survival time from first docetaxel usage.[40] Specifically, median overall survival was 29 months from the time of first docetaxel use in patients receiving subsequent cabazitaxel therapy compared with 25 months in patients receiving subsequent mitoxantrone therapy. Furthermore, a survival benefit was seen in subgroups that discontinued use of docetaxel therapy for progression and in subgroups that discontinued use of docetaxel therapy for other reasons (eg, adverse events, intolerance).[41] The findings in patients with progression while on docetaxel underscore the distinction between docetaxel and cabazitaxel.

As in earlier experiences with cabazitaxel, the most common adverse event noted in the phase III study was neutropenia, with grade greater than or equal to 3 neutropenia occurring in 82% of patients and 8% of patients developing febrile neutropenia.[24] One factor that may account for the high frequency of neutropenia and related events seen in TROPIC was the prohibition of prophylactic growth factor use. With the first cycle of therapy with cabazitaxel, patients were not allowed to use these agents, although they could be implemented subsequently. Recommendations accompanying the FDA approval of cabazitaxel recommend use of growth factor support in at-risk groups, including (1) older patients (age >65), (2) recipients of extensive prior radiation, (3) patients with poor nutritional status, (4) patients with prior documented episodes of febrile neutropenia, (5) patients with poor performance status, and (6) patients with other serious medical comorbidities.[42] It is foreseeable that these criteria encompass most patients in a typical prostate cancer clinic. A retrospective subset analysis of patients who received prophylactic growth factor support from cycle 2 of cabazitaxel therapy onwards did suggest a dramatic decline in grade greater than 3 neutropenia (23.7% vs 57.7%; $P<.0001$).[43] These data support the more aggressive use of growth factors in many patients receiving cabazitaxel therapy today in the clinic.

Other notable toxicities associated with cabazitaxel include diarrhea—several deaths secondary to treatment-related diarrhea were seen in the TROPIC study. Recommendations accompanying the publication of the TROPIC data suggest vigilant monitoring for dehydration, with prompt administration of antidiarrheals and fluids if this toxicity is incurred. Other frequent nonhematologic toxicities include fatigue and asthenias. With the caveats of cross-trial comparisons, several toxicities (ie, neuropathy and alopecia) seem less prevalent with cabazitaxel therapy.

ABIRATERONE

Ketoconazole has been used for patients with CRPC since the 1980s when it was noted to decrease testosterone in patients being treated for antifungal indications.[7] The mechanism of the testosterone decline is enzymatic inhibition of several enzymatic steps (**Fig. 2**) in the androgen synthetic pathway, most notably 17-α-hydroxylase/17,20-desmolase (CYP17). Because inhibition of the 17-α-hydroxylase is associated with decreased cortisol synthesis, ketoconazole at doses of 600 to 1200 mg per day is typically given

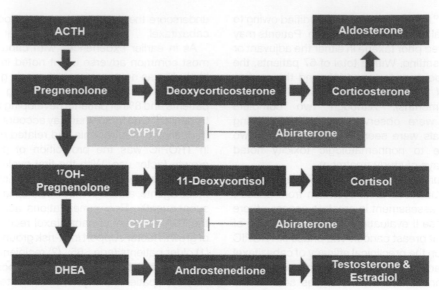

Fig. 2. Mechanism of abiraterone. Abiraterone inhibits critical steps in the biosynthetic pathway of glucocorticoids and testosterone-estradiol.

with glucocorticoids such as prednisone, hydrocortisone, or dexamethasone.

Newer CYP17 inhibitors such as abiraterone also require glucocorticoids, not only to replace cortisol but also to feedback on the pituitary to diminish the corticotropin stimulation, which stimulates increased production of mineralocorticoids.[44] Abiraterone was initially developed by scientists at the Institute for Cancer Research in London. De Bono and colleagues[44] were the first to test the abiraterone-prednisone in prostate cancer clinical trials and excellent initial results were reported for both tolerability and PSA declines. Abiraterone results in a relatively complete inhibition of androgen and estrogen synthesis and substantially decrease, even in castrate men, serum levels of testosterone, estradiol, dehydroepiandrostenedione, and androstenedione.

Oral abiraterone with 5 mg twice a day prednisone is now FDA approved based on a phase III trial with 1195 patients in the mCRPC postdocetaxel ketoconazole-naïve setting.[21] This trial was stopped at an interim analysis after meeting the primary end point of overall survival. This trial randomized patients to receive prednisone 5 mg twice a day plus 1000 mg of abiraterone acetate as compared with patients receiving prednisone-placebo. At 12.8 months median patient follow-up, overall survival in the abiraterone-prednisone arm was 14.8 months compared with 10.9 months in the prednisone-alone arm (hazard ratio [HR] 0.65; P<.001). Secondary end points, including time to PSA progression (10.2 vs 6.6 months; P<.001) and PSA response rate (29% vs 6%, P<.001), also favored

the abiraterone-treated patients. The agent was well tolerated though mineralocorticoid side effects (fluid retention, hypokalemia, and hypertension) were clearly more common in the abiraterone-treated patients.[21] Another phase III abiraterone interim result from asymptomatic or minimally symptomatic ketoconazole-naïve patients conducted in the predocetaxel setting has recently been reported by the sponsor in a press release.[25]

MDV3100

Of the three FDA-approved antiandrogens (bicludamide, nilutamide, and flutamide), bicludamide has the highest affinity for the androgen receptor by a factor of two to four.[45] MDV3100 is a novel androgen receptor inhibitor that has 5 to 8 times the affinity for the androgen receptor compared with bicalutamide. Furthermore, unlike bicalutamide and flutamide, the agent has no agonist activity. MDV3100 also inhibits the androgen receptor nuclear translocation, DNA binding, and cofactor activation.[46]

MDV3100 was evaluated in a phase I-II clinical trial whereby 140 patients with CRPC were given escalated doses of the drug form 30 to 600 mg oral daily.[47] Of the patients studied, 54% had previous treatment with chemotherapy and 78% had bone metastatic disease. Time to radiographic progression (TTRP) was 47 weeks in the intent-to-treat population, and was 29 weeks in the subset of patients with prior chemotherapy exposure. The time to PSA progression by PCWG2 criteria was 32 weeks for the entire population, 21 weeks for the patients with a history of prior chemotherapy, and 41 weeks for the chemotherapy-naïve population. The percent of patients with a maximum PSA decline greater than or equal to 50% was 56% for the entire cohort. The most common grade 2 adverse events were fatigue, nausea, dyspnea, and anorexia. Two of the 140 patients had a seizure and the most common cause of dose reduction or discontinuation was fatigue.

These encouraging data lead to phase III placebo-controlled trial in which 1199 patients who had received less than or equal to two docetaxel-based regimens were randomized 2:1 to receive MDV3100 at 160 oral daily or placebo.[23] The primary end point of the study was overall survival. Secondary end points included TTRP, time to PSA progression, and PSA response. There was found to be an overall survival benefit of 4.8 months, with median overall survival of 13.6 months in placebo-treated patients, and 18.4 months MDV3100-treated patients (P<.001). TTRP was 8.3 months for MDV3100 versus 2.9 months for placebo and the time to PSA progression was 8.3 months for MDV3100 versus 3 months for placebo (P<.0001 for both). There was also a significant improvement in PSA response, with 54% and 1.5% of patients having PSA reductions greater than or equal to 50% from baseline in the MDV3100 and placebo arms, respectively. The most common adverse event was fatigue, with 33% of patients in the MDV3100 group and 29% of patients in the placebo group reporting fatigue of any grade. This trial should lead to the FDA approval of MDV3100 in the near future. The phase III PREVAIL trial comparing MDV3100 with placebo in chemotherapy naïve men is enrolling patients as this article goes to press.

BONE-TARGETED THERAPY

When metastatic, prostate cancer involves bone in approximately 70% of cases.[48] Thus, the concept of bone-targeted therapy has long been considered an attractive and logical concept. These agents are appropriate in the predocetaxel or the postdocetaxel space. FDA-approved bone-targeted products for bone mCRPC include zoledronic acid, denosumab, strontium-89 and samarium-153 lexidronam.[49,50] Zoledronate and denosumab were approved by regulatory agencies as a consequence of trials demonstrating decreased rates of skeletal-related events (SREs), including pathologic fractures, radiation to bone, surgery to bone, or spinal cord compression.[49,50] The radionuclides were approved as a consequence of meeting various palliative end points.[51–53] To date, however, none of these agents have improved overall survival in a phase III trial.

RADIUM-223

In contrast, radium-223 is a novel bone-targeted alpha-emitter recently shown to improve overall survival in a very recently reported large phase III study.[22] Strontium-89 is a calcium homolog that binds to the stroma as a consequence of calcium being deposited in the newly formed bone of osteoblastic metastases. Radium-223 also functions as a calcium homolog and binds avidly to regions of osteoblastic lesions (**Fig. 3**). Instead of releasing a beta particle as an emission, radium-223 emits an alpha-particle. Alpha particles comprise two protons and two neutrons and are approximately 7300 times larger than an electron. Alpha particles are efficient in causing DNA double-strand breaks, which are highly lethal given their propensity to cause nonreparable DNA double-strand breaks.[54] Despite their destructive nature, the distance traveled in tissues is discrete. Whereas beta particles travel millimeters in tissue, alpha particles typical travel only microns. Thus the combination of high lethality and short range of action are typical of targeted alpha-emitters such as radium-223.

In initial clinical trials, radium-223 was associated with minimal toxicities and a suggestion of tumor responses.[55,56] A randomized phase II trial with four doses of radium-223 suggested a survival advantage with minimal toxicity,[56] this leading to a randomized phase III trial (ALSYMPCA) that

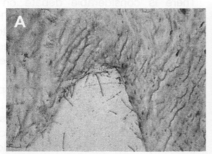
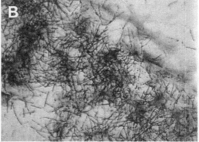

Fig. 3. Normal bone (*A*) compared with osteoblastic lesions (*B*) in a canine model. Note that agents such as radium-223 demonstrate preferential uptake in osteoblastic lesions.

Table 1
FDA-approved agents for the treatment of mCRPC

Agent	Year	Disease State	Primary End point
Estramustine	1981	mCRPC	Disease responses
Strontium-89	1993	mCRPC	Pain reduction
Mitoxantrone-prednisone	1996	mCRPC	Pain reduction
Samarium-153	1997	mCRPC	Pain reduction
Zoledronic acid	2002	mCRPC (to bone)	SRE reduction
Docetaxel-prednisone	2004	mCRPC	Prolonged survival
Sipuleucel-T	2010	mCRPC (asymptomatic)	Prolonged survival
Cabazitaxel-prednisone	2010	mCRPC (postdocetaxel)	Prolonged survival
Denosumab	2010	mCRPC (to bone)	SRE reduction
Abiraterone/prednisone	2011	mCRPC (postdocetaxel)	Prolonged survival

enrolled more than 900 patients.[22] Patients were required to be either postdocetaxel or be unsuitable for docetaxel. Unsuitability was determined by the treating physician instead of by objective criteria. In addition, the eligibility criterion for the phase III was bone-metastatic symptomatic CRPC with no visceral metastases and no lymph nodes greater than 3 cm. Patients refusing docetaxel were also allowed to participate. Standard hematological and biochemical parameters were required for trial entry. Performance status 0 to 2 was required. Patients were randomized 2:1 to radium-223 or placebo. Best supportive care was allowed in both arms. This could consist of various secondary hormonal manipulations. Glucocorticoids, estrogens, and antiestrogens were typically used. Concomitant chemotherapy or hemibody irradiations were not allowed. Patients were stratified by prior docetaxel use, alkaline phosphatase greater or less than 220 U/L, and bisphosphonate use (yes or no). The primary end point was overall survival; secondary end points included both SREs and a variety of biochemical parameters including PSA. The SREs were clinically relevant events. Unlike zoledronate and denosumab, asymptomatic bone survey–detected fractures were not tabulated. Interestingly, no imaging was required and TTRP was not captured.

The ALSYMPCA trial was ended at the first planned interim analysis (after 314 deaths out of 809 enrolled patients) as a consequence of meeting or exceeding a prespecified overall survival threshold for early termination.[22] The early termination threshold for overall survival was $P = .00306$ and the observed P value was 0.00185. The median survival was 11.2 months in the placebo arm versus 14.0 months in the isotopic arm (HR = 0.695, 95% CI 0.552–0.875). The secondary end points, including

SREs and PSA progression-free survival were also positive.[57] The SRE rate was reduced by 31% (HR = 0.61, 95% CI, 0.461–0.807, $P = .00046$). Three of the four prespecified components of SREs were improved in the radium treatment arm; irradiation to bone (HR 0.65, $P = .0038$), spinal cord compression (HR 0.44, $P = .016$), and pathologic fracture (HR 0.45, $P = .013$). This is the first trial in the authors' knowledge to decrease rates of spinal cord compression in prostate cancer.

Toxicity was low in the radium-223 arm.[22] The overall adverse event rate and the serious adverse event rate were lower in the isotopic arm than placebo. Grade 3-4 thrombocytopenia was 4% in the radionuclide arm and 2% in placebo. Grade 3-4 neutropenia was 2% in the radium arm and 1% in the placebo arm. The radium-223 submission to various national regulatory agencies in ongoing as this article goes to press; however, given the overall survival end point results and the toxicity profile, it is anticipated that radium-223 will be part of the armamentarium in the near future.

SUMMARY

There is considerable debate on the optimal sequence of mCRPC therapies. This debate is not based on clinical trials but, instead, on inferences and various biases. No sequence of treatments can be recommended based on clinical trial data but, as mentioned above, both cabazitaxel and abiraterone are only approved in the postdocetaxel mCRPC patient.

Perhaps the current state of affairs in mCRPC is best understood from the historic perspective (**Table 1**). Before 2004 and the randomized docetaxel trials (TAX327 and SWOG 9916), no treatment had been demonstrated to improve overall survival in a large phase III trial. After 2004, the concept of the predocetaxel and postdocetaxel space has defined the regulatory and clinical approach to mCRPC. Such a definition is rational but not biologically based. In 2010, sipuleucel-T was approved for men with asymptomatic or minimally symptomatic mCRPC. A small percentage (roughly 18%) of patients in the phase III sipuleucel-T were docetaxel pretreated. The two most recent FDA-approved agents, cabazitaxel and abiraterone, are specifically approved in patients with prior docetaxel exposure and both prolong survival. Toxicities vary considerably between abiraterone and cabazitaxel and this can form the basis for treatment selection in some patients. The finding that abiraterone-prednisone prolong survival in the postdocetaxel mCRPC disease state clearly indicates that these patients remain sensitive to hormonal manipulations. Agents that do not prolong survival may also be appropriate in the postdocetaxel CRPC patient. Strontium-89 and samarium-153 lexidronam are bone-targeted agents appropriate for bone-pain palliation. The zoledronic acid and denosumab indications are clear and can reduce the risk of SREs.

REFERENCES

1. Huggins C, Hodges CV. Studies on Prostatic Cancer. I. The effect of castration, of estrogen and of androgen injection on serum phosphatases in metastatic carcinoma of the prostate. Cancer Res 1941;1:293–7.

2. Huggins C, Stevens RE Jr, Hodges CV. Studies on Prostate Cancer: II. The effects of castration on advanced carcinoma of the prostate gland. Arch Surg 1941;43:209–23.

3. Labrie F, Dupont A, Bélanger A, et al. Treatment of prostate cancer with gonadotropin-releasing hormone agonists. Endocr Rev 1986;7(1):67–74.

4. Nobel Prize Lecture by Charles Huggins Transcript. Available at: http://www.nobelprize.org/nobel_prizes/medicine/laureates/1966/huggins-lecture.pdf. Accessed March 21, 2012.

5. Klotz L, O'Callaghan CJ, Ding K, et al. A phase III randomized trial comparing intermittent versus continuous androgen suppression for patients with PSA progression after radical therapy: NCIC CTG PR.7/SWOG JPR.7/CTSU JPR.7/UK Intercontinental Trial CRUKE/01/013. ASCO Meeting Abstracts 2011;29:3.

6. Hussain M, Tangen CM, Higano C, et al. Absolute prostate-specific antigen value after androgen deprivation is a strong independent predictor of survival in new metastatic prostate cancer: data from Southwest Oncology Group Trial 9346 (INT-0162). J Clin Oncol 2006;24:3984–90.

7. Small EJ, Halabi S, Dawson NA, et al. Antiandrogen withdrawal alone or in combination with ketoconazole in androgen-independent prostate cancer patients: a Phase III Trial (CALGB 9583). J Clin Oncol 2004;22:1025–33.

8. Tannock IF, Osoba D, Stockler MR, et al. Chemotherapy with mitoxantrone plus prednisone or prednisone alone for symptomatic hormone-resistant prostate cancer: a Canadian randomized trial with palliative end points. J Clin Oncol 1996;14:1756–64.

9. Tannock IF, de Wit R, Berry WR, et al. Docetaxel plus prednisone or mitoxantrone plus prednisone for advanced prostate cancer. N Engl J Med 2004; 351:1502–12.

10. Petrylak DP, Tangen CM, Hussain MHA, et al. Docetaxel and Estramustine Compared with Mitoxantrone and Prednisone for Advanced Refractory Prostate Cancer. N Engl J Med 2004;351:1513–20.

11. Available at: http://www.cancer.gov/cancertopics/druginfo/fda-docetaxel. Accessed July 14, 2012.

12. Kelly WK, Halabi S, Carducci MA, et al. A randomized, double-blind, placebo-controlled phase III trial comparing docetaxel, prednisone, and placebo with docetaxel, prednisone, and bevacizumab in men with metastatic castration-resistant prostate cancer (mCRPC): survival results of CALGB 90401. J Clin Oncol (Meeting Abstracts) 2010;28:LBA4511.

13. Ortholan C, Durivault J, Hannoun-Levi JM, et al. Bevacizumab/docetaxel association is more efficient than docetaxel alone in reducing breast and prostate cancer cell growth: a new paradigm for understanding the therapeutic effect of combined treatment. Eur J Cancer 2010;46:3022–36.

14. Available at: http://www.astrazeneca.com/Media/Press-releases/Article/0022011AstraZeneca-halts-phase-III-trial-of-ZIBOTENTAN. Accessed July 14, 2012.

15. Available at: http://investor.regeneron.com/release detail.cfm?releaseid=661995. Accessed July 14, 2012.

16. Scher HI, Jia X, Chi K, et al. Randomized, open-label phase III trial of docetaxel plus high-dose calcitriol versus docetaxel plus prednisone for patients with castration-resistant prostate cancer. J Clin Oncol 2011;29:2191–8.

17. Nelson JB, Fizazi K, Miller K, et al. Phase III study of the efficacy and safety of zibotentan (ZD4054) in patients with bone metastatic castration-resistant prostate cancer (CRPC). ASCO Meeting Abstracts 2011;29:117.

18. Quinn DI, Tangen CM, Hussain M, et al. SWOG S0421: phase III study of docetaxel (D) and atrasentan (A) versus docetaxel and placebo (P) for men with advanced castrate resistant prostate cancer (CRPC). J Clin Oncol 2012;30(Suppl) [abstract: 4511].

19. Small E, Demkow T, Gerritsen WR, et al. A phase III trial of GVAX immunotherapy for prostate cancer in combination with docetaxel versus docetaxel plus prednisone in symptomatic, castration-resistant

prostate cancer (CRPC) [abstract: 7]. Presented at the 2009 Genitourinary Cancers Symposium in San Francisco, February 26, 2009.

20. Kantoff PW, Higano CS, Shore ND, et al. Sipuleucel-T immunotherapy for castration-resistant prostate cancer. N Engl J Med 2010;363:411–22.

21. de Bono JS, Logothetis CJ, Molina A, et al. Abiraterone and increased survival in metastatic prostate cancer. N Engl J Med 2011;364:1995–2005.

22. Parker C, Heinrich D, O'Sullivan JM, et al. Overall survival benefit and safety profile of radium-223 chloride, a first-in-class alpha-pharmaceutical: results from a phase III randomized trial (ALSYMPCA) in patients with castration-resistant prostate cancer (CRPC) with bone metastases. ASCO Meeting Abstracts 2012;30:8.

23. Scher HI, Fizazi K, Saad F, et al. Effect of MDV3100, an androgen receptor signaling inhibitor (ARSI), on overall survival in patients with prostate cancer post-docetaxel: results from the phase III AFFIRM study. ASCO Meeting Abstracts 2012;30:LBA1.

24. de Bono JS, Oudard S, Ozguroglu M, et al. Prednisone plus cabazitaxel or mitoxantrone for metastatic castration-resistant prostate cancer progressing after docetaxel treatment: a randomised open-label trial. Lancet 2010;376:1147–54.

25. Kawasaki Y, Ito A, Withers DA, et al. Ganglioside DSGb5, preferred ligand for Siglec-7, inhibits NK cell cytotoxicity against renal cell carcinoma cells. Glycobiology 2010;20:1373–9.

26. Madan RA, Pal SK, Sartor O, et al. Overcoming chemotherapy resistance in prostate cancer. Clin Cancer Res 2011;17:3892–902.

27. Caplow M, Zeeberg B. Dynamic properties of microtubules at steady state in the presence of taxol. Eur J Biochem 1982;127:319–24.

28. Kumar N. Taxol-induced polymerization of purified tubulin. Mechanism of action. J Biol Chem 1981; 256:10435–41.

29. White J, Rao G. Effects of a microtubule stabilizing agent on the response of platelets to vincristine. Blood 1982;60:474–83.

30. Bissery M-C, Bouchard H, Riou J, et al. Preclinical evaluation of TXD258, a new taxoid. Proc Am Assoc Canc Res 2000;41 [Abstract: 1364].

31. Vrignaud P, Lejeune P, Chaplin D, et al. In vivo efficacy of TXD258, a new taxoid, against human tumor xenografts. Proc Am Assoc Canc Res 2000;41 [Abstract: 1365].

32. Stone KR, Mickey DD, Wunderli H, et al. Isolation of a human prostate carcinoma cell line (DU 145). Int J Cancer 1978;21:274–81.

33. Mita AC, Denis LJ, Rowinsky EK, et al. Phase I and pharmacokinetic study of XRP6258 (RPR 116258A), a Novel taxane, administered as a 1-Hour infusion every 3 weeks in patients with advanced solid tumors. Clin Cancer Res 2009;15:723–30.

34. FDA clinical pharmacology and biopharmaceutical reviews (Application 201023). Available at: http://www.accessdata.fda.gov/drugsatfda_docs/nda/2010/201023s000ClinPharmR.pdf. Accessed March 22, 2012.

35. Dieras V, Limentani S, Romieu G, et al. Phase II multicenter study of larotaxel (XRP9881), a novel taxoid, in patients with metastatic breast cancer who previously received taxane-based therapy. Ann Oncol 2008;19:1255–60.

36. Metzger-Filho O, Moulin C, de Azambuja E, et al. Larotaxel: broadening the road with new taxanes. Expert Opin Investig Drugs 2009;18:1183–9.

37. Scher HI, Halabi S, Tannock I, et al. Design and end points of clinical trials for patients with progressive prostate cancer and castrate levels of testosterone: recommendations of the Prostate Cancer Clinical Trials Working Group. J Clin Oncol 2008;26:1148–59.

38. Di Lorenzo G, Buonerba C, Autorino R, et al. Castration-resistant prostate cancer: current and emerging treatment strategies. Drugs 2010;70:983–1000.

39. Available at: http://www.cancer.gov/cancertopics/druginfo/fda-cabazitaxel. Accessed July 14, 2012.

40. Sartor AO, Oudard S, Ozguroglu M, et al. Survival benefit from first docetaxel treatment for cabazitaxel plus prednisone compared with mitoxantrone plus prednisone in patients with metastatic castration-resistant prostate cancer (mCRPC) enrolled in the TROPIC trial. ASCO Meeting Abstracts 2011;29:4525.

41. De Bono JS, Oudard S, Ozguroglu M, et al. A subgroup analysis of the TROPIC trial exploring reason for discontinuation of prior docetaxel and survival outcome of cabazitaxel in metastatic castration-resistant prostate cancer (mCRPC). ASCO Meeting Abstracts 2011;29:4526.

42. Available at: http://www.accessdata.fda.gov/drugsatfda_docs/label/2010/201023lbl.pdf. Accessed July 14, 2012.

43. Ozguroglu M, Oudard S, Sartor AO, et al. Effect of G-CSF prophylaxis on the occurrence of neutropenia in men receiving cabazitaxel plus prednisone for the treatment of metastatic castration-resistant prostate cancer (mCRPC) in the TROPIC study. ASCO Meeting Abstracts 2011;29:144.

44. Attard G, Reid AH, A'Hern R, et al. Selective inhibition of cyp17 with abiraterone acetate is highly active in the treatment of castration-resistant prostate cancer. J Clin Oncol 2009. http://dx.doi.org/10.1200/JCO.2008.20.0642.

45. Kolvenbag GJ, Furr BJ, Blackledge GR. Receptor affinity and potency of non-steroidal antiandrogens: translation of preclinical findings into clinical activity. Prostate Cancer Prostatic Dis 1998;1:307–14.

46. Tran C, Ouk S, Clegg NJ, et al. Development of a second-generation antiandrogen for treatment of advanced prostate cancer. Science 2009;324:787–90.

47. Scher HI, Beer TM, Higano CS, et al. Antitumour activity of MDV3100 in castration-resistant prostate cancer: a phase 1-2 study. Lancet 2010;375:1437–46.

48. Wang C, Shen Y. Study on the distribution features of bone metastases in prostate cancer. Nucl Med Commun 2012;33:379–83.

49. Fizazi K, Carducci M, Smith M, et al. Denosumab versus zoledronic acid for treatment of bone metastases in men with castration-resistant prostate cancer: a randomised, double-blind study. Lancet 2011;377:813–22.

50. Saad F, Gleason DM, Murray R, et al. Long-term efficacy of zoledronic acid for the prevention of skeletal complications in patients with metastatic hormone-refractory prostate cancer. J Natl Cancer Inst 2004;96:879–82.

51. Lewington VJ, McEwan AJ, Ackery DM, et al. A prospective, randomised double-blind crossover study to examine the efficacy of strontium-89 in pain palliation in patients with advanced prostate cancer metastatic to bone. Eur J Cancer 1991;27:954–8.

52. Porter AT, McEwan AJ, Powe JE, et al. Results of a randomized phase-III trial to evaluate the efficacy of strontium-89 adjuvant to local field external beam irradiation in the management of endocrine resistant metastatic prostate cancer. Int J Radiat Oncol Biol Phys 1993;25:805–13.

53. Sartor O. Overview of samarium sm 153 lexidronam in the treatment of painful metastatic bone disease. Rev Urol 2004;6(Suppl 10):S3–12.

54. Ritter MA, Cleaver JE, Tobias CA. High-LET radiations induce a large proportion of non-rejoining DNA breaks. Nature 1977;266:653–5.

55. Nilsson S, Franzen L, Parker C, et al. Bone-targeted radium-223 in symptomatic, hormone-refractory prostate cancer: a randomised, multicentre, placebo-controlled phase II study. Lancet Oncol 2007;8:587–94.

56. Nilsson S, Strang P, Aksnes AK, et al. A randomized, dose-response, multicenter phase II study of radium-223 chloride for the palliation of painful bone metastases in patients with castration-resistant prostate cancer. Eur J Cancer 2012;48:678–86.

57. Sartor AO, Heinrich D, Helle SI, et al. Radium-223 chloride impact on skeletal-related events in patients with castration-resistant prostate cancer (CRPC) with bone metastases: a phase III randomized trial (ALSYMPCA). ASCO Meeting Abstracts 2012;30:9.

Index

Urol Clin N Am 39 (2012) 593–599
http://dx.doi.org/10.1016/S0094-0143(12)00087-0

United States Postal Service

Statement of Ownership, Management, and Circulation
(All Periodicals Publications Except Requestor Publications)

1. Publication Title	2. Publication Number	3. Filing Date
Urologic Clinics of North America	0 0 0 - 7 1 1 1	9/14/12

4. Issue Frequency	5. Number of Issues Published Annually	6. Annual Subscription Price
Feb, May, Aug, Nov	4	$339.00

7. Complete Mailing Address of Known Office of Publication (Not printer) (Street, city, county, state, and ZIP+4®)

Elsevier Inc.
360 Park Avenue South
New York, NY 10010-1710

Contact Person
Stephen R. Bushing

Telephone (Include area code)
215-239-3688

8. Complete Mailing Address of Headquarters or General Business Office of Publisher (Not printer)

Elsevier Inc., 360 Park Avenue South, New York, NY 10010-1710

9. Full Names and Complete Mailing Addresses of Publisher, Editor, and Managing Editor (Do not leave blank)

Publisher (Name and complete mailing address)

Kim Murphy, Elsevier, Inc., 1600 John F. Kennedy Blvd. Suite 1800, Philadelphia, PA 19103-2899

Editor (Name and complete mailing address)

Stephanie Donley, Elsevier, Inc., 1600 John F. Kennedy Blvd. Suite 1800, Philadelphia, PA 19103-2899

Managing Editor (Name and complete mailing address)

Sarah Barth, Elsevier, Inc., 1600 John F. Kennedy Blvd. Suite 1800, Philadelphia, PA 19103-2899

10. Owner (Do not leave blank. If the publication is owned by a corporation, give the name and address of the corporation immediately followed by the names and addresses of all stockholders owning or holding 1 percent or more of the total amount of stock. If not owned by a corporation, give the names and addresses of the individual owners. If owned by a partnership or other unincorporated firm, give its name and address as well as those of each individual owner. If the publication is published by a nonprofit organization, give its name and address.)

Full Name	Complete Mailing Address
Wholly owned subsidiary of	1600 John F. Kennedy Blvd., Ste. 1800
Reed/Elsevier, US holdings	Philadelphia, PA 19103-2899

11. Known Bondholders, Mortgagees, and Other Security Holders Owning or Holding 1 Percent or More of Total Amount of Bonds, Mortgages, or Other Securities. If none, check box ☐ None

Full Name	Complete Mailing Address
N/A	

12. Tax Status (For completion by nonprofit organizations authorized to mail at nonprofit rates) (Check one)
The purpose, function, and nonprofit status of this organization and the exempt status for federal income tax purposes:
☐ Has Not Changed During Preceding 12 Months
☐ Has Changed During Preceding 12 Months (Publisher must submit explanation of change with this statement)

PS Form 3526, September 2007 (Page 1 of 3 (Instructions Page 3)) PSN 7530-01-000-9931 PRIVACY NOTICE: See our Privacy policy in www.usps.com

---

13. Publication Title	14. Issue Date for Circulation Data Below
Urologic Clinics of North America	August 2012

15. Extent and Nature of Circulation		Average No. Copies Each Issue During Preceding 12 Months	No. Copies of Single Issue Published Nearest to Filing Date
a. Total Number of Copies (Net press run)		1641	1309
b. Paid Circulation (By Mail and Outside the Mail)	(1) Mailed Outside-County Paid Subscriptions Stated on PS Form 3541 (Include paid distribution above nominal rate, advertiser's proof copies, and exchange copies)	706	657
	(2) Mailed In-County Paid Subscriptions Stated on PS Form 3541 (Include paid distribution above nominal rate, advertiser's proof copies, and exchange copies)		
	(3) Paid Distribution Outside the Mails Including Sales Through Dealers and Carriers, Street Vendors, Counter Sales, and Other Paid Distribution Outside USPS®	467	526
	(4) Paid Distribution by Other Classes Mailed Through the USPS (e.g. First-Class Mail®)		
c. Total Paid Distribution (Sum of 15b (1), (2), (3), and (4))	▲	1173	1183
d. Free or Nominal Rate Distribution (By Mail and Outside the Mail)	(1) Free or Nominal Rate Outside-County Copies Included on PS Form 3541	78	80
	(2) Free or Nominal Rate In-County Copies Included on PS Form 3541		
	(3) Free or Nominal Rate Copies Mailed at Other Classes Through the USPS (e.g. First-Class Mail)		
	(4) Free or Nominal Rate Distribution Outside the Mail (Carriers or other means)		
e. Total Free or Nominal Rate Distribution (Sum of 15d (1), (2), (3) and (4))	▲	78	80
f. Total Distribution (Sum of 15c and 15e)	▲	1251	1263
g. Copies not Distributed (See instructions to publishers #4 (page #3))	▲	390	46
h. Total (Sum of 15f and g)		1641	1309
i. Percent Paid (15c divided by 15f times 100)	▲	93.76%	93.67%

16. Publication of Statement of Ownership

If the publication is a general publication, publication of this statement is required. Will be printed in the **November 2012** issue of this publication.

☐ Publication not required

17. Signature and Title of Editor, Publisher, Business Manager, or Owner

[signature]
Stephen R. Bushing – Fulfillment/Inventory Specialist

Date
September 14, 2012

I certify that all information furnished on this form is true and complete. I understand that anyone who furnishes false or misleading information on this form or who omits material or information requested on the form may be subject to criminal sanctions (including fines and imprisonment) and/or civil sanctions (including civil penalties).

PS Form 3526, September 2007 (Page 2 of 3)

Printed and bound by CPI Group (UK) Ltd, Croydon, CR0 4YY

03/10/2024

01040344-0012